The Complete Idiot's Reference Card

Ten Risk Factors Reduced by Regular Exercise

1. Premature death
2. Cardiovascular disease
3. Coronary heart disease
4. High blood pressure
5. Colon cancer
6. Obesity
7. Osteoarthritis
8. Osteoporosis
9. Non–insulin-dependent diabetes mellitus
10. Mood disorders

Ten Activities That Burn the Most Calories

1. Bicycling more than 20 miles per hour
2. Running at a seven-minute-mile or faster pace
3. Vigorous cross-country skiing, including uphill
4. Bicycling 16 to 19 miles per hour
5. Playing handball
6. Swimming (crawl, butterfly, or treading water vigorously)
7. Vigorous stationary bicycling (for example, spinning)
8. High-impact step aerobics
9. Martial arts
10. Rope jumping

Ten Common Fitness Mistakes

1. Not stretching enough before and after a workout
2. Lifting too much weight too soon
3. Running too far too soon
4. Not warming up before and cooling down after a workout
5. Exercising too intensely for weight loss to occur
6. Not drinking enough water
7. Leaning heavily on the stairstepper
8. Not working out within the target heart rate range
9. Not using controlled movements during weight training
10. Consuming too many high-calorie energy bars and sports drinks

alpha
books

Ten Fitness Web Sites

1. American Council on Exercise (ACE), www.acefitness.org
2. Aerobics and Fitness Association of America (AFAA), www.afaa.com
3. *Prevention* magazine, www.healthyideas.com
4. Fitness Partner Jumpsite, www.primusweb.com/fitnesspartner/
5. FitNews, www.fitnessworld.com
6. Physical Activity and Health News (PAHNet), www.pitt.edu/~pahnet/
7. iVillage Better Health, www.betterhealth.com
8. ThriveOnLine, www.thriveonline.com
9. National Strength and Conditioning Association, www.nsca-lift.org
10. Women's Sports Foundation, www.gogetfit.com
    *From IDEA, a trade organization of training professionals

Ten Secrets for Successful Strength Training

1. List your goals and plan to achieve them over time.
2. Don't try to do too much, too soon.
3. Change your exercise program every four to six weeks.
4. Change your exercise order.
5. Change the number of sets.
6. Vary your recovery time between sets.
7. Change the combination of reps and sets.
8. Keep a log and evaluate your progress every four to eight weeks.
9. Be flexible with your training.
10. Give purpose to every workout.

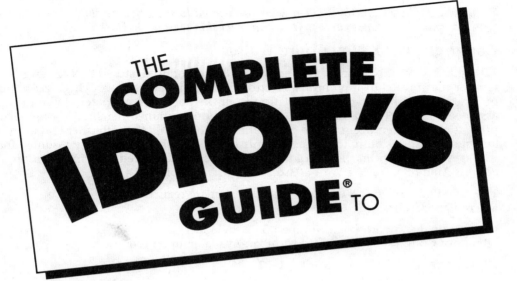

THE COMPLETE IDIOT'S GUIDE® TO

Fitness

by Claire Walter
with Annette Tannander Bank

alpha
books

Macmillan USA, Inc.
201 West 103rd Street
Indianapolis, IN 46290

A Pearson Education Company

To my son, Andrew Cameron-Walter, whose dedication to strength and fitness has helped the New Hampton School football team to a championship season. Go Huskies!

Copyright © 2000 by Claire Walter

International Standard Book Number: 0-02-863658-9
Library of Congress Catalog Card Number: Available upon request.

02   01   00   8   7   6   5   4   3   2   1

Interpretation of the printing code: The rightmost number of the first series of numbers is the year of the book's printing; the rightmost number of the second series of numbers is the number of the book's printing. For example, a printing code of 00-1 shows that the first printing occurred in 2000.

Printed in the United States of America

Publisher
Marie Butler-Knight

Product Manager
Phil Kitchel

Associate Managing Editor
Cari Luna

Acquisitions Editor
Amy Zavatto

Development Editor
Nancy D. Warner

Production Editor
Christy Wagner

Copy Editor
Amy Lepore

Illustrator
Jody P. Schaeffer

Cover Designers
Mike Freeland
Kevin Spear

Book Designers
Scott Cook and Amy Adams of DesignLab

Indexer
Lisa Lawrence

Layout/Proofreading
Fran Blauw
Lisa England

Contents at a Glance

Contents

Introduction

Fitness means different things to different people. For some, it means running a marathon or having a buff, muscular bodybuilder's physique to show off at the beach. For others, it's just the ability to carry a baby or a bag of groceries up a flight of stairs without panting. For the purposes of this book, fitness means having a healthy, *functional* body—one that enables you to lead a comfortably active life. The book also will touch on activities such as Tae Bo, tai chi, yoga, and advanced training tips that might not interest you now, but they might gain new appeal as you get into shape.

Fitness is not only an end unto itself. It also is a major component of wellness, which includes physical and mental health and emotional well-being. A physically active child can be on the right road to a lifetime of fitness. A fit teenager will have a wholesome body image, an ability to compete in sports, and enhanced self-esteem. An adult with a workout program can better combat work-related stress, and fit women usually have more comfortable pregnancies, easier childbirth, and quicker recovery than out-of-shape women.

Fit people are more likely to stay well, active, and productive through their middle years when heart disease, cancer, cardiovascular problems, and other health issues begin to crop up. People who retain, or even build, their fitness late in life can remain active and vital for many years. As we age as a population, such quality-of-life issues are not trivial; they are becoming more important to us as individuals and as a nation and society that is living longer and becoming more conscious of quality of life. Fitness should not be a fling but a lifetime commitment. When you get into a regular program, exercise can become addictive, and it's the best addiction you can have.

Inactivity—a National Crisis

So much has been written about exercise and diet that millions of Americans are quite knowledgeable about these subjects and how they relate to healthy living. But how many people really act on this knowledge? Far too few. Americans are fat and frustrated. According to recent statistics, some 34 percent of the adults in this country are overweight and close to 20 percent are dangerously obese. At the same time, about half of them are trying to reduce. They'd better.

In 1996, the U.S. Surgeon General issued a massive report that concluded, among other things, that inactivity kills about a quarter of a million Americans every year—far more than automobile accidents, shootings, and AIDS combined. The results of inactivity and obesity creep into many corners of our collective life. Ferry boats across Washington State's Puget Sound used to carry 250 passengers; these days, only 230 commuters can scrunch their posteriors onto each boat. Airlines are required to carry seat-belt extenders on every plane, and many are raising the tray tables to fit over passengers' tubby tummies. Even toilet seats are getting bigger—by customer demand!

The national standard for public seating space used to be 18 inches. Now, some sports stadiums and theaters are installing 24-inch seats. Isn't it pathetic that the stands are full of overweight people who fuel up on fatty foods and beers as they watch million-aire sports stars play games? People also sit in movie theaters and ingest buttered pop-corn, humongous sodas, and brick-size boxes of candy as svelte, overpaid movie stars cavort onscreen. What is wrong with this picture? Everything.

We are not the only fat-afflicted society in the industrial world. According to Marks and Spencer, Britain's biggest clothing retailer, the average Englishwoman is now a size 16 as compared to the average size of 12 in the 1950s. Women have steadily added inches to their waistlines and hips. The culprits? A more sedentary lifestyle and fast food—the same as in America.

Many studies have shown that exercise, in combination with a wholesome diet, is the only effective, permanent way to get weight under control—and to enjoy good health and a life of activity and fun. As the baby boom generation continues to bulge, so do the cases of high blood pressure, heart disease, and some kinds of cancer that have been statistically linked to obesity.

Boomer women also are coping with issues ranging from late-life pregnancy and menopause to the specter of osteoporosis. Doctor-sanctioned exercise is now known to be key to an easier pregnancy, quicker postpartum recuperation, milder meno-pause, and escape from osteoporosis. As life expectancy increases, the quality of life ought to keep up. Who wants to live a long but inactive and perhaps painful life full of restrictions and problems? People who are lean, fit, and flexible live longer and get more out of the long life they live.

Making Fitness an Attainable Personal Goal

People are always making resolutions to get in shape. To lose some weight. To tone up. To firm up. They say they'll start the diet on Monday. After the first of the year. With swimsuit season coming up. They say they'll sign up at a health club next week. Next month. Next time there's a membership special. After the first of the year. Perhaps after Memorial Day. Maybe they've already signed up but have gone only once, a couple of times, or not at all.

Other than sheer procrastination, one of the main reasons many people don't really get started on a program is that they are seeking a sure cure or fast fix for flab—or, at the very least, the most efficient way to get in shape. Others don't work out because they don't believe they can do it; being afraid of failure, they don't start at all. But everyone can get stronger and healthier. This book will compare and contrast what's out there in terms of both targeted workout programs and participant sports.

Diet books and, worse, potentially harmful weight-loss formulas sell like proverbial hot cakes (hold the butter and use low-sugar syrup, of course), but many studies have shown that exercise, in combination with a healthful diet, is the only effective, per-manent way to lose weight and keep it off—and also to enjoy good health. This is so true that it cannot be repeated too often. "The only place where success comes before work," Vidal Sassoon once said, "is in the dictionary."

Intake is just part of the answer to the obesity question. Most modern research shows that diet is not the route to long-range success. Diet plus exercise is important in body reshaping, not simply for good looks but, more important, for good health. Specialized books, magazines, and videos abound to help people begin to exercise to get and stay in shape. Not a month goes by without some major women's magazine or general-interest publication doing a cover story on shaping up. Television infomercials promise a sure route to leanness. Common wisdom indicates that yo-yo diets and impulsive, short-lived plunges into workout programs are doomed to fail, yet people keep trying this and that. They spend money, realize disappointing results, and try still another fast fix. The urge for better health resides in many people, however, and this is a good beginning because the seeds of success have to sprout within your mind.

How to Use This Book

Perhaps you are among the people who have gobbled up a great deal of information—so much, in fact, that it's difficult to sort out the promises and decide which ones can work for you. *The Complete Idiot's Guide to Fitness* sorts it out for you. This is not an in-depth analysis of any one approach to fitness. Rather, it's a smorgasbord of options so you can decide which ones you can fuse into a program that will make you stronger, more attractive, and above all, healthier.

This book begins with goal-setting, motivational issues, and tips and tricks to start off on the right foot. It lays out the wide array of workout options and how they compare. When picking a program, the important thing is to find something that works *for you,* something that you can stick with. This book covers working out at home, at a gym, and while you're traveling. It outlines a vast array of classes and tools to help you slim down, tone up, increase your strength and endurance, become healthier, and remain happier. It talks about sports and everyday activities that are easier once you are more fit, because strength and fitness are not necessarily ends unto themselves but tools to help you live a better and more fulfilling life.

Each chapter is seasoned with insights, tips, and cautions to light your route to fitness:

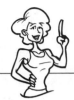

Fitness Fact

These boxes contain interesting statistics and researchers' findings about fitness, wellness, and other health issues.

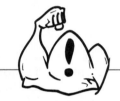

Fit Tip

Here you'll find helpful hints about specific exercises, apparatus, or other steps you can take on the road to getting into shape.

Quote, Unquote

Observations, comments, and inspiration from others about fitness and well-being come in these boxes.

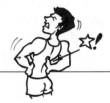

Achtung!

Achtung is a German word signaling an "alert." These cautions and warnings help you avoid injury or other common exercise errors.

Acknowledgments

Immense appreciation goes to all the people who created this book. I am deeply grateful to the valiant warriors on the fitness front who do daily battle to help Americans find their way to fitness and good health—exercise instructors, trainers, nutritionists, authorities in the growing realm of the mind-body connection in being fit and healthy, equipment innovators, physiologists, physicians, and all the others who have shared their knowledge and permitted me to quote their words. Dr. Surasvati Berman of the Rocky Mountain Institute of Yoga and Aryuda cast a knowledgeable eye on Chapter 9, "Other Paths to Stretching and Toning."

My greatest debt of gratitude goes to my three wonderful partners in the project: Annette Tännander Bank, trainer extraordinaire, whose expertise and dedication to this project have been exceptional; photographer Anne W. Krause, who is responsible for the best images in this book; and Lisa DeYoung, a conscientious researcher and fine writer who helped put the pieces together. Without them, this book would not have been possible. Not only has our collaboration been professionally gratifying, but we've become firm friends as well. Thanks also to my careful editors at Alpha Books— Gary Krebs who assigned this book; development editor Nancy D. Warner, production editor Christy Wagner, and copy editor Amy Lepore. Their conscientiousness has enhanced this project, but the responsibility for any errors or omissions is mine.

—Claire Walter

Trademarks

All terms mentioned in this book that are known to be or are suspected of being trademarks or service marks have been appropriately capitalized. Alpha Books and Macmillan USA, Inc. cannot attest to the accuracy of this information. Use of a term in this book should not be regarded as affecting the validity of any trademark or service mark.

Part 1
Start Smart

According to an ancient Chinese proverb, "A journey of a thousand miles begins with a single step." And so it is with fitness. To get in shape, drop inches and pounds, and most important, be fit and healthy, you need a plan, steady work, and dedication.

Televiewers who order quick-weight-loss products demonstrate little planning or stick-to-itiveness. Some products might provide fast results, but they usually are not permanent—and some pills and potions eventually prove to be harmful. At best, most of them don't work over the long run, and the only thing lighter is your wallet.

Such a mind-numbing amount of health information and fitness knowledge is out there that some people who want to shape up, who need to shape up, who must shape up for immediate health reasons give up instead. Building the foundation of a solid workout regime requires strategic planning. This means assessing where you are now and what your realistic goals are.

"People are not lazy by choice. They are forced into it by the abundance of fitness information that is available."

—Dr. Ellington Darden, fitness authority and author

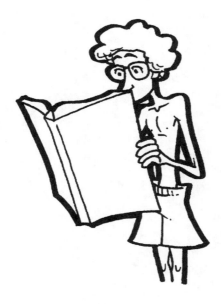

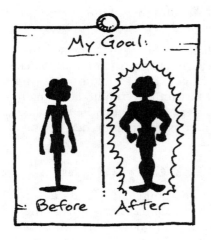

Chapter 1

The Name of the Game Is Goals

In This Chapter

➤ The three basic body types

➤ Can a person be both fat and fit?

➤ Fitness and good health—your cheapest health insurance

➤ How to set fitness goals

"I'm going to lose weight." "I'm planning to get in shape." "I can't stand the way my clothes fit." "I can't zip up my favorite jeans." "My back hurts." "I feel like a slug. I've got no energy. I just have to get up and do something." How many times have you heard these comments? How many times have you said them?

Losing weight, shaping up, looking good, and feeling good are the general goals shared by millions of Americans and others. You probably are one of them, or you wouldn't have picked up this book. Every one of these common resolutions falls into the general category of "getting fit," which includes physical activity, healthful eating, and a commitment to changing the way you've been conducting your life.

Goal-setting gives purpose and direction to any training program and helps promote the motivation, self-confidence, positive attitude, and sense of responsibility to succeed. There's nothing exotic about the means of achieving these goals, but it requires more of a commitment than many people are willing to make. We appear to be a nation of individuals who demand instant solutions to problems, and many of us have the attention span of a flea. Of the top 10 television infomercials, half promote weight-loss or exercise products. Most make grandiose promises of quick, easy results. An old saying that applies here is "If it sounds too good to be true, it probably is."

The truth is that transforming yourself from a sedentary, out-of-shape person to someone fit is not instant. Many people think they can change their bodies quickly, but fitness and good health don't come about overnight. That should be no surprise. After all, we didn't add those extra pounds or become unfit overnight. Shaping up is a process that has to start with a few fundamental steps. Figure out where you are, set realistic goals, and try to determine how you can accomplish them. Then begin.

"Today is the first day of the rest of your life."

This slogan might date back to the era of flower power, smiley faces, and tie-dye shirts, but it's held up better than all those fads. The slogan is as true now as the day it was coined. Make today the day you take charge of your body. Many people play the "tomorrow" tune: *"Tomorrow I'll start working out." "Tomorrow I'll join the gym." "Tomorrow I'll go for a walk at lunch time."* And so on. Quit procrastinating. Don't turn the calendar to any more tomorrows. Start on your fitness quest today. After all, inertia never caused anyone to get thinner or stronger. Details follow, but here's a list of some things you can do right now:

➤ Make a doctor's appointment for a medical evaluation and to get his or her go-ahead for you to start a fitness program.

➤ Sign up for a fitness evaluation with a local gym, community recreation center, or personal trainer.

➤ Go through your refrigerator and pantry and be merciless, discarding high-sugar, high-fat foods.

➤ Go to a gym and sign up for a basic workout program.

➤ Starting today, make a daily walk part of your routine.

➤ Set your fitness goals.

In addition, buy a specially designed workout planner/logbook or a notebook in which you can log your motivation, your specific goals, your workout routine, your daily eating, and your emotions. Be sure to include the positive feelings you get from exercising, such as feeling strong, relaxed, challenged, slimmer, fitter, or any other. If you skip a day of your workout schedule, mark that down, too, along with the reason why you didn't exercise and how it made you feel, such as tired, lazy, guilty, relieved, or any other.

Mark today on your calendar because it is, indeed, the first day of the rest of your new life.

The Big Picture: What's Your Motivation?

You are the general in command of your life. As you embark on your fitness quest, it might help you to think of motivation as the strategy in your battle to become fit forever and to think of your specific goals as the tactics you will have to employ to accomplish what you set out to do. Like all wars, however, you need to know what you are fighting for and keep your goals firmly in sight.

As you begin to plan your get-in-shape program, ask yourself some questions. When you have answered them, jot down those major motivations in your notebook—perhaps in big, bold letters on the first page. You can add your feelings about your "before" self, too. Here are some questions that might help get you started:

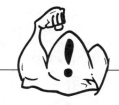

Fit Tip

When you're shopping for a notebook, you can select a loose-leaf binder and can easily add relevant articles from magazines and newspapers to create your own personal handbook. Everything you add should reinforce your determination.

➤ Do you want to be fit to live a long, healthy life? You might want to see your grandchildren grow up, enjoy an active retirement, or avoid some of the health problems you see plaguing older relatives.

➤ Do you want to be fit to look better? If you are tired of waddling when you walk, jiggling when you move, and oozing over the chair when you sit, your motivation for slimming down and shaping up might be mainly for aesthetic reasons.

Quote, Unquote

"We are always getting ready to live but never living."

—Ralph Waldo Emerson

➤ Do you want to be fit to improve your love life? If you believe you haven't found a mate because of your appearance, if you fear your partner is losing interest because you've let yourself go, or if your spouse has left you for someone thinner, you might want to shape up for this most personal of reasons.

➤ Do you want to be fit to take up a sport? Perhaps the ski slopes, the tennis courts, or the golf courses look good to you. You probably feel the need to get in shape to enjoy a new sport and have a reasonable chance of becoming competent.

➤ Do you need to get fit because of serious health concerns? When your doctor tells you that you need to get some exercise and gives you the reasons, it can be a more powerful motivator than your own general notion of being healthy or living longer.

Regardless of which motivations on this list match yours, you'll have to get into gear and change your life to reach them. Keep them in mind as you begin and proceed. Because the most important goals are long-haul, you need to count on a long-range commitment to get there.

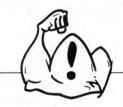

Fit Tip

Tell someone important to you what your fitness goals are to help solidify your commitment—to yourself and to that person.

Can't Do Much About Biology

Before you think about what you want your fitness program to do for you, keep in mind what it *can't* do. Genetics play the leading role in creating the basic shape of your body, and you have to start out being realistic so you can do the best you can with what you have. People are programmed from birth to be tall and long-limbed, petite and short-limbed, small-framed or big-boned, or whatever. By adulthood, you've hopefully accepted the immutable things about your body type, even if you don't like them.

Genetics also determine where you are likely to gain weight, and you might not be quite as cheerful about accepting that. No matter what you do, you might find that any extra pounds you carry appear around your middle, on your hips and thighs, or below your belt line.

Physiologists have divided people into three basic body types, though most people's bodies are a combination of two:

➤ **Ectomorphs** are lean, long-limbed, and often tall. These reed-like people have long torsos, slim hips and shoulders, and small bones in proportion to their height. They often excel as runners. Guys nicknamed "Stretch" or "Slim" are ectomorphs.

➤ **Endomorphs** are short of limb and torso with more rounded bodies. They tend to store body fat easily and might also be big-boned. When they gain weight, it usually is in the lower body. Endomorph women can be curvaceous like Madonna or Pia Zadora. In reality, many endomorphs spend their lives fighting fat.

➤ **Mesomorphs** have square, sturdy bodies and often are fairly big-boned. They are athletically built and can bulk up their muscles more easily than other body types. When they gain weight, it generally is in the abdomen.

People tend to pack extra weight in specific patterns. The names of these patterns are less Latin-rooted than the three morphs just mentioned. Overweight mesomorphs become "apple people" who carry their extra weight around the midsection. Their problems are big bellies and "love handles" on the sides of their torsos. Endomorphs who put on weight become "pear people" and carry their extra weight below the belt on the hips, abdomen, buttocks, and thighs. Fortunately, ectomorphs don't readily gain weight, but they generally can't gain big muscles either. You won't find many ectomorphs bodybuilders.

Stand Tall, Stand Proud

Remember your mother telling you to sit or stand up straight and not to slouch? She was right. Once you decide to shape up, be conscious of the way you carry yourself. Not only will you look better with your shoulders straight and your head held high, you also can avoid problems of the shoulders and upper spine. The routine of checking and adjusting your posture can be a prelude to the new body awareness you will be developing along with your new workout program.

Rounded, hunched shoulders are said to be "protracted"; when they are pulled back, they are said to be "retracted." Many people who hold down desk jobs and sit at a computer all day lapse into a state of "chronic protraction," which is bad. Debbie Horn, a Boulder, Colorado, fitness instructor with a Master's degree in kinesiology from the University of Colorado, has developed a small program to help with posture and to ward off shoulder problems. She suggests setting a timer or stopwatch to go off every 15 or 30 minutes. When you hear the alarm, check your posture. If you are slouching, retract your shoulders—in other words, sit or stand up straight and pull your shoulders back. After a while, this readjustment will become automatic.

Just Weight a Minute

Is it possible to be both fat and fit? Yes, to a limited degree. Five-hundred–pound sumo wrestlers, three-hundred–pound football defensemen, and some long-distance or endurance swimmers are both strong and overweight. However, they

Quote, Unquote

"The thin, lean look is a media invention. There is a range of body types and weights and what is healthy for you might be totally different than the next person."

—Monique Ryan, Personal Nutrition Designs

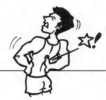

Achtung!

If your slouching dates back to your teen years when you were taller than your peers, it's a habit (technical name: postural roundback) that can be cured by making a point to stand and sit straight and by developing your upper back with such exercises as seated rows, pull-downs, and butterflies. If hunched shoulders developed later in life, however, it could be a sign of osteoporosis that requires a medical evaluation.

cannot be described as completely fit. They are functionally fit for their chosen sports. For most people, balanced fitness leads to a long, healthy life.

Glenn Gaesser and Steven Blair from the highly regarded Cooper Aerobics Center in Dallas studied 20 years of statistics about the relationship between body weight and fitness. Their conclusion was that being active rather than sedentary is the critical factor in health and longevity. This means that naturally thin nonexercisers can be less healthy than overweight people who are physically active. Other studies have backed up these findings. In other words, for most people in the real world, obesity and fitness are mutually exclusive.

The Cooper study ranked physical inactivity and smoking at the top of the list of factors that put people at medical risk. It concluded that men who are the least fit have one-and-a-half times the mortality rate as men who are the most fit, and women who are the least fit have twice the mortality rate of women who are the most fit. It is important to know, however, that the researchers noted that it isn't necessary to be a super athlete to dramatically cut risk factors. Even being moderately fit and physically active can do the trick, and that's what most beginning exercisers are looking for.

The *Journal of the American Medical Association* in late 1999 reported on a government study that underscored the problem and made headlines around the country. Researchers in the Behavioral Risk Factor Surveillance System conducted by the Centers for Disease Control and Prevention announced that the percentage of obese Americans (those who are overweight by 30 percent or more) skyrocketed from 12 percent in 1991 to 17.9 percent in 1999. The biggest change for the worse was among 18- to 29-year-olds and among Hispanics, but this weight increase cut across state lines, age groups, and gender barriers, as the entire country seemed sedentary and to be on one communal eating binge.

Take a Giant Stride Toward Good Health

Fitness and good health are not as instant as boil-in-the-bag meals. There is one thing you can do, however, that will immediately start you on the right road to feeling better, looking better, and becoming healthier: If you smoke, quit. Now. Participate in the Great American Smokeout, an annual nationwide stop-smoking initiative. Do whatever it takes. Plaster a patch on your body, join a support group, undergo hypnosis. Not only will quitting be good for you, it will show you that you can accomplish anything you set your mind to.

Smoking has been proven to be an addiction. You probably know that. If you smoke, you also know that it pollutes your lungs and predisposes you to such horrific diseases as emphysema, cancer of the lung or throat, heart disease, and stroke. Do you realize, however, that young children in a smoking household are more likely to suffer from asthma, bronchitis, pneumonia, and even ear infections than children of nonsmokers? Is that fair?

Even if you and your family dodge the disease bullet, smoking drains your pocketbook, causes wrinkles, stains your teeth, and in the growing community of fit nonsmokers, makes you a social outcast. No other decision, adhered to firmly, can do so much to improve your life. When you begin to reshape yourself by reshaping your life, you will find workouts to be easier and more enjoyable if you become a nonsmoker.

Quick Fix or Fitness Forever?

Sometimes the motivation to lose weight is simply cosmetic because your calendar shows a special occasion coming up for which you want to look trim. Sure, you can go on a crash diet, dump some weight (so that you *look* less dumpy), shine for the special event, and probably feel hungry and horrible. If you do something radical, try using it as a springboard for *real* fitness.

Such quick weight loss has nothing to do with fitness. In fact, virtually all experts agree that people who diet without exercising will quickly regain the lost weight plus some extra. The slow, steady road to fitness and eating sensibly, on the other hand, will result in long-term weight loss and good health. In our fat-obsessed, instant-gratification culture, many people would rather take a pill or undergo surgical procedures—risks and all—than set a course to fitness and stick to it.

The key to keeping weight off and staying healthy is activity. Scheduled exercise should be part of the program, but incorporating activity into your life every single day is the not-so-secret route to long-term success. The Centers for Disease Control, the American College of Sports Medicine, and the Surgeon General's office recommend at least 30 minutes of physical activity every day to have a positive impact on health. A "positive impact on health" is not the same as "lean and fit," but it is a start or a supplement to a regular workout program.

The power of positive thinking also impacts shape-up success. A University of Maryland study followed 54 women who embarked on a nine-month diet and exercise program. Before they started, 28 percent believed they would lose weight and 26 percent did not. At the end of the study period, those who believed lost 30 percent more weight than the doubters. Hallelujah!

Quote, Unquote

"You have to think of physical activity and exercise as being on a continuum. Something is better than nothing. More is definitely better than something. Physical activity is something. Exercise is better."

—Dr. Harold Kohl, Director of Research, Baylor Sports Medicine Institute, Houston

The President's Council on Physical Fitness issued five principles to think about when you begin an exercise program and to keep in mind as you embark on it:

1. Success requires commitment.

2. Patience is essential.

3. Don't try to do too much, too soon.

4. Don't quit before you've given yourself the opportunity to experience the benefits of exercise.

5. Stay convinced of the benefits of fitness and the health risks of unfitness.

Fitness: Your Cheapest Health Insurance

The American Heart Association and its affiliated American Stroke Association are worried. Cardiovascular disease, including stroke, is the number-one killer of women over 25—half a million every year. The AHA believes that at least 30 minutes of daily physical activity will reap untold health dividends and shave that dismal statistic.

Recognizing that many people—especially women pressured by family, job, and community demands—find it difficult to make time, the AHA developed the Choose to Move program. This free, 12-week program is like a correspondence course to help you lift yourself from the sedentary lifestyle. It begins with 10 minutes of easy-to-moderate exercises a day and progresses to the half-hour you need. It also offers fitness tips and invites you to submit a biweekly progress report. For more information, contact the AHA at 1-888-694-3278 (toll-free) or www.americanheart.org.

Think about all the problems obesity can cause and exercise can alleviate. As previously noted, excess weight and a sedentary lifestyle are linked with heart disease, stroke, and diabetes in both genders. Women who do not exercise are vulnerable to a host of other chronic problems. From the age of 40 on, most women lose one half to one third of a pound each of muscle and bone every year and often gain body fat in its place. In perimenopause, which precedes menopause, these changes accelerate. More than one third of American women aged 30 to 49 are already overweight, and by age 50, that figure jumps to more than 50 percent. That's half the female American population inviting osteoporosis, broken bones, fatigue, frailty, depression, and more from lack of exercise.

Not only can exercise alleviate many current health problems and ward off future ones, it also can reveal various disorders. (Remember that cardiologists regularly use a stress test to help diagnose heart and lung problems.) Serious athletes, who tend to be in tune with their bodies, often notice changes in their performance that can signal a medical problem. Even casual exercisers and recreational athletes should be alert to such changes. They might be nothing, or they might help pinpoint such problems as anemia, heart problems, and seizure disorders.

Writing in *The Physician and Sportsmedicine*, Dr. E. Randy Eichner of the University of Oklahoma Health Sciences Center and Dr. Warren A. Scott of Kaiser Permanente in

Santa Clara, California, reported anecdotal evidence of the diagnostic by-product of exercise. They wrote about a 57-year-old man who reported headaches just five to 10 minutes into vigorous swimming or walking. An angiogram revealed severe blockage in three coronary arteries. A 72-year-old softball player who could no longer make it to first base turned out to have Parkinson's disease. A 25-year-old runner who found his 5-kilometer race times eroding from 15 to 18 minutes was found to be anemic.

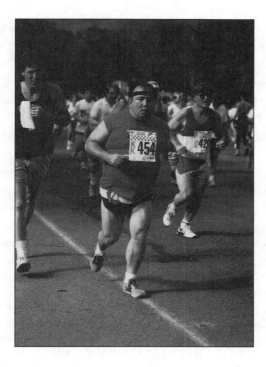

No matter where you start, you never know what you can do until you set a goal and work toward it.

(Photo: Anne W. Krause)

Fitness Starts with Setting Goals

Would you plan a dinner party without a menu or recipes? Would you begin a woodworking or sewing project without a plan or a pattern? Would you head out on a vacation without an itinerary and some maps? Probably not. You can view your dinner party, your project, or your vacation as your goal.

When you decide that *now* is the time to get fit, set some goals for yourself at the outset. Be realistic and make them achievable. If you are a middle-age woman who has given birth to three children and packed on 40 pounds, it's not realistic to think you'll be a size seven as you were when you graduated from high school. If you are a man with a sedentary job and a lardy middle, it is unlikely that you will become the totally muscular GI you were when you finished basic training. Don't even think you'll look like Vanna White or Arnold Schwarzenegger. In fact, if all you focus on is the number on a scale or being the physical clone of some celebrity, you are doomed to frustration.

Instead of dreaming about the unachievable body, think about improving, not perfecting, the body you have. Here are some examples of goals you can set:

➤ You can set general goals such as slimming down, trimming your belly, toning your thighs, or building your upper torso in relation to your body *now*.

➤ It is even more effective to set a specific goal such as losing 25 pounds, going down two sizes, or fitting into an outfit you outgrew five years ago.

➤ You can set an exercise goal such as being able to do 25 pushups, bench press 50 pounds, sustain an hour on a stationary bike or treadmill, or make it through an aerobics class without having to stop.

➤ You can set a functional goal such as running or walking in a race, hiking up a high mountain, or refereeing your child's soccer game without practically collapsing as the final score is posted.

➤ You can set a health goal such as reducing your blood pressure or lowering your cholesterol level.

➤ You can set a scheduling goal such as working out at least three but preferably four times a week for a month or every other day until you've used up every session on a membership card at the gym.

➤ You can sign up for a class that runs for a certain number of weeks and see it through such as a beginner weight-training course, a low-impact aerobics course, a water fitness course, a beginning yoga class, or planned walking sessions with a coach.

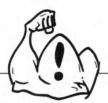

Fit Tip

Write down your goals and post them in a prominent place such as next to your bathroom mirror, on a door you use daily, or on your refrigerator. Set up your computer's calendar program at work so that your goal flashes onscreen when you start your computer every morning.

You might do better breaking down your goals into short-, medium-, and long-term goals. Instead of vowing to lose 25 pounds in four months, for example, you might set incremental goals. A man might aim to lose 10 pounds in the first month, another 10 within two months, and five more in the third month. A woman might try for eight pounds in the first month and five to six pounds during each of the next three months. As your long-term goal, you might select a race distance such as 10 kilometers, which is 6.2 miles. To prepare for the race, set a short-term goal of walking or jogging 1 mile around a local school track without stopping. Your medium-term goal could be 3 or 4 miles on the track or on the road, and then you can begin aiming at 5 miles or more to train for that 10-kilometer run.

Couples or friends often are successful if they embark on a shape-up program together. This can work splendidly for motivation. After all, someone is depending on you for that daily walk or visit to the gym. The goals don't need to be the same. In fact, because men and women lose weight at different rates and build muscle differently, they can't be identical even for the most devoted couple.

Reward yourself for achieving a goal. If you are a woman, when you've succeeded in going down two sizes, buy a sleek new outfit or perhaps a daring swimsuit to show off your new body; or treat yourself to a massage, a facial, or a "day of beauty" at a local spa. If you are a man who has hankered for a particular tool, gadget, or sporting-goods item, buying it is a suitable reward for achieving a goal. If you and your spouse or significant other have both reached some kind of shape-up milestone, reward yourselves with a lovely, low-cal candlelight dinner or a getaway to a romantic inn. The one reward that would be counterproductive is a dinner in your favorite, filling restaurant.

Expect the Start-Up to Feel Strange

The first steps on the road to fitness can be bumpy, but if you know what to expect, you can install some emotional shock absorbers to smooth the way. You can assume that the first few sessions of whatever plan you make will seem really strange and difficult. You also can expect to feel self-conscious, even if you are working out in front of the television in the privacy of your own home. If you join a gym or an exercise class, you very likely will feel as if everybody but you knows what to do and how to do it. Everyone was once a beginner, however, and your fellow exercisers are probably so focused on themselves that they are paying no attention to you. If you register for a class, try to find one aimed at beginners. Not only will everyone be at a similar level, everyone will be equally confused.

Emotions aside, if you haven't been exercising, you might be downright uncomfortable physically. The early sessions can be something of a struggle. After all, getting your rusty body parts moving is an unfamiliar sensation, and you might worry that you are doing too much and straining yourself or doing too little and not benefiting. You will be surprised how quickly the discomfort—both emotional and physical—fades. That's because every time you work out, you are remaking yourself into an exerciser, and you soon will learn how to feel what's right for you.

Be prepared for a new you—not an instant new you but a new you refined over time. You'll notice small changes. At first, you might find yourself having greater endurance or noticing that you no longer get out of breath easily. Your clothes might be looser. It might be easier to get into and out of your automobile. These are better indications of increased fitness than the weight on the scale. With every shred of progress, remind yourself that you are doing the right thing for your health and body shape. Soon, you might also realize that, no matter how much you dread starting to exercise, the negative feeling quickly melts away once you start moving. Be aware that you'll feel physically better very quickly. Note, too, that the feelings of pleasure and satisfaction from a job well done (and a goal that is closer to accomplishment with every workout session) last after you've stopped working out.

The Least You Need to Know

➤ The first step is figuring out what your motivation is for shaping up.

➤ When you set your fitness goals, make sure they are realistic.

➤ If you are a smoker, do whatever it takes to quit—now.

➤ Be prepared to feel uncomfortable when you first begin working out.

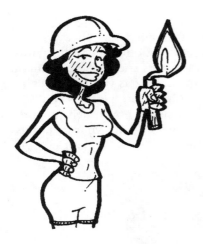

Laying the Groundwork

Once you set yourself up with a slim-down, shape-up goal and decide to get going, it's tempting to join a health club, buy a wardrobe full of cool workout clothes, go on a fast-fix diet, and order exercise videos and gadgets. Some people—okay, women—even use their about-to-start workout program as an excuse to buy a whole wardrobe in the size they plan to be, claiming that the new duds are *incentive* to slim down. Too often, new exercisers tend to start with a burst and get sore or discouraged. The combination of impossible expectations and an out-of-tune body is a formula for fitness failure, and then the expenditure seems like an indictment that deepens the disappointment and discouragement.

Success is not serendipity. It is the result of a good grasp of your starting point, good planning, and a good attitude. Be positive in your approach to sticking with your program, but be realistic about what you can accomplish and in what time frame. Begin with an honest assessment of where you are starting from in order to figure out where you want to go and where you *can* go. Start modestly and sensibly, remembering to reward yourself as you progress.

Be Your Body's Best Friend

Think of what you do for your friends. You motivate them, encourage them to achieve their goals, support them when they've had setbacks, offer practical solutions for thorny problems, and praise them to the skies for progress and accomplishment. You can apply every one of these supportive actions to yourself as you go through various stages in your quest for fitness. Your friends can help you (perhaps you'll even go at it with a workout buddy), but in the end, no matter how much support you have, no one else can make you get into shape. Only you move your own muscles. Only you control what food you put into your mouth.

Being your own best friend will help you through the good times and the challenging parts of your new fitness program.

(Photo: Anne W. Krause)

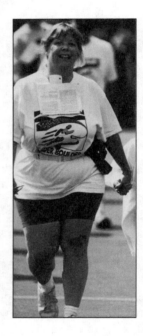

Look in the mirror. The person looking back at you is your best friend. There's all sorts of help out there for you, but you need to get out and walk. You need to get to the gym. You need to watch your diet. Even if you sign on with a personal trainer or join a support group like Weight Watchers as a motivational mechanism, you have to take charge and get there. *You* are the only constant in your life. If *you* take care of your body and treat it the very best way you can, it will repay you with interest. Encouragement and expertise are available from outside sources, but in the end, only you can set some reasonable goals, monitor your own progress, work through disappointments, and reward yourself for your gains. And wherever you go, you will be with your body's best friend.

Analyzing Where You Are Now

It's one thing to vow to "get in shape" or to "lose some weight" (as discussed in Chapter 1, "The Name of the Game Is Goals") but to be successful, you need to set specific goals and make a real plan. The foundation on which any plan should be built is an evaluation of where you are now, both fitnesswise and healthwise.

Because you certainly don't want to harm yourself more than help yourself, pay a visit to your doctor before you start your program. He or she might even have some specific workout suggestions for you or point you to a suitable health club or trainer where your needs will be addressed appropriately. In addition to a medical assessment, there are two basic categories of evaluation:

Quote, Unquote

"Never underestimate your power to change and improve yourself. You are a good person with wonderful qualities, and you have the ability to reach your goals."

—Denise Austin, television and video fitness host and author of several fitness books

➤ Where you are now (body weight, body-mass index, and so on)

➤ What you can do (strength, endurance, and flexibility)

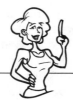

Fitness Fact

In a recent survey of 20,847 adults in a cardiovascular disease prevention program, nearly 75 percent of those who were advised by their physicians to exercise did so, compared to 55.6 percent of those who did not receive a doctor's counsel.

If you begin your fitness quest by joining a gym or a health club, your current health and physical condition will be evaluated. At the very least, you will be asked to fill out a questionnaire about your age, weight, medical history, tobacco use, eating and drinking habits, and the amount and type of exercise you do. Generally, when you join a gym, you will be offered a fitness test as a routine or optional service for new members. A fitness or spa vacation generally starts with a baseline assessment and gives you and any fitness professional you work with a starting point. Remember, to judge how far you've come once you're on a program, you need to know where you started.

Typically, the tester will put you through several steps. You may have to lift weights to evaluate your strength or use a treadmill or do a step-up, step-down test for a specific amount of time to assess your cardiovascular conditioning. You will be weighed on a medically accurate scale and perhaps be measured for body composition (that is, the percentage of fat mass in your body). Details on various assessments and how to interpret them follow in this chapter.

If you decide to embark on your own program, you still can have a professional fitness assessment. If that's not possible, you still should become knowledgeable about areas of concern and should definitely seek medical advice if necessary. No matter what you want to achieve, it is good to get a sense of your starting point. This is true whether you have some identifiable risk factors or are perfectly healthy. Professional fitness testers evaluate several major factors, and you can do some yourself, too.

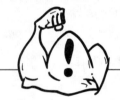

Fit Tip

If you choose to do your own baseline assessment, record such data as the results of your initial evaluation in your notebook. If you have a professional test done, ask for a copy and put that in your notebook.

Weight a Minute

Fitness experts concur that your body-mass index and other factors we've discussed (and will cover in more detail in this chapter) are better indications of fitness than just your body weight, but most of us can't resist stepping on the scale. If you use a scale, you might as well do it right. Take your clothes off, step on the scale, look at the number, and record it in your notebook. It's as simple as that. Your height will remain constant, and your height-to-body-weight ratio is a basic measure of your starting point and your progress. You know what you weigh now, and it's a small matter to reweigh yourself, preferably at the same time every time. Experts suggest weighing in no more than once a week, but many people compulsively do it daily or every few days anyway.

Weight itself should not become a fixation, but having said that, body weight is one significant factor in health. Insurance actuaries and government health officials have calculated healthy body weight/height ratios for adults with small, medium, and large frames. These tables do not take into account body-mass index or other variables, but they are another useful starting point to use as benchmarks if you are trying to lose weight.

The following data is extracted from the Metropolitan Life Insurance Company's height and weight tables (www.metlife.com) for adults aged 25 to 59 with the lowest mortality. Consider these to be normal weight ranges. To see where you fit in, compare your body weight to a recommended range for the same height and build. The weights are given in pounds and include three pounds of indoor clothing and shoes. If you weigh yourself unclothed, subtract about four pounds to match up with the tables that follow.

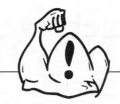

Fit Tip

Weigh yourself at the same time of day every few days using the same scale and wearing the same clothes—or no clothes.

Male Body Weight Chart

Height	Small Frame	Medium Frame	Large Frame
5'2"	128–134	131–141	138–150
5'3"	130–136	133–143	140–153
5'4"	132–138	135–145	142–156
5'5"	134–140	137–148	144–160
5'6"	136–142	139–151	146–164
5'7"	138–145	142–154	149–168
5'8"	140–148	145–157	152–172
5'9"	142–151	151–163	155–176
5'10"	144–154	151–163	158–180
5'11"	146–157	154–166	161–184
6'0"	149–160	157–170	164–188
6'1"	152–164	160–174	168–192
6'2"	155–168	165–178	172–197
6'3"	158–172	167–182	176–202
6'4"	162–176	171–187	181–207

Female Body Weight Chart

Height	Small Frame	Medium Frame	Large Frame
4'10"	102–111	109–121	118–131
4'11"	103–113	111–123	120–134
5'0"	104–115	113–126	120–134
5'1"	106–118	115–129	125–140
5'2"	108–121	118–132	128–143
5'3"	111–124	121–135	131–147
5'4"	114–127	124–138	134–151
5'5"	117–130	127–141	137–155
5'6"	120–133	130–144	140–159
5'7"	123–136	133–147	143–163
5'8"	126–139	136–150	146–167
5'9"	129–142	139–153	149–170
5'10"	132–145	142–156	152–173
5'11"	135–148	145–159	155–176
6'0"	138–151	148–162	158–179

Body Composition

The body-mass index (BMI) is a number reflecting the percentage of body fat in proportion to lean body mass (bone, muscle, tissue, organs, and blood). Experts say it is a better indication of what shape you're in than simple by-the-scale weight. Tests for BMI can be done in several ways, but it is virtually impossible to do any of them, except the tape-measure test, yourself:

> ➤ **Pinch test (technically, anthropometric test).** The tester uses a tong-like skinfold caliper to pinch the skin, fat, and underlying adipose tissue away from your muscles in about half a dozen places on your body. The numbers displayed on the caliper translate into your BMI.

> ➤ **Tank test.** You sit on an underwater scale in a large tank. You exhale until there is no more air in your lungs and then submerge completely for five seconds until your weight is recorded on the scale. Your underwater weight is plugged into a formula that calculates your BMI.

> ➤ **Bioelectrical impedance analysis.** Electrodes are attached to your foot and hand. A painless signal between the two electrodes can determine your BMI because the signal travels at different rates through fat and muscle. The margin of error is greatest in people who are very overweight or underweight.

➤ **Analyzer scale.** This calculates various personal data from a statistical input and a 10-second weigh-in. The unit was developed by a Japanese company called Tanita. Input includes your weight, height, gender, clothing weight, and mode (adult, adult athlete, or child). The printout provides your actual body weight, body-mass index, impedance, fat mass, lean body mass, and percentage of body weight from fat and water.

➤ **Tape-measure test.** This does not measure your BMI, but it's an easy way of checking how many inches you've lost. You can do it yourself at home. Use a tape measure on the places where fat is stored: waist, widest part of the hips, chest, upper arm, and thigh.

Another way to evaluate how close you are to a normal weight range is to look at your body-mass index, as expressed in percentage of body fat, and see where it falls. The lower the percentage of body fat, the lower the BMI number.

Body–Mass Index (in percentages)

	Males	Females
Slightly underweight	<20.7	<19.1
Normal weight	20.7–26.4	25.8–27.3
Slightly overweight	26.4–27.8	25.8–27.3
Overweight	27.8–31.1	27.3–32.2
Very overweight	31.1–45.4	32.3–44.8
Morbidly obese	>45.5	>44.8

Each body-composition test has a statistical margin for error, so select one test as a baseline. To track your progress over time, have the test done by the same person at the same place to provide the best indication of changes in your BMI.

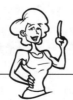

Fitness Fact

Here's another good health reason to slim down, and it takes just a tape measure to assess your risk. University of Glasgow researchers found that women with waists larger than 34½ inches and men with waists larger than 40 inches are at serious risk of weight-related health problems.

Aerobic and Cardio Fitness

Your aerobic capacity and your cardio conditioning are related because the heart and lungs work together to draw oxygen into the body, to send it out through the bloodstream, and to reprocess it. The cardiovascular system refers to the organs involved in this whole process, and your endurance is a function of your cardiovascular health. The entire heart-lung system is referred to as the cardiopulmonary system. To test the efficiency of your heart and lungs, the trainer will measure your heart rate.

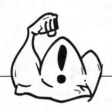

Fit Tip

To take your own pulse, rest your middle and index or ring finger on the artery of the other hand (at the base of the wrist) or on the artery in your neck (under the side of your jaw). Count the beats for a full minute.

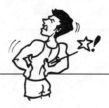

Achtung!

Caffeine can elevate your heart rate, so lay off coffee and caffeinated teas and soft drinks before a fitness evaluation.

Heart rate is fitness-speak for pulse—in other words, the number of times your heart beats each minute. Your resting heart rate is your pulse before you even get out of bed in the morning. (Because trainers don't make early-morning house calls, they get an approximation by checking clients' heart rates when they are sitting down quietly.) The normal adult heart-rate range is 60 to 90 beats per minute. If you already are in reasonable shape, your pulse probably will be at the lower end of the range. If you are sedentary or overweight, it probably will be at the upper end of the range. When you begin working out, your heart rate will rise; when you stop, it will return to its resting rate.

To determine your aerobic fitness, a trainer or exercise physiologist will put you through a submaximal test, or submax for short. You might use a stationary bicycle or a treadmill for about 15 minutes while your heart rate and blood pressure are monitored. The intensity at which you work will be increased every few minutes until you are working at 75 to 85 percent of your maximum. A simpler test requires you to step on and off a 10- to 12-inch-high step and take your pulse after three to five minutes.

Strength and Power

These two are related. Strength is the muscles' ability to exert force, and power is the time it takes to do the work. Generally, fitness assessments include lifting weights to test both the maximum weight you can lift and your muscular endurance. In other words, the tester will find out how many pounds you can lift and how many times you can lift that weight. You might be asked to do a bench press—lying on your back while lifting and lowering a barbell.

Lower-body strength is similarly evaluated on the basis of how much weight you can lift and how many times you can lift it. A common test uses a leg-extension apparatus, which resembles a narrow, armless chair with a weighted bar at the bottom. You hook your ankles under the bar and straighten your legs to lift the weight attached to the bar. As with the bench-press test for the upper body, the combination of the maximum weight you can lift and the number of repetitions is the indicator of lower-body strength.

Pushups are another common upper-body strength test. The weight you lift is your own. The more pushups you are able to do, the fitter you are. Men usually do full-body pushups, supporting their weight on their toes and hands. Because women have significantly less upper-body strength than men, their standards are lower. They usually do half-pushups, supporting their weight on their hands and knees. Both full-body and half-pushups involve raising and lowering the entire torso. For both genders, the number of pushups a person can be expected to do declines markedly with age.

Males—Pushups*

Fitness Level Age	Poor	Fair	Average	Good	Excellent
<29	<20	20–24	35–44	45–54	>55
30–39	<14	15–24	25–34	35–44	>45
40–49	<11	12–19	20–29	30–39	>40
50–59	<7	8–14	15–24	25–34	>35
>60	<4	5–9	10–19	20–29	>30

Note that some authorities feel that these standards are somewhat high.

Females—Pushups*

Fitness Level Age	Poor	Fair	Average	Good	Excellent
<29	0–5	6–16	17–33	34–49	>50
30–39	0–3	4–11	12–24	25–39	>40
40–49	0–2	3–7	8–19	20–34	>35
50–59	0–1	2–5	6–14	15–29	>30
>60	0	1–2	3–4	5–19	>20

Note that some authorities feel that these standards are somewhat high.

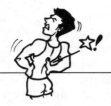

Evaluating mid-body strength also is a counting game. Sit-ups are the key test of the body's core section, and traditional evaluation systems such as the one the YMCA has used for decades require them. Very fit people, especially men, can do the full-body version. The motion starts at the hips, and the entire upper body is lifted from a lying to a sitting position in one fluid motion.

Most women and out-of-shape men are asked to do crunches instead, in which the head, shoulders, shoulder blades, and lower back are lifted off the floor. In a crunch, you do not raise your torso to near vertical from the floor. Instead of sitting up all the way, raise your head, shoulders, and upper back but leave your lower back pressed to the floor. In other words, you reach the highest position with your lower back remaining on the floor and your shoulder blades off—that is, in more of a horizontal than vertical plane. Ratings again are related to age and gender.

Males—Crunches

Fitness Level Age	Poor	Fair	Average	Good	Excellent
<29	<20	21–35	36–45	46–70	>70
30–39	<15	16–20	21–40	41–60	>60
40–49	<10	11–15	16–35	36–49	>50
50–59	<5	6–10	11–15	26–39	>40
>60	0	<5	6–15	16–30	>30

Females—Crunches

Fitness Level Age	Poor	Fair	Average	Good	Excellent
<29	<15	16–30	31–40	41–60	>60
30–39	<10	11–15	16–35	36–50	>50
40–49	<5	6–10	11–30	26–39	>40
50–59	<3	3–5	6–10	21–29	>30
>60	0	1–3	3–5	10–19	>20

Flexibility

This crucial fitness factor often is overlooked or ignored by exercisers who want maximum results in minimum time. As dancers and athletes—such as gymnasts, figure skaters, and high divers—prove, however, flexibility is an important element of being in shape. Runners regularly stretch before a training run or race, and even muscle-sports athletes such as football players and boxers add flexibility training to their regimes. Pilates, yoga, and stretch classes are among the most popular disciplines that focus specifically on helping with flexibility.

You can assess the flexibility of each part of your body by performing a simple motion and seeing how far you can go. If you get into the habit of warming up with light cardiovascular activity for at least five minutes before your new workout and stretching during the cool-down afterward, your flexibility will improve and you will reduce the risk of injury. To check the flexibility of your

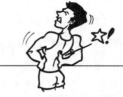

Achtung!

Although this is rarely a problem for beginning exercisers, too much flexibility can increase the risk of injury just as too little flexibility does.

➤ **Hamstring and lower back**, stand with your feet shoulder-width apart and your knees slightly flexed. Roll down from the waist, reaching your fingertips toward the floor. If you can easily reach the floor, you have good flexibility in these locations. If you can touch your toes, you are moderately flexible. If you're not even close, you need to work on this. If you have lower-back problems, it's best not to attempt this at all.

➤ **Shoulders and upper back**, raise one arm and reach back behind your shoulder and neck in a downward direction. Then place the other hand behind your back and raise it. With your forearms on a diagonal across your back, try to clasp your hands together behind you. If you can do so easily, you have flexible shoulders. If you can bring your fingertips close without touching, you are moderately flexible. If your hands can't come close, you might experience stiffness and discomfort in your neck and shoulders so you need to work on this.

➤ **Calves**, sit squarely on the floor and extend your legs straight out in front of you. Flex your feet. If your toes exceed the perpendicular angle and point slightly back toward you, you have very flexible calf muscles. If your toes are perpendicular to the floor, your calf muscles are moderately flexible. If you can't get your toes comfortably toward perpendicular, you might be susceptible to ankle problems so you need to work on this.

➤ **Quadriceps and hip flexors**, lie on your stomach with one leg straight and bend the other toward your rear. If your heel easily touches your buttock, you have good quad flexibility. If it comes close but doesn't touch, you are moderately flexible. If you can't even come close, you might be prone to knee problems so you need to work on this.

➤ **Hips and buttocks,** lie on your back and bring up one knee. Keeping your other leg straight on the floor, hug the knee close to your chest. If you can do this but your straight leg rolls toward the outside of the hip, you are moderately flexible. If you can't bring your knee close without your straight leg rising from the floor, you might have hip or back problems so you need to work on this.

A Simple Analysis for Cardio Fitness

Instead of administering a series of exercise tests to measure fitness, some trainers have taken to assessing their clients' fitness by creating simple categories and having their clients assign a number to each category. They refer to this as the PA-R. The higher the number, the fitter the person is. You can use the first part at home to come to a reasonable assessment of where you are on a scale of current activity. Here are the rankings:

0   Avoids walking or exertion

1   Walks for pleasure, occasionally engages in activity that results in elevated breathing, uses stairs instead of elevators

2   Participates in an organized recreational activity or work that requires moderate physical activity (household chores, yard work, weightlifting, golf, and others) for 10 to 60 minutes per week

3   Participates in an organized recreational activity or work that requires moderate physical activity for more than one hour per week

4   Regularly participates in a difficult physical activity (running, swimming, aerobics, tennis, cycling, and others) for less than 30 minutes per week

5   Regularly participates in a difficult physical activity, such as running 1 to 5 miles or participating in a similarly difficult activity, for 30 to 60 minutes per week

6   Regularly participates in a difficult physical activity, such as running 5 to 10 miles or participating in a similarly difficult activity, for one to three hours

7   Regularly participates in a difficult physical activity, such as running more than 10 miles or participating in a similarly difficult activity, for more than three hours per week

Trainers take another step by plugging this PA-R into a more complicated calculation that also includes body-mass index (BMI) and several other figures to come up with a client's oxygen utilization capacity.

Fitness Fact

Fitness assessment assistance is available on the Internet as well. The Aerobics and Fitness Association of America (AFAA), for example, developed Fitness Triage to help people identify various factors that might have an impact on the safety and effectiveness of specific exercise programs. Upon completion of a registration form and profile, Fitness Triage provides a red, green, and yellow advice screen with go-aheads and cautions based on your profile. To register, log on to www.afaa.com. For other Web sites with fitness assessments, see Chapter 4, "Using All the Help You Can Get."

Another Form of Assessment

How old is your body? You know how old you are. Your chronological age is right there on your driver's license. Depending on how out of shape you are, however, your body might be old beyond your years. When you seriously undertake a fitness program, you will find that your body's age actually gets younger as you progress.

Exercise experts know this in theory, but a company called FitnessAge puts it into easily understandable numbers. This system, introduced in 1999, takes your cardio, BMI, flexibility, and strength evaluations and plugs them into a computer (along with other factors such as your age, height, weight, and medical risk factors). The computer program compares your information to a YMCA national database of 60,000 other evaluations. It determines your body's age, compared to those 60,000 people, in each of the four areas and also as a total.

The program guides you to the area or areas you need to work at most if you want to become functionally younger. A retest every six to eight weeks will show you how well you are doing. Some health clubs offer FitnessAge assessments through their trainers. For information about where to find these, call 1-888-4-FIT-AGE. You also can get information and a do-it-yourself evaluation at www.fitnessage.com.

Medical Caveats

The first stop on your road to fitness needs to be your doctor's office. After all, you want your new program to make you healthier and fitter, not to put you at medical risk. Many gyms require that you see a doctor if they feel there might be a problem. Exercise can help combat these medical conditions, and your physician can prescribe a suitable program for you or send you to a suitable physiologist or trainer.

Every fitness authority, every exercise video, every TV workout show, and every book strongly suggests consulting your physician before starting any new workout program. This not only is the result of our litigious society, it also makes good sense. If you are under 35 and in good health, authorities feel it might not be necessary to get a doctor's okay before you start working out. It is imperative, however, to get a medical exam if you are over 35 and have been inactive, if you have a family history of conditions that might require precautions, or if you yourself have certain medical conditions.

According to the President's Council on Physical Fitness, you should consult with a doctor if you have *any* medical concerns, particularly heart disease, high blood pressure, elevated cholesterol levels, frequent dizzy spells, extreme breathlessness after mild exertion, arthritis or other bone problems, severe muscular or ligament problems, back problems, obesity, or a family history of such diseases.

Take a Before Picture—for After

The day you decide, once and for all, to set out on the path to fitness, put on a leotard or a nonconstricting bathing suit, stand in front of a nondistracting background, and ask someone you know and trust to take a series of photographs from every angle—front, rear, and side views. You also could strip naked, put the video camera on a tripod, and film yourself. Be merciless—no flattering light, no sucked-in gut—and just let it *all* hang out. Take a quick look, which might be all you can stand at the beginning of your fitness quest, date the visuals, and lock them away.

Later, when you are well on the road to your fitness goal, take another set of photos or a video. In fact, if you have a long way to go and are on a program that will take a lot of time, do so every three months as you progress. When you've reached your goal, look at these visuals and be very proud of what you've accomplished. This optional trick can be either motivational or discouraging. It works wonders for some people but depresses others. The reward can be comparing before, during, and after pictures after you've reached your goal.

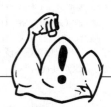

Fit Tip

Instead of photographs, you can take chest, waist, hip, thigh, and upper-arm measurements and record them. When you remeasure, the comparison will help you track your progress.

The Least You Need to Know

➤ It's up to you to take charge of your life.

➤ Check with your physician for medical clearance and advice.

➤ Get a baseline assessment of your endurance, strength, cardio fitness, and flexibility.

➤ "Before" photos, videos, or measurements will help you compare your results.

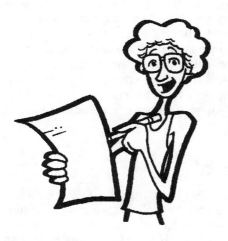

Chapter 3

Drawing Up a Fitness Plan

> **In This Chapter**
>
> ➤ Fitness comes in many forms
>
> ➤ Calories do count in a fitness plan
>
> ➤ Select a program you can live with
>
> ➤ Consistency and motivation are the keys to success

Would you start on a long trip without a destination or a road map? Probably not. The same is true for the road to getting fit. After you've set your goals and looked honestly at your starting point, it's time to draw up a specific plan for reaching them. If you are young, somewhat active, not significantly overweight, and in good health, your ambition might be to run a half-marathon, to participate in a bicycle tour, or to go on a long backpacking trip. You have set a lofty goal, but it is a realistic one, considering that you are taking off from a pretty good starting position. You can probably handle a significant workout to begin with and can build from that quickly. In contrast, if you are not in the first flower of youth, if you are sedentary, overweight, and perhaps have some medical concerns, you must start with a substantially lower level of intensity. On an absolute scale, your goals are more modest, but in relation to where you are now, they are just as ambitious—and your fitness program will be equally challenging.

No matter where you start and where you want to go, the most effective fitness and weight-management program combines aerobic exercise, resistance training, and stretching—and, of course, eating the right kinds of food. Aerobic exercise burns calories, provides cardiovascular and cardiorespiratory conditioning, and improves endurance. Resistance training, primarily working out with weights, builds and tones muscles. Stretching increases flexibility and helps prevent soreness and even injury. There are numerous ways to pursue each of these components. The beauty of a fitness plan is that you can tailor it to your tastes and time frame by mixing and matching the elements in your routine. If something doesn't work for you or you get tired of it, you can change the mix. As you get fitter, you will increase the challenge of your activities, but you will find it easier to add new ones.

"But I just want to lose weight."

Many people think that, if they just want to lose weight, dieting, crash dieting, fasting, or some other reduction of food intake will do the trick. In fact, dieting without exercising can be counterproductive, especially for women, who have less muscle and bone in proportion to their body weight than men have. If you stop eating or take in extremely few calories each day to lose weight, the opposite soon happens. Your body thinks it is starving, reverts to its natural defense against famine, and holds on to what it has as if it's a matter of life or death.

In contrast, exercise helps control weight. Scientists, nutritionists, and physiologists studying the relationship between diet and exercise have drawn conclusions that point to exercise as a weight-loss enhancer, not a detractor. When you exercise, you build muscle and become both fitter and leaner. More on this in Chapter 6, "Tune Up That Muscle Machine."

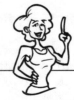

Fitness Fact

According to a University of Michigan study, when women diet without exercising, 25 to 30 percent of the weight they lose is water, lean tissue, muscle, and even bone. Corroborating the Michigan findings is a Tufts University study, in which 10 overweight women were put on customized food plans. Five did strength training just twice a week; the other five did not. The women who dieted but did not exercise lost an average of 13 pounds during the study period, but 2.8 percent of that was lean muscle mass. The exercisers lost an average of 14.6 pounds, while gaining 1.4 pounds of lean tissue.

Calories Do Count

If you're just out of shape but not overweight, working out to build your strength and endurance might be your formula for fitness. Most people are not only unfit, however; they also are overweight—and losing weight is the number one reason people resolve to get into shape. Landing the one-two punch—weight loss and conditioning—takes a change in eating habits as well as a workout program. Diet plans come and go, but one of the constants in weight management is the principle of burning more calories than you consume. Diet controls caloric intake, but exercise controls how many calories are burned in a process called *metabolism*. This complicated biochemical process sustains life. At its simplest, you can think of metabolism as the process used by your body's engine (your digestive, cardiorespiratory, and circulatory systems) to burn fuel (food or fat) to keep you going. Regardless of the food source (fat, carbohydrate, or protein), when it comes to metabolism, a calorie is a calorie. According to the *Journal of the American Medical Association,* 35 percent of American men and 40 percent of women who said that they are trying to lose weight are not tracking their caloric intake. Although they may be eating less fat, which is, on balance, good, they may be taking in so many calories that weight loss is not possible without a substantial increase in exercise.

The exact number of calories that you, or any other individual, will burn for any given exercise period depends on your body weight, your metabolic efficiency, the intensity of a specific aerobic activity, and even the air temperature during the workout. When you're reaching for that cookie or you decide to skip the walk, figure that a surplus intake of just 100 calories a day can add 10 pounds a year to your body weight. By contrast, a brisk 20- to 30-minute walk can burn 100 calories.

As a guideline when evaluating different activities, you can use the following chart, which compares the number of calories that various fitness activities burn during 45 minutes of exercise. Your caloric burn may, of course, vary. This chart has been adapted from Fitness Partner's Activity Calendar. To calculate your calorie-consumption rate based on your body weight and the time allotted for these and other activities, log on to www.primusweb.com/fitnesspartners/jumpsite/.

In the Gym

	110 lbs	150 lbs	180 lbs
Stationary bike (vigorous)	416	459	454
High-impact step aerobics	396	540	648
Cross-country ski simulator	376	513	616
Elliptical trainer	356	486	583
Rowing machine (vigorous)	337	459	551
Calisthenics (vigorous)	317	432	518

continues

In the Gym (continued)

	110 lbs	150 lbs	180 lbs
Circuit training	317	432	518
Stationary bike (moderate)	277	378	545
Low-impact step aerobics	277	378	545
High-impact aerobics	277	378	545
Rowing machine (moderate)	277	378	545
Weightlifting (vigorous)	238	324	389
Stairstepper	238	324	389
Low-impact aerobics	218	297	359
Rider (moderate)	198	270	324
Calisthenics (moderate)	178	243	292
Water aerobics	158	216	259
Stretching	158	216	259
Hatha yoga	158	216	259
Weightlifting (moderate)	119	162	194

Keeping a Workout Log

Remember the notebook that you started after reading Chapter 1? Make the core of it a workout log, which is like an exercise diary. You can track every exercise and sports activity you do, how long your walks or swims are, and anything else regarding physical activity. You can make it as simple or as detailed as you like, but you'll find it both informative and rewarding as you proceed with your program. Having to put pencil to paper often serves as a great motivator when you don't feel like working out. After all, you have that page to fill.

In addition to being motivational, a log helps you track your progress. Even if your scale doesn't show the weight loss you might like, the fact that you can lift heavier weights, do more repetitions, or put another riser under your aerobic step is encouraging.

To get the most out of your workout and your log, be sure to write down everything as soon as you've completed it. If you are working with weights, note each exercise, the number of sets and reps, and the weights. If you are walking, jogging, or cycling, record your distance and time. If you take a class or work out with a tape, put that down, too. You can even jot down your goals in the margins to remind you what you are shooting for.

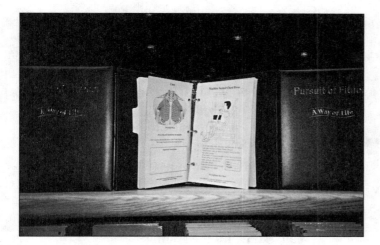

Workout log.

Finding Activities You Enjoy

After you establish where you are (point A) and set your sights on where you want to be (point B), it's time to decide how to get from point A to point B. If you have been inactive and want to begin a workout program, a good way to start is by combining a light weight workout to build your strength, walking and/or using a stationary bike or treadmill in a gym to increase your endurance, and stretching before and after each session to become more limber. Yoga also might be your cup of herbal tea. It can make you stronger and more flexible and can even help your respiratory system through controlled breathing. If you already work out some but want to be more active, you have a greater array of options. Subsequent chapters will tell you more about these forms of conditioning.

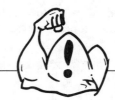

Fit Tip

In addition to raw numbers representing time, weight, and the like, you can add a column to the log to note whether a workout was easy or hard for you. This will also help you track your progress.

Options for Enhancing Your Fitness

There are so many options to help you get in shape and stay that way that sorting through the choices becomes a challenge. To try to sort them out, ask yourself some basic questions to determine what kind of activity might be most suitable:

➤ Do you want a sport or exercise you can do by yourself, as part of a twosome, or with a group? Some solo activities also can be enjoyed with a group of companions, and some group activities also work for lone eagles and couples. These are just examples, not rigid rules:

35

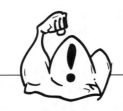

Fit Tip

Before you sign up for a long-term program, sample what's available. Visit health clubs in your area. Check out the local Y, adult education, and local recreational centers. Take a sample class or buy a punch card. After you've settled into a groove and have made working out a habit, sign on for a longer membership period.

Solo. Aerobics, running and jogging, in-line and ice skating, bicycling, swimming, kayaking, Alpine and cross-country skiing, snowshoeing, swimming

Twosome. Tennis, badminton, tandem cycling, racquetball, fencing, martial arts, rock climbing

Group. Volleyball, softball, snowshoeing, Ultimate Frisbee, touch football, soccer, ice and roller hockey

➤ Do you prefer indoor or outdoor activities?

Indoors. Dancing, squash, racquetball, aerobics, and other gym activities

Outdoors. Trail running, skiing, bicycling, softball, skiing, in-line skating

Indoors or Outdoors. Tennis, swimming, rock climbing, ice skating

➤ How much risk, or perceived risk, are you comfortable with in sports?

Low. Tennis, dancing, walking, jogging, aerobics

High. Rock climbing, kayaking, in-line skating, downhill skiing, snowboarding

➤ How important are convenience and proximity, especially if you live in a city or a suburb?

Convenient. Tennis, racquetball, handball, dancing, walking, jogging, in-line skating, swimming, bicycling, softball, climbing in a gym, aerobics

Inconvenient. Rock climbing, skiing, mountain biking, kayaking

Pace Yourself or Push Yourself?

We all know the fable about the hare and the tortoise, in which the hare bounds from the starting line energetically, hops about erratically, gets distracted frequently, and all but loses interest in the finish line. The tortoise, meanwhile, plods methodically forward, never loses sight of the goal, and eventually wins the race.

Many people who vow to begin working out have all the good intentions in the world but are hares at heart. They purchase a long-term membership at a gym or buy expensive home equipment. They start working out frantically, trying to compensate for a long period of inactivity. Although they start strong, they tend to fade fast. In fact, observers of the fitness scene say that half of all beginners quit within two months. Sometimes they drop out because of injury, sometimes because of exhaustion, sometimes out of boredom, and sometimes because they haven't geared themselves up for the long haul. The goal is to be a tortoise, building your fitness steadily and consistently, step by step, and making it part of your routine.

Fitness Fact

According to the Consumers Union, beginning exercisers are the most likely not to use two thirds exercise equipment they buy. Nearly two thirds of fitness-machine purchases are made by people who are not physically active but presumably intend to be, and they are more likely to stop using them.

When the U.S. Surgeon General's office began taking serious notice of the American public's need to exercise, the original modest recommendation for maintaining cardiovascular health was to undertake three high-intensity workouts per week. More recently, the recommendation has changed to daily exercise but on a more moderate level such as a brisk walk, a bike ride, or climbing stairs. Consistency, this medical authority has concluded, is the most important element of a fitness program.

Beyond the Comfort Zone

After you get into workout mode, it's important to keep pushing yourself to reach your goals. If you get to a certain point in your program and don't increase the challenge and/or duration, it's like putting your car into cruise control. You'll make a journey, but you won't be revving up the engine.

Quote, Unquote

"You cannot learn to fly by flying. First you must learn to walk, and to run, and to climb, and to dance."

—Friedrich Nietzsche

Exercise experts have long agreed that revving up the engine is important in getting leaner and fitter, but there have been long-running debates about what type of exercise and what intensity are the most effective at burning fat. Settlement of this issue is on the way. The *Journal of Strength & Conditioning Research* reported on a preliminary study in which eight men and 12 women, aged 18 to 50, completed fitness tests on two different aerobic apparatus, a treadmill and a stationary bicycle.

The test subjects were monitored when they worked out at submaximal and maximal intensity. The researchers found that fat oxidation was virtually identical between the two pieces of equipment for each level of intensity. This is encouraging for exercisers on a weight-loss program who, say, prefer rowing to the stairstepper, prefer riding a stationary bike to running on a treadmill, and so on. If these preliminary findings are correct, it means you can achieve your goals on whatever kind of apparatus you would like to use.

Quote, Unquote

"Laziness may appear attractive, but work gives satisfaction."

—Anne Frank

A Wealth of Options

According to the American Council on Exercise (ACE), more people are finally wising up and exercising for health instead of for some kind of ideal or perfect body. At the dawn of the twenty-first century, ACE has identified the following dozen hot trends in getting fit and staying active. Surely, even the most languorous couch potato can find something on this list to love. (This book discusses all of these in subsequent chapters.)

➤ **Personal trainers.** They're not just for the rich and famous anymore. Services are now increasingly available for moderate-income clients, perhaps spreading consultations over a period of several months to help people establish and maintain a safe, effective course of exercise. In addition to working in clubs, trainers make house calls and office visits for client convenience.

➤ **Box-aerobics and kickboxing classes.** Built on a martial arts foundation, these classes emphasize strength and endurance, and they frequently include self-defense training, too.

➤ **Children's fitness.** Gyms and fitness centers are adding programs to get kids moving.

➤ **Body pump.** Group strength-training classes set to music help fight the tedium that some people find in solo weight work.

➤ **Boot camp.** Intense workout sessions are patterned after military fitness training including the awesome Navy Seals. Another type of program is modeled after firefighters' training.

➤ **Studio cycling classes.** Also known as Spinning, the best known program of this kind, this superheated fitness trend of the late 1990s continues into the next millennium with new bike designs and specialty classes for beginners, seniors, and other target groups.

➤ **Outdoor activities.** Hiking, mountain biking, rock climbing, and other adventure sports are high on many people's lists of active sports interests.

➤ **Indoor treadmill classes.** Another ennui-fighter, such classes are modeled after studio cycling classes. They are called trekking or treading. Group rowing classes also are appearing on the fitness horizon.

➤ **Sport-specific workouts.** Get-in-shape-for-skiing classes are a staple on the class calendar of health clubs, Ys, and community recreational centers—ski clubs sometimes offer them for members, too. Now, similarly specialized training programs are designed to increase performance in such sports as rock climbing, tennis, and even golf.

➤ **Programs for older adults.** Senior centers and even nursing homes are offering exercise and strength-training programs designed especially for older people.

➤ **Elliptical trainers.** The longest lines at many top fitness centers are for this new generation of aerobic machine. It combines the benefits of a stairstepper and a treadmill but is easier on the joints.

➤ **Interactive cardio machines and Web-connected interactive fitness machines.** High tech enters the gym with smart workout machines.

➤ **Specialty classes.** No longer is Jazzercise the only class around set to specialty music. Now, aerobic workouts are choreographed to hip-hop, African rhythms, gospel music, and big-band beats.

➤ **Office workouts.** As more employers come to realize the value of fit, healthy employees to their bottom line, state-of-the-art exercise facilities and even classes are popping up in the workplace.

Reality Check

Changing your inactive lifestyle into an active one is not easy, but it is possible. Because so many New Year's resolution-makers and beginning exercisers quit before they see any results, take a look at the pattern of your life and try to start when you'll have the best chance for long-term success in making fitness part of your life. Just as it is important to know your body, it is important to analyze your patterns and see how you can make them work for you.

Does your job have seasonal peaks and valleys? Would a new workout program help you cope with the stress of peaks? Or are you better off starting during a valley when you are less pressured and might also have more time? Are you a procrastinator who needs to schedule an activity specifically? Or can you generally plug it into your day? Would it make sense to start a workout program when your kids start the school year, go off to summer camp, or spend time with the other parent if you are divorced? There are many factors to consider.

Examine your own rhythms. If you are a morning person, schedule your workouts early in the day so you'll have the best chance to succeed. Some people get up early for a walk, run, or swim to jump-start the day. Do you like to load activities at the end of the workday? If so, evening is the time when you can make fitness a habit that will stick. Can you break away at lunch to get some outdoor exercise or to spend time at the gym? It's a more productive way to spend your midday break than chowing down.

When you decide to do something, what's your willpower level? Do you put things off? Or do you easily stick to a plan after you've made it? If you tend to procrastinate, figuring that you'll go for a walk "later," select activities that are scheduled for specific times. These activities might include aerobics and other classes, a regular appointment with a personal trainer, tuning in to a TV exercise program that comes on at a certain time, or making a workout date with a friend. If having a workout log that you *must* fill in every day suffices, you can go for a walk or run at your leisure, plug an exercise tape into the VCR, or go to the gym and lift weights at your convenience.

What about seasons? If you live in the North and love being outdoors when the weather is mild, spring or fall is the ideal time to start walking, jogging, bicycling, or playing tennis. If you live in the sunbelt, outdoor activity might be tolerable only in the winter. Although the weather may be mild, the rainy winters that characterize the climate of the Pacific Northwest inhibit many people from outdoor activities. In any case, joining a gym during the season of maximum outdoor discomfort might work for you. You can take advantage of northern winters and take up snowshoeing or skiing or enjoy sunbelt summers by swimming laps or joining an aqua fitness class at an outdoor pool.

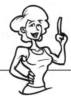

Fitness Fact

Many people make New Year's resolutions to get in shape, and more people join gyms in January than any other month of the year. No matter how long a membership they sign up for, by February, many of them already have dropped out.

The Least You Need to Know

➤ Dieters who also exercise lose more weight than sedentary dieters.

➤ A workout log is the best way to track progress and to provide further motivation.

➤ Moderate daily exercise, done consistently, is the best route to overall good health.

➤ Exercisers are less vulnerable to a variety of chronic health problems.

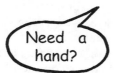

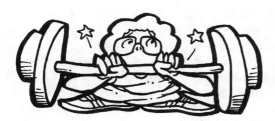

Chapter 4

Using All the Help You Can Get

In This Chapter

➤ Join a gym for classes, equipment, and professional advice

➤ Exercise videos and TV fitness shows can guide at-home workouts

➤ Can you afford a personal trainer?

➤ Exercise with your mate or a workout buddy

"Walk Your Way to Fitness." "Cardio Quickie." "Get Your Body Ready for the Beach." "Trim Your Thighs." "Work Your Abs." "Ten Minutes to a Better Butt." "Punch Away Pounds." "Look Great Naked—Build a Ready-to-Bare Body." "Yoga Shapes You Up and Calms You Down." "Target Those Trouble Zones." "Look Leaner Now." These are the types of messages screaming from magazine covers month after month. Written to lure us to buy new issues, these short, punchy phrases extol this workout or that and make them all seem like quick solutions to your body's shape, weight, or stress problems.

As you embark on your fitness regime, you—like many beginning exercisers before you—might think that someone has developed a magic formula to give you the body you want, the energy you need, or the tranquillity you crave. Magazines, books, and television infomercials abound with promises of magic slimming, toning, weight loss, and more. For every magic exercise, there's also a magic diet plan. By combining magic exercise with magic eating, you think you can create a magic new you quickly, almost automatically. The media, books, and the Internet do provide a lot of good information, and if you use it wisely, you will see good results.

Fitness is so wrapped up in issues of body, mind, and motivation, however, that tapping into personal help might be the most effective way to reach your fitness goals. This includes professional expertise as well as the support of family and friends, supplemented by workout, diet, and general health advice from media sources. Take a sample class at a local health club for a workout that is energetic, motivational, and fun. For effectiveness, however, you have to be conscientious about following a program.

In short, there's a lot of good fitness information. The problem for many beginners—and often experienced exercisers, too—is sorting it all out. Precious few people have unlimited time and resources to do nothing but get in shape. The media, the people who work at the gym, and your personal interaction with a wider support system can help you sort out all this information and hone in on a program that works for you. All these resources can act as a support system, but remember that you are the captain of your workout ship. Think of the other resources as your crew, but only you can actually move your body to make it fit and healthy.

Finding a Workout That Works for You

Even after you've resolved to get in shape, set a realistic goal, figured out your baseline, and started your logbook, you still face a bewildering array of possible activities. Some new exercisers and returnees to the workout world easily find a program they can stick with until they've achieved a goal. Others might try several combinations of aerobic and strength training before they hit on a combination they can live with. Still another type—let's call them "fashion-forward exercisers"—wants only the latest workout trend: Jane Fonda in the '70s, step aerobics in the '80s, studio cycling and Tae-Bo in the '90s. When you are trying to select your workout, shop around, try some options, and then get going. Thinking about exercising doesn't shape you up. You need to start something and stick to it.

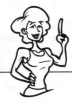

Fitness Fact

Respondents to a 1999 poll conducted by Fit-Net, an online health and fitness resource, were asked what kind of cardio workouts they do. The most popular cardio workout was treadmill/running (57 percent). This was followed by biking or spinning (37 percent), "sports" (36 percent), stairsteppers (22 percent), cross-training and aerobics (tied at 19 percent each), and step classes (9 percent). "Other" was selected by 18 percent of the respondents.

Joining a Gym

Health clubs and gyms provide not only equipment but also on-staff experts to get you working out and to keep you coming back. In an increasing number of communities, Ys and public recreation centers offer similar facilities and programs. A typical gym offers locker rooms, at least one aerobics room, an array of aerobic apparatus, and a weight room with multifunction weight machines and free weights. Many also have studios for dance, martial arts, or yoga, a swimming pool, and perhaps hot tubs, saunas, or steam rooms. For details about what to expect at a gym, see Chapter 21, "A Primer on Gyms."

This is a good time to remind you that gyms are not just buildings made of brick and mortar and filled with fitness toys. They are places where exercising *feels* right. In addition to equipment and atmosphere, they offer expertise. Someone usually is on duty to teach you how to use free weights, weight machines, and aerobic apparatus such as fitness riders, treadmills, stairsteppers, and so on. These people can show you how to use a specific apparatus and can help you use each device properly. Such basic assistance and advice is part of the fee you pay to use the facility. If you need more guidance, you can book time with the gym's staff of personal trainers, either for an ongoing program or just to help get you started.

Gyms also offer an array of group classes from aerobics to yoga and often at various levels from "fit over 50" to "high-energy steppers" or some comparable range. Some classes are offered for a specific number of weeks and you need to sign up; others are drop-in classes you can take at your convenience. Instructors lead classes with cheerleader-like enthusiasm to motivate you to get moving and to keep you coming back. Don't let classes intimidate you. No one was born knowing all the moves, all the steps, and all the combinations. Everyone was once a beginner.

When you get into a class with the music going, the instructor shouts encouragement as well as directions, and like the other exercisers, you will get into the spirit. When you first join a class, you might not have the stamina to go the distance even in a fairly easy class. The contagious group energy is sure to pump you up, however, and you'll be able to do more than you might have expected. Studies have shown that people feel better and get more out of fitness classes led by an instructor who tries to learn and use participants' names, who provides frequent individual attention, and who gives positive feedback to the class and to individuals.

Quote, Unquote

"Nothing is so contagious as enthusiasm. It moves stones. It charms brutes."

—Edward Bulwer-Lytton

Videos Can Work

Videos are great for at-home exercisers, especially beginners who might feel self-conscious in a gym. You can pop a tape into the VCR at the most convenient time for you, and it needn't be the same time every day. You can exercise first thing in the morning, before or after work, late in the evening when it's dark outside, on stormy days, while the baby is napping, while older children are at school, or any other time you want.

Hundreds of videos are available, and many of them are moderately priced. Working out with videos presents many options and offers both variety and flexibility. Working out with videos has several other advantages as well. You can do one or more routines a day. You can turn the volume as high or low as you want. You don't have to get dressed to go out, you don't have to figure into your workout schedule the time it takes to drive to and from the gym, and your shower is right there. You can slip a video into your VCR and make it your main exercise routine, or you can use it to supplement walking, running, classes, or a gym membership.

Select your videos as you would classes at a gym. Ask yourself some basic questions. Your answers can help steer you to the appropriate videos.

➤ **What are your goals?** There are videos for general conditioning, aerobic videos for fat-burning, strength-training videos, yoga videos that enhance flexibility and relaxation, tai-chi videos that are ideal for older exercisers, and more.

➤ **Do you like simplicity or glamour?** Videos using simple studio sets and a trainer who is not a star might appeal to some people, while others might prefer to work out with a big-name trainer whose program is captured in a glamorous location.

➤ **Are you a beginner or do you have some experience?** Videos aim at all exercise levels. If you are just starting an aerobics or step program, for instance, you'll want a simple program that you can do easily. If you are intrigued by kickboxing, be sure to start with a basic program to get the moves right and prevent injury.

➤ **What are your musical tastes?** Hip-hop, rock, jazz, New Age? Find a video you can gladly listen to as well as watch.

➤ **How much space do you have for your workout?** If you have a lot of room, you can accommodate an aerobics or dance workout that covers a lot of floor space. If space is a problem, select a workout suitable for a small area.

You can test-drive videos before you buy something you may or may not use. Many video stores stock exercise tapes. Rent the ones that interest you before investing. Also, keep an eye out for used tapes that the video store might be selling.

Some people play one video day after day. Others have a virtual library of videos for different purposes. Videos run the gamut from general workout tapes to those that help strengthen and tone specific body parts, from easy intro programs to fairly demanding aerobic routines. Certified trainers and all sorts of celebrities have made videos. The most important thing is to *use* the videos you've bought and to follow the instructions as if you were taking an exercise class with a live instructor.

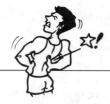

Achtung!

Videos only work when you use them as regularly as you would a scheduled class. An unplayed or rarely played tape does nothing to enhance your fitness.

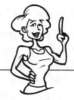

Fitness Fact

Kathy Smith has made more fitness videos than anyone. Her first aerobics video came out in 1980; her twenty-sixth, a kickboxing tape, came out in 1999.

The Complete Guide to Exercise Videos is a free, comprehensive mail-order catalogue of current exercise videos, as well as motivational tapes for walking, and exercise accessories. It categorizes each offering by length, level, and emphasis, and also summarizes the philosophy and spirit behind each. To order the catalogue, call Collage Video Specialties at 1-800-433-6769 or log on to their Web site, www.collagevideo.com.

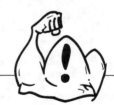

Fit Tip

To combat boredom from an oft-repeated workout, you and your friends can trade or exchange exercise videos.

Tune Your TV for Fitness

If you like the idea of working out at home, but never seem to put the tape into the VCR, a television exercise show might be just the ticket. It comes on at the same time every day, so you get the same built-in scheduling that a fitness class offers but with the convenience of scheduling it at home. If you like a particular instructor, you can make your own tape and play it whenever you like. A number of half-hour shows can fit on one tape, and you can even pause during the taping to delete commercials. As with other videos, you then can play it at your convenience. If one segment deals with a problem area you particularly want to tone, such as abdominals or glutes, you can work with that show more often than the others.

These television programs are like half-hour, on-air exercise classes. Most programs that focus on aerobics or weight training begin with warm-ups and end with cooldowns, just as a good instructor does in a live class. The shows never repeat the same exercises or sequences two days in a row, so your interest will stay high. Each program tends to remain at the same level, however, and often is geared toward novice exercisers. Some shows include demonstrations at various levels of challenge, but others don't increase the difficulty level. This can stall you as your own level of fitness improves, and you might not continue to challenge yourself if you do nothing but work out with the same TV show. Still, exercise shows are convenient and can be really good for maintaining a fitness routine when you just can't get out to a gym.

In addition to aerobics, weight training, and toning shows, you might find alternatives such as yoga and tai chi on one of your offered channels. Fitness programs are concentrated on weekday mornings, especially on ESPN2 and stations affiliated with the Public Broadcasting System (PBS). You can find a current list of shows on www. thriveonline.com. Some cable and satellite systems also receive a channel that provides nothing but workouts and fitness information. Remember, however, that infomercials for fitness products are not the same thing as instructional shows. Their purpose is not to help people get fit but to sell products.

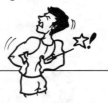

Achtung!

When you follow an onscreen instructor, you have no one to watch you and correct your form as necessary. Listen for the instructor's tips on correct form, and work out in front of a mirror to check yourself.

Teaming Up with a Workout Buddy

If you have trouble getting to the gym or going out for that walk or run, make a standing date with a friend. It'll be harder to procrastinate or to skip a workout if you know someone is depending on you. If you and a neighbor become workout buddies, you can meet for a walk or a jog every day. You can visit each others' homes to work out with that video or with the television fitness shows. This will provide both of you with companionship as well as a safety element for those short winter days when it might be dark when you get in your exercise. You also can carpool to the gym. This not only helps you both stay on track, it makes environmental and economic sense, too.

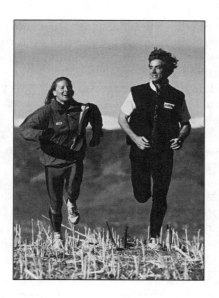

Workout partners can keep each other motivated and have fun together.

(Photo: Claire Walter)

If you and your buddy have similar goals, you also will serve as a mutual support system. You'll be able to notice if your buddy is getting leaner or faster or stronger—and he or she will notice the same about you. You might even have such a revelation about your shared workouts. Complimenting your buddy and hearing compliments about notable progress boosts you both.

Your spouse or partner can be the ideal workout buddy. It is better for both of you when you share the goal of fitness and good health than when one person is in the mindset and mode of getting fit and the other is "televeging" on the couch munching snacks.

Quote, Unquote

"Exercise with a friend. Instead of having a cocktail party and dinner, plan a tennis mixer and picnic with your eight closest friends."

—Denise Austin, television and video fitness host and author of several fitness books

Personal Trainer: Yes or No?

Hiring a personal trainer might seem like the ultimate extravagance, like something only Oprah or Madonna can afford, not you as a beginning exerciser. Beginners and perennial fitness dropouts, however, might need a trainer's help more than experienced exercisers who already are in tune with their bodies and have made a commitment to staying in shape. In addition to offering encouragement, a trainer can make sure you don't overdo the beginning stages in your zeal to get fit and show you proper techniques so you'll remain injury-free.

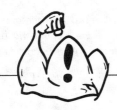

Fit Tip

If you and a friend or mate are thinking about joining a health club, be on the lookout for two-for-one membership offers and other incentives for two people to sign up rather than one.

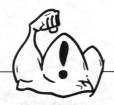

Fit Tip

If you can't quite afford a trainer, find a fitness partner to share the time and the fee. One-on-one training can't be beat for personal attention, but one trainer with two clients is still a very good ratio.

Such one-on-one training isn't necessary every time you work out. Sure, some people do turn it into a long-term relationship, but more likely, you'll derive sufficient benefits from an occasional session. You can schedule two or three sessions to assess your fitness, to design a program, and to get you started. Then sign up for another session after you've been working out for a few weeks to monitor your progress. You can meet with your trainer again two or three times when you've hit a plateau. If you hit a mental wall because you're bored, the trainer can remotivate you and can suggest another program that will pique your interest again. If you've reached a maintenance level with your routine, your trainer can ratchet it up to an appropriate higher level. Your trainer also can determine whether just one or a combination of these elements built the plateau.

A personal trainer provides one-on-one guidance for your fitness program. In addition to expertise in designing a program and tweaking it as you progress, a trainer can fulfill other roles that are important to keeping you on track. It's like having a coach, a guru, and a confessor all in one. One Boulder, Colorado, training studio elegantly refers to its services as "personally guided exercise." Your trainer will do initial and follow-up fitness assessments, help you focus your goals, motivate you when you are flagging, cheer your resolve and hard work, and redesign your program when the time comes.

For many people, the bottom line that makes it worthwhile to pay between $25 and $100 for an hour of a personal trainer's time is that a good trainer will figure out what it takes to push you to work harder and more efficiently than you could on your own. He or she also will make sure you have a balanced program to help all aspects of fitness—not just the ones you enjoy most. With knowledge of both the psychology and physiology of exercise, a good trainer will set reasonable limits for you that also are effective in helping you reach your goals—then, he or she will set higher ones.

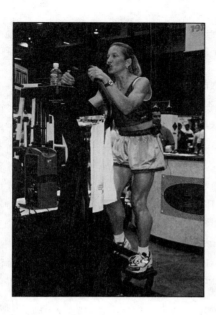

Keep on stepping with motivational words from an instructor.

(Photo: Claire Walter)

At one time, becoming a personal trainer was an on-the-job, learning-by-doing career, but now trainers themselves are trained. Education at schools such as the American College of Sports Medicine can be tilted toward personal training, and organizations such as the National Federation of Trainers have set certification standards. In addition to credentials such as education, certification, and experience, important traits in a trainer include enthusiasm, congeniality, and communication skills. It's crucial to the success of your relationship that he or she can get through to *you*.

Some people sign up for a preliminary training session at a health club or respond to an ad in a local paper. If there's good rapport, they have found *their* trainer. IDEA, a trade association for fitness professionals, suggests an interview rather than the trial-and-error approach. Here are IDEA's suggestions for questions to ask a prospective trainer to see whether his or her philosophy and approach match your needs:

Quote, Unquote

"You can't give yourself the workout a trainer will give you. When you think you can't do one more [rep], your trainer will say, 'Okay, do three more.' The motivation and the results double—you work harder because the trainer pushes you."

—Cameron Macdonald, Aspen Athletic Club, Colorado

➤ What is your exercise and educational background?

➤ Are you certified by a nationally recognized organization?

➤ What is your current level of training experience?

➤ How do you keep current on the latest training techniques, research, and trends?

➤ Will you keep track of my workouts, chart my progress, and make sure my medical history is updated periodically?

➤ Do you carry liability insurance?

➤ Do you provide clear-cut, written policies regarding cancellations, billing, and so on?

➤ What is your rate per session?

➤ Do you offer any discounts or package pricing?

➤ What hours are you available to train?

➤ Will you help me set reasonable goals, not unattainable results?

➤ Do you have a network of physicians, dietitians, physical therapists, and other fitness and health professionals?

Many people who work with a trainer, on whatever schedule and budget they can afford, find it the wisest fitness investment they can make.

Working Out with the Web

The Internet is shaping up and so can you. As with many fields, the astonishing amount of available fitness and health information means that sorting through it can be a Herculean task. Organizations that promote fitness, manufacturers of fitness products, online magazines by recognized fitness authorities, magazines that focus on fitness topics, mail-order sources for fitness products, and medical organizations that do physiological research all have Web sites. In addition, you will find fitness forums and chat rooms where you can do everything from swap training tips to get (or give) recommendations for gyms in your community.

Several Web sites feature quizzes you can take to get an instant fitness program that would be generally suitable for individuals with particular characteristics. Questions include your age, height, weight, specific or general types of activities you enjoy, and/or the time you have available to work out. Enter your answers and a suggested program pops up on your screen, often at no cost. On other sites, you can sign on with a cybertrainer, who tailors a more customized exercise and diet program to your needs. You can e-mail your progress and any questions you might have. Your trainer will send suitable motivational messages via e-mail and will even provide personal responses to your specific questions. Such services run $15 to $20 a month.

TV exercise personality Covert Bailey offers personalized exercise and diet counseling on the Net (or over the phone). The Fitness Quickie is one session designed to jump-start a program and to provide guidelines to follow. Telecoaching is a six-session program in which clients speak to a personal coach once a week to help them stay on track, receive encouragement, and get answers to their questions. You can reach Covert Bailey Fitness at 1-800-657-7571, via e-mail at info@covertbailey.com, or on the Web at www.covertbailey.com.

Interactive CD-ROM fitness information is in its infancy. FitnessAge began with a CD-ROM that was marketed as a fitness-assessment tool but more recently moved over the Web. In 1999, Reebok introduced *Powered by You,* which it bragged is "a bold new fitness initiative: the first interactive CD-ROM featuring detailed, personalized fitness and nutritional information." The CD-ROM was packaged with its top-of-the-line women's training shoe. Undoubtedly, more companies will follow in Reebok's steps.

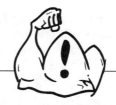

Fit Tip

Here are some Web sites that currently provide free online fitness quizzes or assessments of some sort: www.afaa.com, www.coryeverson.com/, www.fitnessage.com, www.fitnet.com, www.healthyideas.com, primusweb.com/fitnesspartner/, www.chsnet.com/YourHealth/BodySmart/, www.thriveonline.com/fitness/, www.trulyhuge.com

The Printed Word on Fitness

Bookstores' shelves overflow with books on the topics of losing weight and shaping up. Many are step-by-step workout and eating plans accompanied by instructional illustrations, recipes, and more. Books cover topics from aerobics to yoga, outline specific workouts from organizations as diverse as the New York City Ballet Company and Navy Seals, and offer different philosophies from drill-sergeant regimentation to mind-body-spiritual connections in fitness. If your local bookstore doesn't have enough of a variety, check www.amazon.com or www.barnesandnoble.com.

Although magazine coverlines on fitness are designed to sell magazines, once you open the magazine, you'll find a wealth of information. Many articles feature one specific topic but cover it in depth and offer fine advice. *Fitness, Men's Health, Men's Fitness, Heart and Soul, Muscle and Fitness, Shape, Vim and Vigor, Walking, Weight Watchers Magazine, Women's Sports and Fitness,* and *Yoga Journal* are just a few of the publications that focus on fitness. Men's and women's general-interest magazines often include a fitness article or two, and sports publications include get-in-shape pieces geared toward that specific sport. You can sample various publications at half off the newsstand price with the Magazine-of-the-Month Club. Through its Female Health and Fitness service, you can try a dozen publications, including *Fitness, Health, Total Health, and Walking.* You can subscribe by calling 1-888-775-6247 or logging on to www.magazineofthemonth.com. You can also find many of these magazines at your local library.

Your local newspaper also probably has a weekly section with fitness, health, and nutrition articles. In 1996, the *Akron Beacon-Journal* of Ohio developed a 26-week exercise and food plan called the Akron Diet, which was widely syndicated to newspapers subscribing to the Knight-Ridder News Service. Thousands of people around the country followed its step-by-step approach to sensible eating and physical activity to shape up.

Free Fairs

Free or low-cost *health fairs* are an annual fixture in many communities. These events often take place on weekends, frequently at local or regional shopping malls. They offer a smorgasbord of health and fitness information and services. For instance, you often can get simple health evaluations, advice about maintaining a healthy lifestyle, recipes and nutrition tips, natural-food samples, and information about fitness equipment and programs. You might have an opportunity to test exercise machines designed for home use or even to take a sample class with an instructor from a local gym. Some local businesses pass out coupons at health fairs or offer good values to attendees who make a purchase at the event. Such health fairs might be of general interest or targeted to the particular needs of women, seniors, or families.

Some retail businesses also get into wellness counseling as a customer service. Wild Oats, a Colorado-based chain of natural-foods supermarkets, for example, has installed "wellness centers" adjacent to some of its stores. They are staffed by acupuncturists, chiropractors, massage therapists, lifestyle counselors, and nutritionists, all of whom offer reasonably priced services. The centers also have lending libraries where customers can check out books, videos, and audio tapes about health and wellness. "We encourage healthy choices that reflect the needs of the whole individual: body, heart, mind, and spirit." This is the Wild Oats' stated motive for creating such centers.

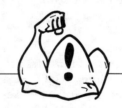

Fit Tip

An experienced salesperson can give you tips about using an exercise machine and a more realistic estimate of what to expect than other information sources. An advertisement or commercial might lead you to believe that anyone can burn, say, 500 or 1,000 calories using a particular piece of equipment. In reality, a well-conditioned athlete using the apparatus at top resistance levels or speed might get that much benefit, but you probably won't.

Store-Bought Help

When you begin to work out and participate in sports activities, you'll probably head straight for the nearest discount store for exercise and sports footwear and clothing. You can get some reasonable values there, especially if you have done your homework and know exactly what you want to purchase. Buying at a big general-merchandise store can sometimes be false economy, however, because you can't be sure of the level of merchandise quality or the expertise of the sales staff if you have questions.

If you are having performance problems, you might be wearing the wrong athletic shoes or using the wrong equipment, and specialists who are knowledgeable about fitness products are more likely to diagnose this. Suppose, for instance, you get into running and find that your running shoes wear out quickly, which in turn can affect your comfort. A running or athletic-footwear store might recommend shoes with a long-wearing polyethylene base, which is said to be more wear-resistant than other materials. If you are experiencing discomfort, orthotics might be in order. A discount store would be less likely to make such recommendations.

If you are investing in a big-ticket item such as a new bicycle or a home-exercise machine, it is even more important to go to a specialty store. A bike should fit you right, stand up to the use you intend to make of it, and be the right kind—mountain bike, road bike, or city bike—for your purposes. If you plan to buy home-exercise equipment, again quality pays off. In such cases, it often is worth the extra money to buy from a specialty store with a reputation that relies on selling quality items and providing a knowledgeable sales staff.

The Least You Need to Know

➤ There is no such thing as getting fit instantly.

➤ A lot of good fitness information is available in print, broadcast, and videotape form, as well as on the Web.

➤ A personal trainer can give you one-on-one attention and push you to achieve your goals faster.

➤ Gyms, health clubs, and specialty retailers offer equipment and expertise.

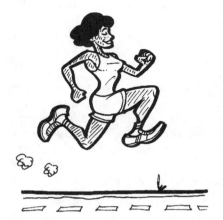

Chapter 5

Rules of the Fitness Road

In This Chapter

➤ Learn to listen to your body

➤ Drink before you are thirsty to prevent dehydration

➤ Warm up at the beginning of every workout and cool down afterward

➤ Flexibility is crucial to fitness, health, and injury prevention

➤ Efficient breathing can influence the success of your workout program

Being active brings about a different mindset than being the proverbial couch potato. You begin to look at what you consume in terms of food and beverages and how it will affect your workout. You know what goals you are aiming for, and you work toward them, taking care not to do more harm than good when you exercise. You gain a core of general knowledge about the human body, in particular about the musculoskeletal system and how it stores fuel and burns energy, and you get to know your own body in particular. You tap into resources such as those outlined in Chapter 4, "Using All the Help You Can Get," you gain experience as an active person, and you build your own wisdom around it. This chapter is a handbook to some of the things you eventually would learn from other sources.

Myriad combinations of aerobic and strength training can make up the basis of a sound fitness program, but physiology and good sense dictate certain fundamental rules for all exercisers. It is important to fuel the body to be physically active.

Avoiding dehydration is crucial, no matter what mix of fitness activities you enjoy. Experts also agree that warming up, cooling down, and stretching are as important as the aerobic and strength-training components.

What Every Body Knows

"Learn to listen to your body." This piece of sage advice is spoken like a mantra by fitness experts, trainers, and athletes from coast to coast. In the beginning of your new way of life, you will sometimes feel sore and sometimes feel fine, with nary a twinge. Sometimes you will be tired after you've exercised and sometimes re-energized. Sometimes you will almost feel yourself getting stronger or leaner, and sometimes as if you have been working out to no effect at all. Eventually, after you have been working out for a while, you will intuitively be able to determine what message your body is sending you.

You will learn to differentiate the *good pain* that signals your increasing fitness from the *bad pain* that means you've overdone it and could even be an injury alert. You'll discover how to know whether you are tired in a good way because you have pushed your personal envelope or you have worn yourself into dangerous exhaustion, which is a bad kind of tiredness. You will learn what you need to do in terms of warming up and stretching to make your workouts work for you. Perhaps most important, your body will tell you that it is missing something when you skip a workout. As you find yourself developing this sense, you will know that it, too, is one of the important stepping stones on the routeto to fitness.

Keys to Good Health

Think "trim" instead of "thin." Think "healthy" instead of "skinny." Think "health" instead of "fashion." These are the thoughts you should keep in mind when embarking on a fitness or weight-loss program. After all, the mind and the brain have a lot to do with how successful you will be. IDEA, a trade association for fitness professionals, offers the follow eight keys to healthy weight (more detailed information about implementing these concepts appears in subsequent chapters):

➤ Don't rely on magic.

➤ Forget the "one-size-fits-all" mentality.

➤ Develop a positive self-image.

➤ Set realistic weight goals.

➤ Learn to play again.

➤ Get stronger.

➤ Harness the power of the [food] pyramid.

➤ Be patient and persistent.

Fueling Up

You wouldn't head out for a drive without gas in the car's tank, so why start your workout when your personal fuel gauge is approaching empty? Because most people work out in the morning, midday, or afternoon, breakfast and lunch are the most important meals of the day, because they provide fuel for the physical exertion to follow. Food fashions ebb and flow, but nutritionists recommend a balanced low-fat diet, high in complex carbohydrates. Nutritionists recommend starting your day with energy-rich complex carbohydrates such as whole-grain bread or hot or cold cereal with fruit rather than sugar if you need a sweetener. Proteins are good, too, but not in the form of fatty breakfast sausages or bacon. At lunch, low-fat bean soups, broth-based soups, sandwiches with a little lean meat and vegetables on whole-grain bread, thick-crust pizza topped with vegetables and reduced-fat cheese, or pasta with fresh marinara sauce are good choices to fuel you through your workout. You'll learn more about eating well in Chapter 20, "You Are What You Eat."

Water, Water, Water

To keep the body humming, drink at least eight glasses of water during the course of a day—more if it's hot or dry, or when you are working out. In fact, it is especially important to drink before you begin exercising, to drink as you go, and to rehydrate after your workout. If you wait until you are thirsty to drink, you have waited too long.

Most experts recommend drinking about 16 ounces of water one to two hours before exercising. One hour is the commonly accepted standard, but if you hydrate two hours before working out, it will allow you to eliminate any excess fluid before you begin, and you won't have to interrupt your workout to use the restroom. (If you work out first thing in the morning, you just have to do the best you can.) You should drink four ounces of water every 15 to 30 minutes while you work out. The harder you exercise and the hotter it is, the more you'll have to drink during your workout. It's a good idea to keep a water bottle handy so that you can sip as you need to.

Camelbak was the first hydration system to hold water in a bladder strapped onto the back. A flexible, on-demand drinking tube makes it especially popular with cyclists. HydroSport is a combination of a strap-on wrist weight and a water bottle,

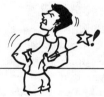

Achtung!

When you exercise outdoors on a hot summer day, drink lots of water but avoid carbonated soda, fruit juices, and caffeinated drinks until you're through working out. Because caffeine is a diuretic, go easy on coffee, caffeinated tea, and cola drinks. In fact, avoid all carbonated beverages before and after a workout. Their acetic acid leaches calcium from bones.

and it's convenient for keeping hydrated while running, walking, or taking an aerobics class. Each one weighs a half-pound and holds 4 ounces of water. Call 1-800-HYDRO-95 for information.

If you're new to working out and drinking as much water as you need, you might have to start both slowly. Just as you progress from lighter weights to heavier ones, from less to more time and tension on an aerobic apparatus, and from a short walk or run to a longer one, up your daily water intake. Drink one additional glass each day until eight is your standard—and remember to drink more when you're working hard or in a hot or dry place.

When you get to the point where your workout lasts longer than an hour—especially if you perspire heavily—consider a sports drink. They not only rehydrate your body, they replace electrolytes (sodium and sodium chloride are the most common) and provide carbohydrates to help you re-energize during a long spell of physical exertion. You lose electrolytes through perspiration, and electrolyte-depletion can cause cramping.

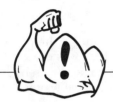

Fit Tip

Some authorities believe that drinking ice-cold water helps you lose some additional weight because you burn calories as it is being warmed up to body temperature. Other experts recommend room-temperature water because they believe it is absorbed into the body more quickly.

Build a Base and Then Get Specific

If you've never worked out before, the concept of different kinds of workouts to accomplish different aspects of your goal might seem totally intimidating. Balancing the need for increased endurance, muscle strength, and flexibility is not instinctive to someone breaking out of a no-exercise lifestyle. Good beginning routines are offered at many gyms and also are available on tape. These programs virtually always begin with a warm-up, include a short aerobic section, feature light weight work, and finish with a stretch and cool-down. "You can do it!" is the major motivational theme of entry-level programs that will help you build a base from which to launch a major assault on weight, conditioning, and stamina problems.

Once you have built that base, you will begin making your workouts longer and stronger. If you like, you can begin to divvy them into aerobic and strength-training days. Not only does this add variety to your workout week, it also gives your muscles time to recover. Some people like a two-day cycle; others prefer a three-day cycle. Workout veterans tend to do these categories on alternate days. Some people like to do a full weight workout one day and an intense aerobics workout the next; others prefer one day of lower-body strength training, one day of upper-body strength training, and one day of cardiovascular work.

Warm Up, Cool Down

The warm-up at the beginning of a workout and the cool-down afterward have a couple of things in common. Both involve relatively gentle movements and some stretching. The purpose of both the warm-up and the cool-down is to enhance flexibility, minimize discomfort, and even prevent injury. The warm-up specifically prepares the muscular system for the harder work to come. It helps you loosen up before your aerobic workout to get the blood flowing and to loosen your muscles for the upcoming exercises. The cool-down allows your body to relax, to discard some of the waste products and lactic acid you might have accumulated, and to return to a resting state after you are finished. Begin your workout with a couple of deep breaths, inhaling through the nose and exhaling through the mouth. If you are planning to walk or run, do a few hundred yards at a slower walk or a gentle jog. Start an aerobics routine with a few minutes of light, dance-like motions to bring your heart-rate up slowly and gradually. This warm-up period is vital in increasing the blood flow to your muscles, which in turn makes muscles and connective tissue more elastic. Before you rev into your routine, do a few gentle calf, hamstring, and hip flexor stretches to limber up.

The cool-down routine is similar, but in reverse—slowing the pace from your aerobic walk, run, or choreographed routine—to enable your heart rate to return to fewer than 100 beats per minute. Soon, your breathing and heart rates will return to normal. Your post-aerobic stretches can be stronger, because muscles are more elastic after a workout than before. Done over time, these stretches help lengthen the muscles and make you more flexible.

The Flexibility Factor

Stretching is the unappreciated stepchild of the fitness family, but it can make or break the rest of your fitness program. Workout veterans, athletes, and dancers know the importance of stretching, but it isn't just for jocks and gym rats. It's for everyone. Especially as people get older, regular stretching can help retain flexibility and a good range of motion, not just for exercising but for everyday activities.

Flexibility also has postural benefits. The key to healthy, natural, and functional posture is a balance of strength and flexibility between opposing muscle groups. Interestingly, being too flexible, even double-jointed, is not good either. When ligaments and tendons are too lax, the results can include instability and risk of dislocation and other injuries. Too little flexibility, however, is far more common than too much.

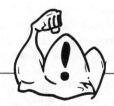

Fit Tip

Some trainers now use the phrase "warm-down" instead of "cool-down" because activity is involved. If you are genuinely pressed for time and can only stretch once during a workout, it is better to stretch at the end. Just try not to make a habit of avoiding a gentle warm-up stretch.

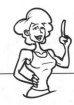

Fitness Fact

The body has several types of joints: ball-and-socket joints like the hips and the shoulders, which are capable of a wide range of motion; hinge joints like the elbows and the knees, which only move one way; the condyloid joints of the wrist, which to some degree move in all directions; the pivot joints of the spinal column; and the gliding joints of the feet.

Ballet dancers often take stretch classes to keep their muscles long and limber, and a few minutes of stretching usually are tacked onto the end of an aerobics class. If you are really tight, you might find it necessary to work with a personal trainer to learn to stretch properly. You also can try yoga, Pilates, and other disciplines that have flexibility and limberness at their core. These activities are discussed in Chapter 9, "Other Paths to Stretching and Toning."

Aerobics instructors routinely finish each session with a cool-down and a stretch, and they do it so seamlessly that it simply becomes an expected part of the program. Don't forget to stretch, however, when you're working out on your own. Some people are naturally more flexible than others, and some people have trained themselves to improve their flexibility, but stretching can increase everyone's range of motion and limberness. It is a gradual process, especially if you have not been stretching. Increasing your body's flexibility by making stretching a regular part of your program contributes to improved posture, better body balance, and an enhanced sense of well-being. As your overall flexibility improves, you will discover many benefits to both your workout regime and the rest of your life. With more flexibility, you will find all movements easier, from hefting a bag of groceries to getting in and out of the car.

Stretching and deep breathing are important parts of the warm-up and the cool-down.

(Photo: Anne W. Krause)

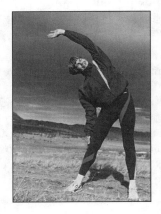

Stretching Basics

Stretching is not only important to overall fitness and often neglected, but the more you stretch the more flexible you will become. However, stretching requires caution to prevent injury. Somehow, it seems easier to get into the habit of stretching some muscle groups than others. Stretching the long leg muscles after a walk or a run comes naturally and feels good, but people tend to neglect other parts of the body such as the knees. In any case, do not stretch to the point of pain.

There are two basic types of stretches: the ballistic (or active) stretch and the static stretch. The ballistic stretch uses momentum and motion to lengthen the muscle. Examples include a leg swing or an arm swing. Light ballistic stretches are an integral part of the warm-up before your workout. With the static (or passive) stretch, the muscle is lengthened as far as it comfortably will go and is held in that position. You can do a light static stretch during your warm-up and then stretch more aggressively after your cool-down while your muscles are still warm. To increase your flexibility, hold each stretch for 15 to 20 seconds or longer, release, and then repeat. You also can breathe deeply, intensifying the stretch as you exhale. There is a very good physiological reason only to stretch lightly during the warm-up and not to overdo your cool-down stretches. When you begin to stretch a muscle, especially a cold one, the muscle automatically reacts in the opposite way, contracting to resist the stretch. This is called the *stretch reflex*. To overcome it, it is important to stretch slowly and smoothly without bouncing or jerking. Breathe evenly throughout the stretch and do not hold your breath.

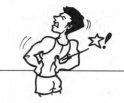

Achtung!

When you warm up and stretch lightly, move for five to 10 minutes to loosen your muscles. Even though movement is involved, don't bounce because bouncing can cause small tears in the muscle fibers.

Cool down from your aerobics workout and then begin stretching, striving for five to 10 minutes of static stretches. Stretch each muscle group you worked, holding each stretch for 15 to 20 seconds. After a weight workout, whether with free weights or machines, be sure to stretch all the muscle groups you worked—legs, arms, shoulders, and back. You can boost a static stretch with external pressure in various ways. Sometimes your trainer will apply pressure to a particular muscle to lengthen it. In some stretches, you can turn your own body against the stretch to provide pressure. You also can quickly contract the muscle to be stretched by pressing it against your trainer, your workout partner, or even the wall. When you release that contraction, you will be able to stretch farther than before.

Fit Tip

If you tend to get stiff, take a hot shower or bath before exercising to increase flexibility.

When stretching, it is just as important not to put the joints or the spine at risk for injury as it is to lengthen your muscles. Several common moves could cause problems. The hurdler's stretch (a favorite among track coaches, a seated stretch with one leg extended straight out and one leg bent and tucked next to the body) and the kneeling quadricep stretch (also called the knee-sit) both could injure the knee joint. The Plow from yoga (lying on your back and stretching both legs up over your head) can pressure the neck vertebrae. Even those relaxing neck circles can be bad for the neck. Circling your head to the back can hyperextend it. You can safely circle your head to the front and sides, however, or tip your head toward your shoulders.

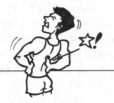

Achtung!

When you begin a workout program or significantly increase or change the one you've been doing, expect to feel sore 24 to 48 hours after you start your new program. You should feel this soreness in the muscles, not in the joints. Muscle aches are a response to a new workload. Joint pain could be a sign of injury.

Every Breath You Take

Breathing is so automatic that you don't even have to think about it, right? Wrong—especially while you are working out. In addition to food and water, your body needs to process oxygen, transferring it from the lungs through the bloodstream to the muscles. There is a growing belief that the effectiveness of any exercise program at any level is impacted by breathing efficiency and technique. In fact, many trendy fitness centers have been adding breathing classes, and athletes seeking peak performance are turning to breathing coaches as part of their training.

In fact, the role of breathing in various body functions is nothing new. Breathing is an integral part of such Eastern disciplines as yoga and tai chi. Weightlifters and bodybuilders exhale so forcefully while they are lifting that they grunt as they lift. Even ordinary people on weight-training programs are routinely instructed to "breathe on the exertion" when they lift.

Lamaze and other childbirth preparation programs use controlled breathing as a way to relax. Oxygen bars flared up as a '90s fad. It has long been known that the lung capacity of well-conditioned athletes exceeds that of ordinary people, but this was generally considered to be an effect of training.

During the course of an ordinary day, adults take an average of 28,000 breaths, most of which are shallow inhalations in which air does not reach deep into the lungs. Such shallow breathing tightens neck muscles, which in turn can cause stiffness and pain in the neck, upper back, chest, and shoulder areas. You might find it ironic to have to relearn, or at least become aware of, proper breathing.

Breathing workshops use the diaphragm to breathe deeply and rhythmically, expanding the rib cage and pulling air down to the bottom of the lungs and deep into the belly. Poses derived from yoga and exercises to enhance awareness of what part of the lungs is filling are part of such classes. Some instructors then move students onto aerobic machines so they can practice their new breathing techniques and at the same time increase their exercise intensity.

You can begin to enhance your awareness of your own breathing with a simple exercise. Lie on your back with your hands on your diaphragm. Begin breathing slowly, deeply, and rhythmically, inhaling through the nose and exhaling through the mouth. Feel your chest and midsection rise and fall with each breath. Move your hands down to your abdomen and try to expand the belly as you inhale.

This exercise is useful when you need to relax, when you need to charge up, or when you need to focus on your body.

Awareness of your breathing patterns leads to the next step, which is applying them to your workouts. Inhale deeply several times as part of your warm-up. This primes your air pump, which is what your lungs are. During aerobics, breathe through your nose as long as you can, because the nose helps humidify the dry air of the gym. When you are breathing hard and your nose can't pull in enough air, open your mouth to fill your lungs.

Quote, Unquote

"Nine out of 10 people are not getting the full capacity that they could. Our lungs are capable of holding a couple gallons of oxygen per breath, and we're settling for only a few pints."

—Pam Grout, author, *Jump Start Your Metabolism With the Power of Breath*

Exhale on the exertion when you are contracting your muscles (as in lifting a weight); inhale as you return to your starting position (as in releasing the weight). Be sure not to hold your breath. For many people, this is a natural reaction to muscular exertion. During the cool-down, your heart rate and breathing will return to normal. Finally, while you are stretching, breathe naturally and evenly, inhaling deeply at the farthest extension of a stretch to lengthen the muscles a bit more.

What does all this deep breathing do outside the gym? There are various opinions, although most authorities believe it is good for you. One school believes that oxygen intake is determined by how much of it the body needs, while another school believes that a regimen including controlled deep breathing actually increases the metabolism. Both sides agree that breathing properly is relaxing and stress-reducing, and it is less taxing on your neck muscles. And, oh yes, it will improve your performance as well.

The Least You Need to Know

➤ As you begin to get fit, you will learn to read your body.

➤ It is important to drink water before, during, and after your workout.

➤ Warm up before you work out and cool down afterward.

➤ Stretching should be part of every workout to increase flexibility.

➤ Become aware of your breathing patterns and learn to control them to enhance your workout program.

Part 2

Strengthen and Tone Your Body

You've made your resolutions. You've gotten your doctor's go-ahead. You've even had a fitness assessment done. Now what? You only have 24 hours a day, and getting in shape probably isn't the only aspect of your life. Sorting out different ways to gain fitness—both upping your cardio condition and getting stronger—can be daunting. There are many options. None is "better" or "worse" than the others. They all help some people to get fit and healthy. The only thing that doesn't work is a broken resolution. Remember, procrastination is not an exercise.

The chapters that follow highlight many exercise programs to help you select what's right for you. The most important aspects of getting fit are to balance your exercise program between aerobic and strength training and to keep at it consistently until you see results. If something sounds good to you, but it doesn't feel right after you've given it a fair chance, you can try something else. Or if you start gradually—as you should—and outgrow your initial regime, you can switch to a different program.

Whatever you select, remember that a workout is work. You have to put effort into getting fit in order to be fit—and to stay fit. "No pain, no gain" was once a popular motivational phrase, and some people still use it. More recent thinking, however, believes that pain needn't be part of any program. The sense of extending your physical horizons, putting in real effort, and stretching your limits is still what makes a workout work.

> *"The way I see it, if you want the rainbow, you gotta put up with the rain."*
> *—Dolly Parton*

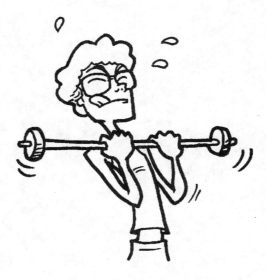

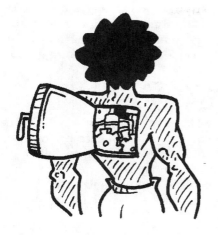

Chapter 6

Tune Up That Muscle Machine

In This Chapter

➤ Weight training makes you stronger, healthier, and more capable of everyday activities

➤ Learn a little about muscles before you begin a fitness program

➤ Feel good about feeling sore when you begin strength training

➤ Free weights and weight machines have pros and cons

If your muscles had a motto, it would be "Use it or lose it." Not original—but true. Unused muscles ultimately atrophy, and even underused muscles quickly lose strength. Muscles that are used are functional, and when they are challenged, they get stronger—quickly. This phenomenon begins in infancy and continues into advanced age. Just think how excited parents are when their baby first lifts his or her head, rolls over, sits up, stands, creeps, crawls, and finally walks. Every one of these small actions demonstrates that the baby's muscles are getting stronger. He or she explores the increasingly accessible world with unbridled curiosity and enthusiasm. At the other end of the spectrum, elderly people who become sedentary are increasingly confined and fragile, and their world shrinks, too.

Most of us are in the great sea of humanity that floats between infancy and old age. We can make and remake ourselves. When we "let ourselves go," we are neglecting to build or maintain muscular strength, and we thereby tilt our bodies unnaturally and prematurely toward the older end of the lifespan spectrum—regardless of our biological age. Assuming that you have no health problems, nothing—but nothing—stops and even reverses the body's clock more than strength training. If you have medical concerns, the shape-up prescription probably will include muscle conditioning, too.

What to Expect from Weight Training

Weight training (or strength training) is one of the key elements of an overall fitness program. When you incorporate it into your life, you not only will become stronger, more capable, and healthier, you also will become more energetic, will feel better, and will look better. Remember that muscle is denser than fat, so a toned body looks slimmer, stronger, and more attractive than a flabby one. Also remember that a toned, slimmer-looking body might actually weigh as much as, or even more than, a flabby, out-of-shape one.

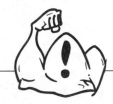

Fit Tip

Visualize the relationship between muscle and bone this way: Muscles work, tugging on your bones and making them stronger. Fat, on the other hand, is dead weight. It just sits on the body, much like a heavy coat sits on a hanger.

For muscles to become stronger, you need to demand more of them than their usual workload. Working them harder in this way is known as *overloading*—that's what you want to do when weight-training. Physiologically, when you lift enough weight to overload your muscles, you cause tiny tears in the muscle fibers. When they regenerate, the muscles become incrementally stronger. Not only will you be able to lift more in the gym, everyday activities will quickly become easier.

In addition to the benefit of muscular strength in and of itself, strong muscles and strong bones are linked. Muscles are attached to bones. When you strength-train, those muscles literally *tug* on bones. Therefore, as you build your muscles, your bones become stronger as a response to the greater force being exerted on them. In a sense, your bones try to "match" your muscles. You can help the process by taking in sufficient calcium and by participating in aerobic activities.

Various studies indicate that weight training reduces various serious health risks. Strength training improves glucose metabolism, for example, which can help control adult onset diabetes. Such training also helps speed the digestive process, or gastrointestinal transit time, and reduces the risk of colon cancer. It can help ease lower back pain and can reduce arthritis pain, both osteo- and rheumatoid. Strength training can even help emotional well-being. A recent report in *Medicine and Science in Sports and Fitness* revealed that male and female volunteers experienced "significantly reduced anxiety" for three hours after a single weight-training session.

The bad news about muscles is that, when they are not used, they lose strength rapidly. The good news, however, is that strength can easily and quickly be recaptured, even by people who have never worked with weights. Muscle tissue burns calories much faster than fat tissue, so even after you've stopped exercising for the day, the "furnace" muscles keep utilizing calories. In other words, strong muscles actually will raise your metabolism. Obviously, the best thing you can do for yourself is not let your muscles become weak and flaccid in the first place. If you are out of shape, be encouraged by the fact that muscles begin to build extremely quickly when you commence strength training.

People differ in their potential strength. This is why some can become bodybuilders and others can't. *Everyone*, however, can become stronger. Some people feel increased strength from weight-training session number one and weight-training session number two. Virtually everyone sees a marked difference after six to 10 weeks of conscientious strength training. When tested, this increase can be anywhere from about 10 percent for a tentative new exerciser to as much as 40 percent for an aggressive person (especially males, who in general, have greater muscle-building capacity than females).

One of America's leading experts in fitness issues has a list of a dozen reasons to strength-train. Dr. Wayne L. Westcott, research director at the South Shore YMCA in Quincy, Massachusetts, found the following after a 12-year study of 1,132 people in YMCA weight-training programs. The following are his 12 reasons why every adult should weight-train:

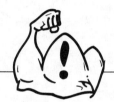

Fit Tip

Start your strength training slowly and then gradually intensify. Even as your muscles become stronger, your ligaments and tendons might still be vulnerable to injury.

> ➤ To avoid muscle loss
> ➤ To avoid metabolic rate reduction
> ➤ To increase muscle mass
> ➤ To increase metabolic rate
> ➤ To reduce body fat
> ➤ To increase bone mineral density
> ➤ To improve glucose metabolism
> ➤ To increase gastrointestinal transit time
> ➤ To reduce resting blood pressure
> ➤ To improve blood lipid levels
> ➤ To reduce low back pain
> ➤ To reduce arthritic pain

In addition to Dr. Westcott's dozen reasons for adults to weight-train, here are three more:

➤ To improve posture

➤ To increase sex drive

➤ To improve overall quality of life

Educate Yourself

Before you embark on your fitness quest, bone up about bones and the rest of the body. Study the exerciser's version of Anatomy 101 so you'll at least know a little about how the body functions. The skeletal system is your body's framework. Because it's what holds everything up, physicians and fitness instructors often talk about "building strong bones" through weight-bearing exercise and sufficient calcium intake. The organs—heart, lungs, stomach, liver, kidneys, and all the rest—take in oxygen, food, and liquid, process them, send them around the system, and eliminate waste. At the most basic level, your muscles enable you to sit, stand, and move. Strengthening, toning, and stretching the muscles should be a major part of any fitness program.

Anterior and posterior muscle chart.

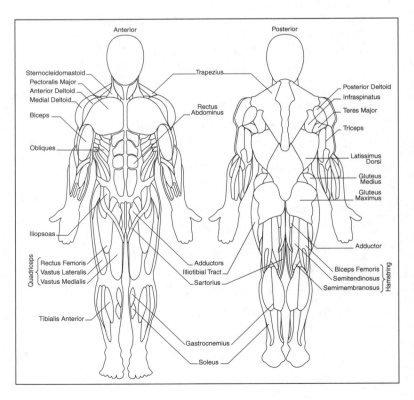

Men and women obviously have some different internal organs, but we all have the same muscles—roughly 650 of them, two thirds of which are skeletal muscles that enable you to move your body. Many are so obscure that only a medical student is likely to know them by name. Astonishingly, no two muscles perform exactly the same function, although groups of large and small muscles function in harmony to enable you to perform specific moves. Of these hundreds of muscles, your exercise program will target roughly two dozen. Simply and briefly, the major muscles and muscle groups are described in the sections that follow.

Lower Body

There are four quadriceps muscles on the front of each thigh (QUADriceps, get it?) and three hamstring muscles on the back. Nicknamed *quads* and *hams,* they respectively enable you to straighten and bend your knee. The two muscles that comprise your calves, on the back of your lower leg, are the gastocnemius and soleus. They are used when you walk, run, stand on your toes, or jump. You use the tibialis anterior, on the front of the shins, when you raise your forefoot while your heel is on the ground.

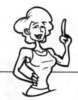

Fitness Fact

The hamstrings are a muscle group with two heads (that is, two attachments). The anatomical names of the three hamstring muscles are biceps femoris, the semitendinosus, and the semimembranosus.

The gluteal muscles, nicknamed *glutes,* are the muscles that shape your backside. You use the gluteus maximus to stand up from a seated position, to climb stairs, to walk up hills, and to extend your leg out behind you. The gluteus medius, more commonly known as the *abductor,* is the muscle that runs along your outer thigh. It is an important hip stabilizer, and it also enables you to step sideways (as you do when playing tennis), to move your leg out to the side (as you do when in-line skating), and to rotate your leg outward or laterally from the hip joint. The adductors are a group of inner thigh muscles that enable you to kick a soccer ball with the inside of your foot, to pressure your legs against the saddle when you are horseback riding, and to skate.

Torso

No muscle group causes more agony and concern than the abdominals (or *abs*). Everyone wants them to be firm and flat. This muscle group runs along the front and sides of your trunk. The rectus abdominus is the big, flat muscle that runs between your rib cage and your pubic bone. It enables you to stand up straight and to bend at the waist. It stabilizes your torso, and when it's toned, it looks terrific. When it is *really* toned so that every muscular ripple shows, it is called washboard abs. The internal and external obliques wrap around the sides of your torso. You use these diagonal muscles to twist your body and to bend at the waist.

The pectoral muscles (or *pecs*) comprise a fan-shaped muscle group on your upper chest below your shoulders. Buff men like to build shapely pecs, and women who work their pecs often find that their breasts appear firmer and sometimes larger. You use your pecs when you push a baby carriage, a shopping cart, or a lawnmower and also for such sports as golf, tennis, and volleyball.

Crunches, done regularly, can help flatten and tone the tummy.

(Photo: Anne W. Krause)

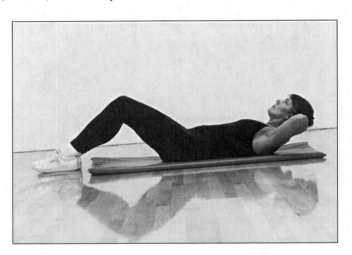

The latissimi dorsi (or *lats*) are the biggest muscles in your back, running from the inside of your upper arm next to the pectoral attachment down to your waist. These muscles are used when you pull something. The erector spinae run down the length of your back on either side of your spine. These postural muscles, along with the abs, enable you to stand up straight. You also use them to straighten up when you are bent over. The rhomboids are fairly small muscles on either side of the spine. These also are postural muscles, located under the trapezius muscles, that allow you to pull your shoulder blades together. If you were in the military, you'd use them a lot— whenever you had to stand at attention.

Shoulders and Arms

The trapezius muscles (or *traps*) run from the base of your skull, down your neck, across your shoulders, and down your upper back. You use them when you raise your arms to the side or shrug your shoulders. You wear your deltoids (or *delts*) like a muscular cap over the tops of your arms and shoulders. This important group of three muscles (front, side, and back) is used to move your arm. You use your deltoids for everything from picking up the telephone or reaching for a light switch to shoveling snow or jacking up a car. The rotator cuff holds your arm in its socket, and it's one of those muscle groups that people pay little attention to until they injure it. You use the rotator cuff to throw a ball, to swing a tennis racquet or a golf club, and to do the breaststroke while swimming.

The biceps is a muscle with two heads (BIceps, get it?) on the front of your upper arm that attaches in two places on your shoulders. You use your biceps to flex your arm at the elbow. When a small child wants to show you how strong he or she is, it's the flexed biceps you'll be asked to feel. The triceps is one muscle with three heads (TRIceps, get it?) on the back of the upper arm that enables you to straighten your arm at the elbow and that also can help you push something. Your forearm is full of small muscles that enable you to wield a tennis racquet, to twist a jar lid or screwdriver, to use a computer keyboard or mouse, and to play the piano. These are the "Popeye" muscles, but even the most ardent weightlifter can't bulk them up the way the cartoon sailor does.

Quote, Unquote

"Long legs. Long hair. Full bust. Full lips. These are style standards currently in vogue. But wait. Aren't the standards of beauty really a burden? After all, how did so many women today start desiring a washboard stomach and a bountiful bosom when so many have a washboard bosom and bountiful stomach?"

—Francine Parnes, Denver *Post* fashion editor

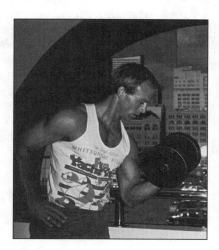

Look at those biceps.

(Photo: Anne W. Krause)

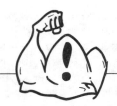

Feel Good About Feeling Sore

When you start a workout program that includes weight training, you can expect to feel sore and tired afterward. You might wonder whether you are doing yourself a favor or actually harming yourself. Keep in mind that, if you have not done anything like this, light weights and modest repetitions are the smart way to start. If you have not been doing any weight training—and especially if your daily routine includes lifting nothing heavier than a cereal box—you *will* feel sore. This is good because it means your muscles are being used.

Experts recommend one day of weight training followed by one day of rest from weight training. (Daily aerobic exercise, however, is fine.) When you strength-train, you actually cause small tears in the muscle fibers. This is what causes soreness the day after you work out. The tears take two days to heal, a process that also results in steadily increasing strength. The initial soreness will go away and be replaced by a feeling of postexercise well-being. As you get comfortable with resistance training and add weight or repetitions, some soreness might return the day after you work out. This is your muscles telling you that you've just gotten a little bit stronger and a little bit fitter than you were when you started.

When it comes to strength training (and aerobic activities as well), remember that staying in your comfort zone won't get you fitter very fast. If you keep using an amount of weight that you can easily lift, you will maintain whatever muscle tone you have, but you won't steadily increase your strength. To do this, you need to challenge yourself. At the same time, you will begin to experience how good you feel when you have worked hard. A little bit of soreness is a small price to pay for the physical and emotional benefits you are getting.

Muscles Burn Fat

If your goal is to reduce weight, think of exercise as the gift that keeps on giving. The calories you burn while you are lifting weights or doing other strength training are only the beginning. When it comes to weight loss and fat reduction, your muscles keep working even after the workout is over. Exercising revs up your metabolism. Researchers have found that a pound of muscle requires more calories, even at rest, than fat does. This means that a fit and strong body uses more calories just to sustain itself than a sedentary body of the same weight.

Every body function requires calories and therefore burns some degree of fat. Muscle tissue requires more fat just to maintain itself than other tissue. There are studies upon studies to determine why this is so and what patterns can be discerned. Various researchers have found strong evidence that weight training helps people become and remain slim. Keep in mind that one pound of fat is equal to 3,500 calories.

The University of Massachusetts Medical School conducted a weight-loss study in which some subjects only dieted, some dieted and participated in aerobic activity, some watched what they ate and participated in strength training, and some did all three. Although the group size was modest, just 65 subjects for the entire study, the most successful group did all three activities, losing weight while also building lean muscle mass.

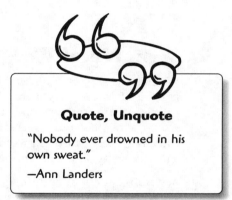

Quote, Unquote

"Nobody ever drowned in his own sweat."

—Ann Landers

Men and Muscles

Men are muscle-building machines. Men's bodies have a higher proportion of muscle than women's, and testosterone, a male hormone, enables them to build muscles faster than women. Men who work out more readily build round, beefy muscles—big shoulders, sculpted pectorals, bulging biceps, and the like. If you want to look as strong as you are, it will only happen if you are not overweight. When a man starts weight-training, some muscles—back, pectorals, biceps, quadriceps—get stronger and firmer faster than others. Because men have the potential to build big muscles, their weight training shows results quickly. Still, fat on top of muscles hides the sculpted muscles that strength training builds. When it comes to muscular strength, size matters. In general, the bigger the muscle, the stronger it is. Men are genetically preconditioned to build big muscles, so they are, in general, stronger than women.

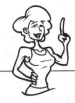

Fitness Fact

Some 25 years ago, Dr. C. Harmon Brown and Dr. Jack Wilmore of the University of California at Davis placed 47 college-age women and 26 college-age men with no prior weight-training experience on a 10-week program. At the end of the study, the men's upper-body strength was 50 percent higher than the women's, and their lower-body strength was 25 percent higher than the women's.

Women Need Weight Work, Too

Women, who are significantly more likely to suffer bone loss, weakness, and fractures later in life, need weight training even more than men. For women, *osteoporosis* should be the scariest word in the English language. This debilitating condition, in which bone becomes less dense and therefore more fragile, afflicts 25 million Americans, 80 percent of them women. Osteoporosis is serious bone loss that comes with age, inactivity, and calcium depletion.

Beginning at about age 35, an adult woman can lose 1 percent of her bone mass every year, which translates to 5 to 7 pounds per decade. During and after menopause, a woman's muscle loss speeds up. Miriam Nelson, a physiologist at Tufts University, studied 40 postmenopausal women. The women in the control group who did not exercise lost 2 percent of their bone mass in a year. Those who weight-trained regained 1 percent of previously lost bone mass.

Think about it this way. Between the ages of 35 and 55, the bone density of a woman who does not counteract this syndrome will be diminished by roughly 20 percent. Because unchecked bone loss accelerates after menopause, by age 75, this same woman will have lost 50 percent of her bone mass, becoming frail, hunched-over, and injury-prone. No wonder many old ladies are frail and ultimately incapacitated. Isn't this reason enough for every woman to weight-train?

As important as strength training is for women—both for present activities and for future health—some women shy away from it because they are afraid of developing big, bulging muscles. Not to worry. Most women are genetically programmed to build long, lean muscles rather than round, bulky ones. Women who begin strength training replace fat with lean muscle. As you work out, you actually will find that you become more toned and slimmer from strength training, even if the number on the scale doesn't drop.

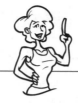

Fitness Fact

Doctors have traced 1.5 million hip, wrist, back, ankle, and other fractures a year to osteoporosis. After age 20, the average woman loses five pounds of muscle and gains 15 pounds of fat per decade, a net increase of 10 pounds of fat every 10 years.

What Kind of Weight Training?

Weight rooms in gyms are equipped with two kinds of weight-training equipment: free weights and weight machines. Free weights are simple, consisting primarily of dumbbells and barbells. Weight machines include various types of complicated-looking apparatus. Multistation machines use a combination of weights, pulleys, and cables to challenge the muscles. The amount of weight is adjustable. Other machines use resistance—either hydraulic or pneumatic—to challenge the muscles. Nautilus machines use spiral-shaped pulleys to provide constant resistance, therefore working the muscles equally as they extend and contract. Various types of apparatus are covered in Chapter 7, "Making Weight Training Work for You," and home versions are discussed in Chapter 16, "Where to Work Out."

Quote, Unquote

"Generally speaking, 99 percent of American women could not develop large muscles if their lives depended on it."

—Dr. Ellington Darden, *Especially for Women*

Some people get hooked on a particular type of strength-training apparatus, while others enjoy workout variety. The good thing is that free weights versus weight machines is not an either-or choice. You can do both at different times. Perhaps you'll use a particular brand of machine at the gym and have a set of free weights at home. Perhaps you'll do different weight workouts for variety, or you'll grab free weights if you are in a hurry and there's a wait for the machines at the gym.

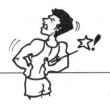

Achtung!

Muscles get stronger more quickly than attachments (that is, tendons and ligaments). If you start lifting weights that are too heavy, too quickly, because your muscles are strong enough, you risk injuring the tendons and ligaments.

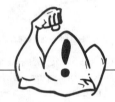

Fit Tip

Many experts recommend that new exercisers, embarking on their first strength-training program, should start with machines rather than free weights. The stabilizing muscles required for free weights can relax because the machine takes over the stabilizing job. Therefore, machines require less coordination and experience. Beyond convenience and personal taste, there are benefits and drawbacks to both basic kinds of strength training.

Good or Bad Ideas?

Electric muscle stimulators, which claim to strengthen muscles and even help weight loss, are bogus at best and harmful at worst. According to a report on MSNBC, the impulse created by the weakest machines is too feeble to do any good at all, while the strongest, cranked up high, is potentially dangerous. Physical therapists do use electric stimulators to aid in muscle rehabilitation. However, unlike the clinical setup, home models do not restrain the limb that contains the muscle being shocked into contraction, and this creates the possibility of injury. Even more seriously, people can misuse the machine by putting the transmission pads on their chests or necks, where blood vessels carry blood to and from the heart and head. Think *heart attack* or *stroke*, and you'll get the idea of why such devices are dangerous.

Weight Machines

The main benefit of weight machines is that they are easy to use and are comparatively safe. They are suited to beginners, because in many ways, the machines dictate the exercise. In many cases, by guiding the movement, they automatically initiate proper form and help prevent injury.

The weight's position and *route* of travel—that is, the body motion required to move it—is controlled, and some trainers believe this helps beginners avoid mistakes in form. Have a trainer or a weight-room staffer set you up for proper alignment on each machine and record the adjustments in your notebook. The discipline imposed by machines also means that, if you follow your program, you will work all the muscle and muscle groups by completing a circuit of all the prescribed apparatus in the gym.

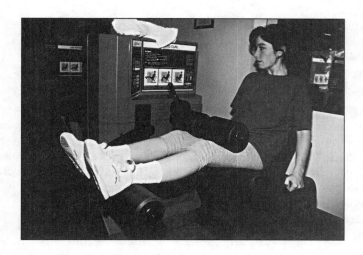

Weight machines are well-suited for beginners and work for most body sizes.

(Photo: Anne W. Krause)

Weight machines are for everybody—sort of. Some brands are not designed to accommodate women under 5'3" or men over 6'2". A bad fit can mean bad form—or possibly even injury. Another drawback to machines is inconvenience. Unless you have a well-equipped home gym, you have to go where the machines are. Sometimes you might feel you don't have time to get to the gym, work out, shower, and get back home or return to the office, so you might skip a workout. At peak times, there might even be a queue for the weight machines.

Another problem some people encounter with machines is boredom. Weight equipment does not always face a television set the way aerobic machines frequently do, weight rooms don't always have music, and you can't read while you are working out. Being tethered to a machine with little diversion can be very tedious for some exercisers.

Free Weights

Free weights are *free* because they are not part of a machine, not because they are gratis. Dumbbells, or hand weights, are designed to be held in one hand but usually are used in pairs. The lightest are just one pound each; the heaviest are Superman-size 100-pounders. Barbells are larger. They consist of a five-foot supporting bar with weights on both ends, and they are designed to be used with two hands. You can customize your barbell by adding or removing weights (the same on each side, of course). The weights range from 2½- to 45-pound plates. Various combinations are affixed to the ends of the bar to achieve the desired weight.

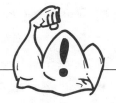

Fit Tip

If your gym is equipped with mirrors, you can watch yourself work out to double-check your form and to relieve boredom as well.

If you like the lightness of hand weights but the balance and control of a barbell, consider a weighted exercise bar. These well-balanced bars are about the length of a barbell, are two inches or less in diameter for easy gripping, and weigh between 9 and 36 pounds. These are especially useful for biceps, triceps, deltoid, and pectoral exercises.

Many experts believe that free weights are biomechanically superior to weight machines because they allow the user to mimic natural movements with the addition of weight rather than impose the machine's alignment. In addition, you get the same workout on both arms because you are lifting the same amount of weight on each side. If you have a weaker side, it doesn't get a *free ride* as it does on a machine. Additionally, if one position doesn't work for you while you are lifting free weights, a slight adjustment often will make the exercise comfortable. Such freedom of movement and position can ease the stress on your shoulders, wrists, and elbows.

When it comes to use, free weights, particularly dumbbells, offer ease and versatility. You just pick them up and start lifting. You can use the same weights to strengthen different muscles, depending on your arm position and body position. Move the weights to any vacant spot in the gym for a workout. Combine light weights with an aerobics or step class for additional cardio benefits as well as light strength training.

Free weights' prime disadvantage is their very freedom. Some beginning exercisers also find that free weights require more coordination than weight machines. Without cables and pulleys to keep the weights where you need them, it is easier to do something wrong and perhaps sustain an injury. (After all, you can't drop a weight machine on your thumb or your toe, but you certainly can do that with free weights.) When people get into lifting heavy weights, stabilization and constant control can be a real problem.

The Least You Need to Know

➤ Weight training reduces a slew of health risks.

➤ To strengthen muscles, you need to work them to overload.

➤ Underused muscles weaken; unused muscles atrophy.

➤ Women as well as men need to weight-train.

➤ Weight training can be done on exercise machines or using free weights.

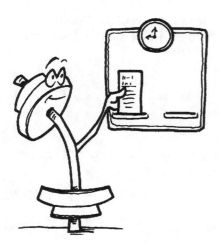

Make Weight Training Work for You

It's one thing to understand the importance of weight training. It's another thing to put that knowledge to work for you. Always keep in mind that—more than the numbers that register when you step on the scale—good muscle tone is what impacts how you look and feel. Never forget that strong muscles mean better health.

To be effective, weight training should be precise and should be done with a purpose. To tone and strengthen your muscles without injuring yourself or stressing your joints, you need to embark on the strength component of your program with particular care. After a few weight-training sessions, the equipment will be familiar to you. Proper form will come easily because your muscles will *know* how to move.

General Guidelines for Weight Work

Weight training is important, no matter which method or equipment you select. As far as your muscles are concerned, it doesn't really matter whether you go to a gym or exercise at home or whether you use weight machines, free weights, or some of the strength-training options described in Chapter 8, "Iron-Free Resistance Training." Regardless of your regime, several principles for weight training have become standard simply because they have been shown to be effective:

➤ Always warm up before your workout.

➤ See a trainer for a program or plan one that works each muscle or muscle group to fatigue.

➤ Start with light weights.

➤ Continue challenging your muscles by making the workout harder as you get stronger.

➤ Add challenge by increasing reps, increasing sets, increasing weight, or decreasing rest time.

➤ Do strength training every other day to allow your muscles to recover after each workout.

➤ Stretch after each workout.

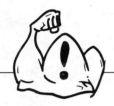

Fit Tip

If you are not a morning person and cannot force yourself to be one, you can take comfort in at least one small, albeit inconclusive, study that shows late evening to be more effective for strength training. According to *Woman's Day* magazine, German researchers found that exercisers who did their weight work at 9 P.M. improved 20 percent more than those who did theirs at 9 A.M.

As with any component of your fitness routine, the best time for strength training is whenever you can plug it into your schedule. If going to the gym or picking up weights at home in the morning before you go to work is most convenient for you, that's when you should be working out. Ditto for lunchtime, late afternoon, or evening.

Reps, Sets, and All That Jazz

Weight rooms have a bit of mystique to the uninitiated, partly because of all the complicated-looking apparatus and partly because of the lingo that flies through the air. Two words you'll hear constantly in the weight room are "rep" and "set." *Rep*, short for *repetition*, refers to one completed movement. *Set* refers to the number of reps performed steadily, without stopping or taking a break. These terms are applied to exercises that use both free weights and weight machines. As an example, people speak of doing "one set of 10 reps" or "two sets of 15 reps" and so on.

Other words also are bandied about the weight room. In fitness-speak, *circuit* has nothing to do with electricity. The word refers to the sequential use of all the machines in a weight room. It developed this meaning because many gyms arrange their weight machines roughly in a circle. In fact, even when a gym arranges machines in a row, the word circuit often is used because you go from one station to the next with little rest in between. When you move between stations without a break between exercises, you keep your heart elevated in addition to strengthening your muscles.

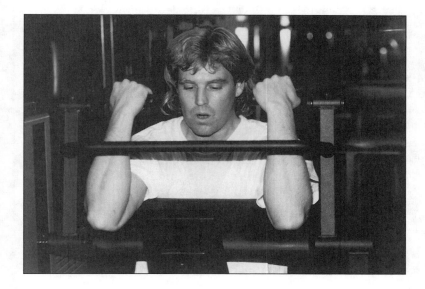

"Whew! Only two more reps to go in this set." Your muscles should be fatigued at the end of a set.

(Photo: Anne W. Krause)

The weights on traditional weight machines are called *plates.* They resemble iron bricks, and they each weigh 5, 10, or 20 pounds, depending on the manufacturer. These plates are placed one on top of the other in a *stack* and are guided by a cable-and-pulley system along a path or track of some kind. To adjust the desired amount of weight, you insert a metal pin into a hole in one of the plates. When you begin using the apparatus, you are lifting that plate and every one above it. Sticking the pin into the bottom plate to capture all the plates in the stack is called *racking.*

Between 1987 and 1998, Americans' use of weight or resistance machines rose by 47.6 percent and use of free weights skyrocketed by 83 percent, according to the Sporting Goods Manufacturers Association.

Weight rooms attract serious body-builders and lifters, as well as those who use weight training as just one component of a fitness program. Even if you are just starting out, don't be intimidated by sharing space with people who lift way more weight than you could ever dream of—and don't feel you have to try to match their abilities.

Designing a Program

If you think you can afford to consult with a personal trainer just once, the beginning of your weight training is the time to do so. If a trainer isn't in the cards at all, keep in mind the principles listed at the beginning of this chapter. Whether you select free weights or machines, start strength-training two or three times a week and work each

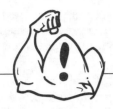

Fit Tip

Whether you work with weight machines or free weights, control the weights throughout the full range of motion to get the maximum benefit. Inhale on the exertion, whether it's a lifting, pulling, or pushing motion, and exhale when returning the weight to the starting position. Do not allow the weights to swing or let momentum take over.

major muscle group every time. As an option, you can weight-train six days a week, alternating upper- and lower-body workouts and taking the seventh day off.

Weight, reps, and sets can be combined in several ways to match your goals. If you want to tone your muscles, make strength training part of a weight-loss program, and make your muscles stronger for your everyday life, start with two sets of 10 to 15 reps per exercise, using relatively light weights. If you want to build big muscles, do fewer reps—no more than 10—with heavier weights. (Experienced body-builders seeking maximum strength gains lift as much weight as they possibly can, but they do six or fewer reps each time they work out.) If you want to build muscles but also maintain a nicely toned, nonbulky body, alternate these routines. Moderate weights and many reps help promote muscular endurance. What constitutes "heavier," "lighter," or even "moderate" depends on the strength you have to begin with. This, incidentally, is why a preliminary fitness assessment helps plan the right program for your needs and goals.

A personal fitness trainer can design a suitable weight-training program.

(Photo: Anne W. Krause)

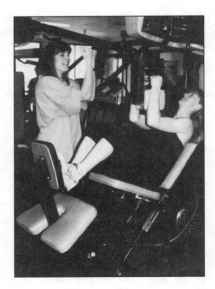

If you are committed to a weight program, your biggest question is probably, "How much weight should I lift?" The answer is, "It depends." It depends on your strength, your age, and other factors. If a trainer plans a program for you, he or she will outline the appropriate amount of weight as well as the number of sets and reps for each exercise. If you put together your own program, you'll have to use the trial-and-error method. Try several different weights and then pick one for each exercise that you can lift between eight and 12 times before fatigue, all while maintaining correct form. The last two or three repetitions should feel hard to do, but they should not be so difficult that completing them causes you to compromise your form or technique.

Whatever the amount of weight you can lift when you start, it won't be long before you are ready to increase the workload. When you are comfortably lifting an amount of weight and are completing the sets with good form, it's time to add more weight. Bump it up using the smallest possible weight increase. Every body part or muscle group won't *graduate* equally. You might be ready to increase weights for one muscle group but not another.

If you hit a plateau and can't seem to lift a heavier weight, you can try what is called eccentric contraction. This means you work with weight beyond what you normally can lift on your own. Your trainer or exercise buddy will help you pull, push, or lift the weight—in other words, by contracting the muscle. You then return it to the starting position on your own—in other words, controlling the weight as the muscle lengthens and returns to its resting length. Most trainers recommend one to three sets of eight to 12 reps in this way.

Managing Weight Machines

The most common weight apparatus in a gym is called a multistation machine. It consists of a strong metal framework, pulleys, handles, seats, ankle cuffs, and adjustable iron weights. Plates are stacked one on top of the other with holes in the sides. To adjust the amount you want to lift, slide a metal pin into the desired hole. When you pull or lift, you are moving the selected stack. Some brands are labeled with clearly illustrated instructions for setting up each machine.

Typically, such weight-stack cable machines have several stations that enable you to exercise various muscles. You will find specific stations for all major muscle groups: shoulders, back, chest, biceps, triceps, outer and inner thighs, hamstrings, and quadriceps. Some exercises require you to stand up, some to sit down, and some to lie down.

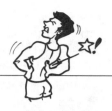

Achtung!

If and when you begin lifting heavy free weights, you need to enlist a spotter to guide you as you lift or lower the weights. A spotter can help protect you if the weight proves too heavy or if your form deteriorates in a way that could cause injury. If you have a workout partner, you can spot for each other.

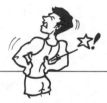

Achtung!

If the weights bang together, you are not in control of the machine—it is controlling you. Crashing plates means you are lifting too fast, using too much weight, or both, and you cannot control each rep fully.

Before you begin each exercise, adjust the seat for your height (if there is an adjustment) and the weight stack for your program. Then begin lifting, pulling, or pressing, depending on the exercise. Try to stay in control throughout the exercise, lifting and releasing evenly and smoothly.

The following chart outlines 10 terrific exercises for weight machines. There are many more exercises and refinements, but these are among the most common that you can expect to be able to do in most weight rooms. As you look at the third column, "Position and Action," keep in mind that no two brands of weight machines are exactly alike. Even different models or vintages of the same brand may be designed and function slightly differently. Therefore, some of the movements may vary. If you have any questions, ask a weight-room attendant for help or set up a how-to session with a trainer to get you started correctly.

Ten Terrific Machine Exercises

Machine or Station	Muscle or Muscle Group	Position and Action	Function	Form
1. Leg Curl	Hamstrings (back of thighs)	Lying: While lying face down, hook your ankles behind a padded bar, press your hips down, and bend your knees to bring your heels toward your buttocks. Straighten your legs to return to the starting position. Seated: While seated, hook your ankles behind a padded bar and lift your lower legs until they are parallel to the floor. Bend your legs to the starting position.	Climbing stairs and hills	A shapely behind
2. Leg Press	Quadriceps and gluteals (front of thighs and buttocks)	While lying on your back with your knees bent, place your feet against a pad and push your legs forward and up, stopping a few degrees short of the straightest possible extension. Bend your knees to return to the starting position.	Jumping, squatting, or lifting heavy objects from the floor	A firm and toned lower body

Machine or Station	Muscle or Muscle Group	Position and Action	Function	Form
3. Triceps Press	Triceps (back of the upper arms)	While seated, grasp the handles at your sides with your elbows bent and straighten your arms, pressing downward and back. Bend your elbows and return to the starting position.	Pushing up from an armchair	Toned triceps that eliminate flapping upper arms, especially in women
4. Arm or Biceps Curl	Biceps (front of upper arms)	While seated with your arms in front of you, grasp the handles and pull them up toward your shoulders, bending at the elbows. On some machines, you stand with your arms lowered in front of you, grasp the handles, and pull them up toward your chest, bending at the elbows. Straighten your elbows to return to the starting position.	Carrying a baby or a toddler, lifting and carrying heavy objects	Sculpted biceps— one of the classic muscles that shows muscle mass
5. Chest Fly	Pectorals (chest)	While seated, raise your forearms to chest level, place them behind padded panels or grip padded handles, and press them together in front of you. On some machines, you lie on your back and grasp handles above your chest, extend your arms out to your sides, and bring them up above your chest. Return to the starting position.	Pushing heavy objects, playing racquet sports	For men, a sculpted chest; for women, breasts appear firmer and sometimes larger

continues

Ten Terrific Machine Exercises (continued)

Machine or Station	Muscle or Muscle Group	Position and Action	Function	Form
6. Shoulder Press	Deltoids (shoulders)	While seated, grasp the handles at chest or shoulder level and push them straight up. On some machines, you sit leaning forward slightly. Lower your arms to return to the starting position.	Lifting heavy objects	Well-developed shoulders that make your waist appear narrower
7. Upright Row	Trapezius, deltoids, rhomboids, and biceps (shoulders and upper arms)	While standing with your arms extended in front of your hips, grasp the handles and—bending and raising the elbows—pull them back and up to shoulder level. Lower your arms to return to the starting position.	Carrying heavy objects, rowing or paddling	Broad shoulders that make your waist appear narrower
8. Chest Press	Pectorals (chest)	While seated, grasp the handles in front of you at chest level and push them away from your body. Bend your elbows to return to the starting position.	Pushing heavy objects	For men, a sculpted chest; for women, breasts appear firmer and sometimes larger
9. Seated Row	Latissimi dorsi, trapezius, rhomboids, biceps, and erector spinea (back)	While seated with your legs bent, grasp the handles in front of you and pull them back, bending the elbows, as if rowing a boat. Return to the starting position.	Pushing heavy objects, helping posture, rowing and paddling	Pulling, lifting, standing, and sitting erect

Machine or Station	Muscle or Muscle Group	Position and Action	Function	Form
10. Lat Pull-down	Latissimi dorsi (back)	While seated, grasp the overhead bar and pull it down in front of your body to chest level, leaning back slightly. The weights will pull your arms upward to return to the starting position.	Lifting and pulling heavy objects, swimming	Well-developed lats that make your hips appear narrower

Some brands of strength-training apparatus use something other than iron plates to create resistance. The exercises often are similar to weight-stack machines, but the mechanics are different. Instead of cables and pulleys to lift and lower weights, some machines have hydraulic (fluid) or pneumatic (air) chambers or cylinders to provide resistance. Proponents of these machines like the even resistance throughout each exercise with this type of equipment. Nautilus equipment was based on a somewhat different principle. The system's spiral pulleys mimic nature's nautilus seashell to provide smooth, full-range-of-motion resistance training.

Working with Free Weights

As you progress and become stronger, you might want to use barbells, but at least at the beginning of your fitness quest, light dumbbells are the free weights for you. Starting with one-pounders, they come in small increments. A typical weight room might be equipped with weights of 1, 2, 3, 5, 8, 10, 12½, 15, 17½, 20, and 22½ pounds—perhaps even more.

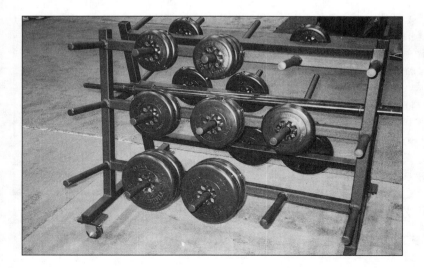

A rack of free weights stores a variety of sizes (and weights) for you to choose from.

(Photo: Claire Walter)

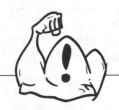

Fit Tip

Whenever you lie on your back while weight-training, make sure your lower back is in contact with the mat, floor, or bench. For some exercises, bend your knees, bring them to your chest, or cross one leg over the other to press the torso down and avoid arching your back.

Hold the weights lightly but firmly in your hands without clutching them in a death grip. Some trainers like people to start light and progress to heavier weights. Under this approach, after warming up for each exercise with light weights, you increase the weight for each new set until you have reached the heaviest comfortable weight. If you haven't completed your planned reps by the time your muscle fatigues and your form begins to go, some trainers recommend that you rest briefly and then switch to the next-lightest weight, or even no weight, for the remainder of the set. Other trainers like people to warm up, begin with the heaviest possible weight, and then move to lighter weights to complete the set.

Early in your exercise career, when you are using very light weights with small-diameter handles, you can crisscross, say, a three-pounder and a one-pounder, holding them both in the same hand to add just a little weight. This can get tricky, however, if you have very small hands or if the handle is large, because it is possible to drop one. Although dumbbells are used primarily for upper-body exercises, they can also be used to add challenge to such lower-body exercises such as lunges, step-ups, or squats.

Scores of variations exist for dumbbell exercises. Here are half-a-dozen basic ones for the upper body. To determine what they do in terms of function and form for specific muscles or muscle groups, see the preceding chart on weight-machine workouts.

The following are six sensational free-weight exercises:

1. **Arm or biceps curl.** Standing with your feet shoulder-width apart, your knees slightly bent, and your arms straight and close to your body, bend your elbows up to your chest. Straighten your arms and lower the weights to the starting position. The term *arm curl* or *biceps curl* is used when you do this exercise with the palms facing the ceiling. When you rotate your forearms so that your thumbs are facing the ceiling, the variation is called a *hammer curl;* when you do it with the palms facing the floor, it is called a *reverse curl*. Each variation strengthens the biceps and the muscles of the forearm in a slightly different way. You also can do these curls while sitting on a bench or using a barbell.

2. **Triceps curl.** You can do this exercise with one weight in each hand or with a heavier weight held in both hands. Standing in the same position as in the preceding exercise or sitting on a bench, raise your arms straight overhead, keeping them close to your ears, and bend your elbows, lowering the weights behind you. Straighten your arms to raise the weights to the starting position.

3. **Forward arm raise.** Standing in the same position as in the first exercise or sitting on a bench, keep your left arm at your side and raise your right arm straight in front of you to shoulder height. Alternate bringing your left arm up and your right arm down and then your right arm up and your left arm down. This exercise strengthens your shoulders.

4. **Lateral raise.** Standing in the same position as in the first exercise with your palms facing each other, raise both arms out to your sides to ear level. Return to the starting position. This exercise strengthens the shoulders, especially the deltoids.

5. **Chest press.** Lie on your back on a bench or a mat with your elbows bent, your hands at chest level, and your palms toward your feet. Press your hands upward and straighten your elbows without locking them. Bend them to return to the starting position. This exercise strengthens the shoulders, triceps, and pectorals. You also can do this exercise with a barbell. When you do it on a bench, which gives you a greater range of motion, it is called a *bench press*.

6. **Fly.** Lie on your back on a bench with your elbows slightly bent and your hands above your chest. (If you are uncomfortable on a bench, you also can do this exercise lying on a mat, but you won't get as much range of motion.) Extend your arms out to the side. Alternately open them and bring them together above your chest. Lying on a bench gives you a greater range of motion. This exercise strengthens the chest.

> **Quote, Unquote**
>
> "Form is most important. Endurance will follow."
>
> —Margaret Richard, *Body Electric* host, Public Broadcasting System

Weight-training accessories for special situations are also available. If arthritis is a problem that makes gripping hand weights uncomfortable, try heavy-duty plastic extenders called EZGrip, which clip onto the weights and provide a larger, more comfortable surface to hold on to. Call 877-439-4747 for details. Body-builders, of course, use support belts to prevent abdominal injuries while lifting heavy weights. Some people like to wear gloves while working with weights (especially if and when they start using heavy weights). If you wear gloves, you can avoid blisters by getting the right size. When your gloves begin to wear out or stretch, it's time for a new pair. These products are readily available where serious exercise equipment is sold.

Let's Hear It for Leg Weights

The most popular wrap-around leg weights are flexible, padded, and have Velcro closures. The most versatile designs feature lead bar weights that slip into pouches and therefore can be adjusted for weight as well as size. Others, such as Lei Weights, contain small, heavy pellets. They are soft and comfortable and can be draped over the leg or used in place of dumbbells in other free-weight exercises. To intensify inner- and outer-thigh toning, hold the last rep of the last set for eight to 16 counts before releasing.

No matter what design you prefer, the following are the two most common lower-body exercises that use leg weights:

1. **Outer-thigh leg lift.** Lie on your left side with your hip bones stacked one above the other, perpendicular to the floor, with your left knee slightly bent. You can lift the right leg up and down, you can lift it and alternately bend and extend the knee, or you can combine these movements so that, on each rep, you lift, extend, bend, and lower the leg. Work up to two or three sets of 15 repetitions of each component of these outer-thigh lifts. You can complete the exercise by elevating your right leg to hip level and pulsing it for one set. Don't lift the right leg any higher than the hip, because you don't want to roll back onto your buttock. The idea is to keep the hip bones stacked. Switch to the other side. This exercise tones your outer thighs.

2. **Inner-thigh leg lift.** Lie on a mat or on the floor, as in the preceding exercise. Bend your top leg and place it on the floor in front of your body. Raise your bottom leg off the floor and lower it to the starting position. Again, be sure to lift your leg without rolling onto your buttock. Your goal should be the same number of reps and sets on each side as for the outer-thigh leg lift. This exercise tones the inner thighs.

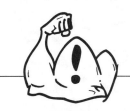

Fit Tip

Putting leg weights on the ankles is more effective weight work because, being low on the leg, the position creates a longer weighted lever. However, for some exercises, it is safer to put the weight above the knee in order to protect the knee joint.

Stretch After Weight Training

Stretching after you have worked your muscles is the key to flexibility, and as you become stronger, you also should concentrate on increasing your flexibility. The two go hand in hand. Not only does stretching feel good, it also helps prevent soreness after weight-training. When you lift weights, your muscles are being shortened. Stretching not only returns them to their resting length, but you also become more flexible if you stretch immediately after strength-training because the muscles already are warm.

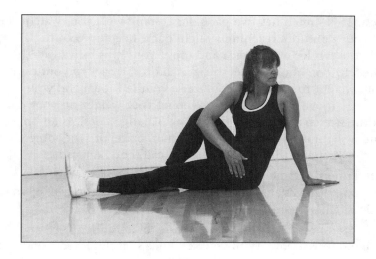

Loosen your hardworked muscles after weight-training.

(Photo: Anne W. Krause)

Here are a dozen basic stretches to follow your strength session. If you include both upper- and lower-body training, do them all. If you do just one or the other, be sure to stretch the muscles you worked. Hold each stretch for 20 to 30 seconds. Do not hold your breath and do not bounce. Instead, inhale when you are at a comfortable stretch, feeling slight tension but not pain. Exhale and try to increase the stretch slightly. Keep breathing throughout each stretch, even after you have reached maximum comfortable extension.

The following are a baker's dozen of super stretches:

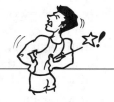

Achtung!

We all have heard about muscle-bound football players or other athletes who emphasize weight training. Being muscle-bound means being inflexible, which is a result of not stretching commensurate with strength training.

1. **Butterfly stretch.** Sit on the floor or on a mat with the soles of your feet together and your knees out. Grab your feet with both hands and, bending from the hips, gently pull your body forward. This stretches the groin area and the lower back.

2. **Modified hurdler's stretch.** Sit on the floor or on a mat with your left leg bent (imagine it as half of sitting cross-legged) and your right leg at a 45-degree angle from your body. Try to keep your right leg as straight as you can, although beginners often need to bend it. Raise your left arm, curve it over your head, and stretch your right arm out as far as you can over the right leg. Change sides. Your goal is to eventually be able to keep your straight leg flat on the floor, flex your foot, and grab onto that foot. This stretches the hamstring, calf, and lower back.

3. **Back-of-leg stretch.** This stretch has two parts. First, stand with your weight on your left foot and your right foot reaching straight back. Keeping your back heel on the floor, bend your left leg at the knee and move your hips forward with your weight on the left foot. You will feel the stretch on the back of your right leg. Next, shift your weight to your right foot, raise your left toe, bend your right knee slightly, and move your hips back, keeping your weight on your right foot. You will feel the stretch in your left hamstring. Change sides. As an option, you can stand a slight distance from a wall, chair, barre, or other object for stability. This exercise stretches the Achilles tendon, calf, and hamstring.

4. **Hip-flexor stretch.** From the same position as in the preceding stretch, keep your weight evenly on both feet and sink straight down, lifting the heel of your back foot off the floor. Change sides. This stretches the hip flexor.

5. **Quadriceps stretch.** Stand near a wall, a chair, a barre, or another object, and hold on with one hand for stability. With your left knee slightly flexed, bend your right leg up toward your buttocks, reach back with your right hand, and grab your foot. Gently pull your right foot toward your body. Change sides. As an option, you can do a cross-stretch version in which you grab your left foot with your right hand and vice versa. Another alternative is to lie on your side on a mat or on the floor, bending the knee of the top leg toward your buttocks and reaching back with the same arm to grab the foot. This stretches the quadriceps.

6. **Runner's lunge.** Kneel on a mat or on the floor with a folded towel under your knees as a cushion. With your hands on either side for support, move your right foot forward until your knee is directly above your ankle at a 90-degree angle to the floor. Do not hyperextend (move the knee of the supporting leg in front of the ankle) or support your body weight on your hands. Change sides. This stretches your hip extensors, lower back, and quadriceps.

7. **William's stretch.** Lie on your back on a mat or on the floor. Bend your left knee and keep your left foot flat on the floor. Bend your right leg and raise it toward your chest. Reach under your knee and support your right thigh with your hands. Pull your leg toward your torso. Change sides. This stretches the lower back, hips, hamstrings, and gluteals.

8. **Lying hamstring stretch.** Begin as in the preceding stretch. Slowly straighten your right leg, pulling it gently toward you. Flexing the foot intensifies the stretch. If you cannot accomplish this by reaching around your leg, loop a small towel or band around your foot and pull it toward your body with both hands. Lower your leg to the floor. Repeat the lift-and-pull sequence eight times. Change sides. This stretches the hamstrings and gluteals.

9. **Glute stretch.** Stand on your left leg in front of a pole that cannot move and grasp the pole firmly with both hands. Place your right foot just above your left knee. Bend the left knee and sit back on that standing leg, holding on to the pole for support. Change sides. This stretches the gluteals.

10. **Reach.** From a seated position with your back straight and your legs bent comfortably in front of you, or while standing with your feet shoulder-width apart, reach both arms upward, interlace your fingers, and turn your palms up toward the ceiling. Push your arms back slightly. This stretches the shoulders, arms, obliques, and back.

11. **Triceps stretch (also called an arm pullover).** From a seated or standing position as in the preceding stretch, raise your left arm over your head with your elbow bent and your hand behind your head. With your right hand, grasp your left elbow. Gently pull your elbow and bend your upper arm gently to the right. Change sides. This stretches the triceps, lats, obliques, and waist.

12. **Rotation stretch.** From a seated or standing position, as in the William's stretch, twist your upper body to the left at the waist and turn your head to look over your left shoulder. Change sides. If you are doing this while standing, simply place your hands at your waist. If you are doing this while seated, it is slightly more complicated. To stretch to the left, bend your left leg comfortably in front of you (again, half of sitting cross-legged), cross your right foot over your left thigh, and place it on the floor. Place your left hand on the floor behind you, grasp your right thigh with your right hand, and twist your upper body gently to the left. Turn your head to the left. This stretches the middle and lower back and your waist. The seated version also stretches the outer thigh.

13. **Full-body stretch (also called an elongation stretch).** Lie on your back on a mat or on the floor. Raise your arms over your head (on the floor, not raised in the air) and keep your legs straight. Stretch your arms and hands up and your legs and feet down, elongating your body. Try to make yourself as tall as you can. Turn over onto your abdomen and repeat. You can do an optional cross-stretch, reaching away from your body first with your left arm and right leg and then switching sides. This stretches the arms, legs, and torso.

Remember that you do not want to stretch to the point where tension becomes pain. Pain means you are overstretching or stretching too quickly, and this can lead to an injury.

The Least You Need to Know

➤ Consult with a personal trainer before you start weight work.

➤ You will strengthen your muscles by lifting weights, whether you use machines or free weights.

➤ To build big muscles, do fewer repetitions using heavy weights, but to tone muscles, do more reps using lighter weights.

➤ It is vital to stretch after a weight workout to increase your flexibility even as you become stronger.

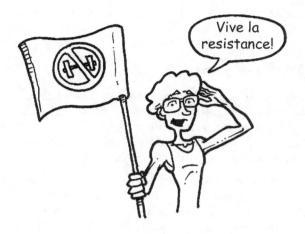

Chapter 8

Iron-Free Resistance Training

Vive la resistance!

In This Chapter

➤ Use your body weight instead of iron for strength training

➤ It's buyer beware for fitness devices hawked on television

➤ Exercise tubes, bands, and balls: simple and effective

➤ Water exercises: low-impact and gentle on the joints

When it comes to strength training, especially for new exercisers, no single method works best for everyone—and you don't have to use a single method all the time. In fact, it often is better to have more than one type of workout in your repertoire and to vary your training. Mixing various kinds of strength training, cardiovascular conditioning, and sports is called *cross-training,* but you can consider varying your strength condition to be targeting cross-training. Not only is it more interesting than doing the same thing all the time, but it also reduces the likelihood of injury. Remember that you will build up and tone your muscles by working against resistance. To strength-train, you need to work your muscles to fatigue. Some people love to pump iron—and you might, too—but you might prefer another method that suits you. No matter how you strength-train, if you do it regularly and properly, you will get stronger and fitter.

There are four basic types of iron-free strength training. The first uses your own body instead of iron to create resistance. The second relies on other types of equipment to provide the necessary resistance for a strength workout. The third type is aquatic exercise, in which the water offers resistance. The final option is to exercise with a partner, because two people can offer strength-building resistance for each other. Trainers often use this technique. The important thing is to start modestly and keep at it—whatever *it* you choose to do.

Pump Your Body Instead of Iron

Exercises that use your own body weight are so fundamental to a strength-training program that they often are lumped in with weight training. They fit in well with the weight-training days on your program. Even the most ardent weightlifters often do push-ups, sit-ups, or crunches along with their ironwork.

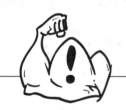

Fit Tip

Exercises that rely on your body instead of other gear have the additional benefit of portability. Wherever you go, along comes the capability to do these exercises—in a hotel or motel room, when you are a house guest in someone's home, or even if you are camping.

Some of these exercises, such as push-ups and abdominal crunches, require you to heft your own body weight. Others are traditional calisthenics that you might have done in a long-ago gym class. They get the joints and muscles moving to provide general toning and mobility conditioning rather than specific strength or aerobic training. Several target the lower body, which many people say they most want to tone. For each of the exercises that follow, begin with a set of eight to 10 reps if you can, rest, and then do another set. When sets of eight or 10 become easy, increase the number of reps in increments of five and then up the number of sets to three or four. The key to success is slow, controlled movement through a full range of motion. Mega-reps are not necessary. Ultimately, you can notch yourself up to more advanced versions of these exercises.

Abdominal Crunches

Crunches are the most basic abdominal exercises in fitness today. There are countless variations on the theme of crunches. In all of them, you begin by lying on your back with your lower back pressed against the mat or floor, your knees bent, and your feet flat on the floor. Begin by contracting the abdominal muscles and then slowly lift and lower your head, shoulders, and upper back. You can select your arm position. If you feel tension in your neck, place your hands behind your head with your fingers interlaced or touching. If your neck does not bother you, you can extend your arms straight in front of you or overhead, or you can place them on your thighs and slide them up as you lift your upper body, shoulders, and head. If you are comfortable doing so, you can cross your hands over your chest. Some trainers advise clients to tuck the chin in; others advise to keep the cervical area straight. *Lightening* your feet off the floor, thus releasing weight from them, as you lift your upper body makes the crunch more challenging. You can feel this effect by alternately raising your right and left toes with each crunch.

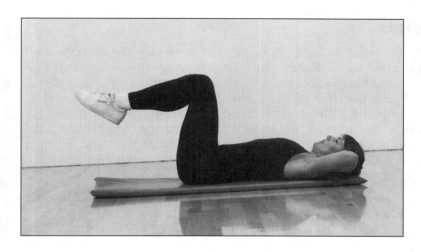

No matter what variation you select on the abdominal crunch theme, keep your lower back flat on the mat.

(Photo: Anne W. Krause)

Protect your back by tilting your pelvis forward so your entire spine is in contact with the floor, and contract your abdominals to keep it that way. To work deeper into the lower section of the rectus abdominus, keep your heels on the floor but alternately raise your left toes and then your right toes as you come up for each crunch.

Fitness Fact

The commonly used word "abdominals" includes the rectus abdominus, a flat, wedge-shaped muscle reaching from the rib cage to the pubic bone; the obliques, which are on each side of the waist; and the transverse abdominus, which wraps around the waist like a cummerbund.

Whichever position you prefer (and this might change over time), suck in your gut so that your lower back presses against the mat or floor. You can visualize pressing your bellybutton *through* your back to the floor. You also can think of this as not pushing your stomach out as you crunch. Work through the entire exercise slowly and steadily, without heaving yourself up or flopping down.

Modified Crunches

Crunches work the entire rectus abdominus, but several other exercises also concentrate on the lower section of the abdominal area. The easiest of these is a crunch with a modification. Lie on your back as you would to start your crunches, but let your knees fall outward, keeping your feet together. When you do your crunches from this butterfly position, you will feel your lower abs handling more of the load. To tone the "love handle" area on the sides of your torso, you need to work your obliques. The easiest version is to place your hands behind your head for support and begin alternating your left shoulder toward your right knee and then your right shoulder toward your left knee.

You also can increase the intensity of your abdominal exercises by doing a pulse set after your regular crunches. Pressing your lower back to the mat or floor, pulse for one set at the top of the exercise and then hold the very highest position for a count of 10. Remember to breathe. Other advanced abdominal exercises involve more challenging positions. For example, you can lift your legs off the floor and cross your ankles when you do your crunches to really work your waist. Reverse curls are the power exercise for the lower abs. Lie on your back, lift your legs straight up (or raise them and cross them at your ankles), and place your hands under your pelvis to support your back. Contract your abdominals to raise your hips off the floor. Be sure to suck in your gut with each lift, or else your back and hip flexors will do most of the work. Finally, when your abs are really strong, you can intensify your exercises further by combining crunches and reverse curls.

After you work your abs, remain on your back to stretch. First, raise your hands above your head and stretch your arms, legs, and torso, elongating your entire body. Next, bring your knees up to a bent position and let them fall to one side of your body. Stretch your arms to the other side. You also can roll over onto your abdomen with your legs stretched behind you. Place your hands, palms down, on either side of your body and raise your upper body. Stop at a comfortable point to protect your back. You do not have to straighten your arms fully for this to be an effective stretch.

Push-Ups

Before septuagenarian Jack Palance accepted an Oscar for his supporting role in *City Slickers,* he got down on the stage and wowed the audience by doing one-arm push-ups. You won't ever have to do this, but it should be motivational to know that someone his age did—in public.

You can start your push-ups very gently and modestly. Get down on your hands and knees on the floor or on a mat. For the most basic push-up, start with your feet and shins on the floor and your hands a little more than shoulder-width apart. Keeping your back straight, bend your elbows to lower your shoulders and upper body until your forehead and nose almost touch the floor. Straighten your elbows to raise yourself. You can even ease into push-ups by starting from a standing position and holding on to a horizontal support such as a sturdy porch or deck railing or a ballet barre. Bend your elbows to angle your upper body toward the support and straighten them to return to the starting position.

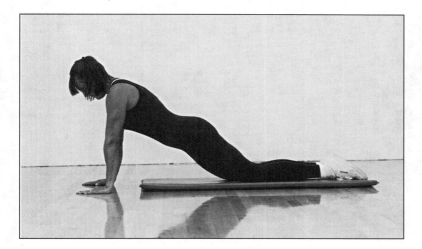

The easiest push-up position requires your shins and feet on the mat, a flat back, and your hands a little more than shoulder-width apart.

(Photo: Anne W. Krause)

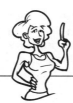

Fit Tip

If your wrists bother you when doing push-ups, you can use special push-up grips that resemble handles on sturdy bases. If you aren't using a mat, place a folded towel under your knees for comfort.

The next level of push-ups is nicknamed "girlie push-ups" because even many fit women, who generally cannot build upper-body strength like men, do them. Begin as in the basic push-up, but cross your ankles to raise your feet off the floor. Keeping your back straight, bend your elbows to lower your torso until your face, chest, and hips almost touch the floor; then straighten your elbows to raise yourself. You can begin with two sets of eight or 10 push-ups and, when you are comfortable doing these, continue until you cannot complete one fully.

For full or military push-ups, which only very fit women and reasonably strong men can do, keep your body straight, supporting your weight on your hands and toes.

Begin bending and straightening your elbows to raise and lower your body. You can do full push-ups to fatigue and then complete the exercise with one of the easier versions. If you ever make it to Jack Palance mode, you can put one arm behind your back!

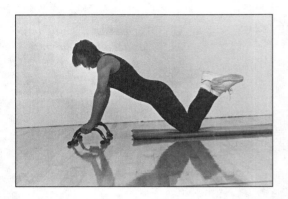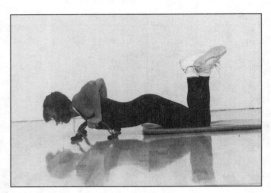

Using push-up grips is easier on your wrists.

(Photos: Anne W. Krause)

Stretching after push-ups relaxes your arms, shoulders, and back. First, stay in a kneeling position with your feet flattened against the floor and shift your hips back until you are sitting on your lower legs. Stretch your arms in front of you. Next, sit with your legs crossed comfortably in front of you and reach behind your back, clasp your hands together, and press them back to stretch your upper arms, shoulders, and chest. Then bring your hands in front of your body, clasp them at shoulder level, and round your back to stretch your arms, shoulders, and upper back.

Triceps Dips

Sit at the edge of a straight chair or weight bench with your feet slightly in front of you and slightly apart. Place your hands on the edge of the seat next to your hips with your palms down and your fingers forward. Slide off the seat, supporting your weight on your hands. Bend your elbows 90 degrees, flexing your knees to lower your hips toward the floor. Then, straighten your elbows to return to the starting position, with your hips level with the seat. Slide back onto the seat to rest between sets or whenever you need to. To stretch, raise your right arm and bend it behind your head. Grasp your right elbow with your left hand and press back against your forearm with the back of your head. Switch sides.

Leg Lifts

Lie on your right side with your hips stacked. You might be comfortable propping your head on your right hand, or you might prefer to extend your right arm out and cushion your head on it. To work your outer thigh, bend your right leg to a 45-degree angle from your body for stability. Raise your left leg from the hip until it is parallel to the floor and then lower it to the starting position. When you are ready for a slightly more advanced exercise, straighten your knee while your leg is raised, bend it, straighten it, and then lower it. When you can easily do two or three sets of each of these, you can add a set of small pulses and hold your leg up at the highest part of the lift for a count of eight and release. Switch to the other side.

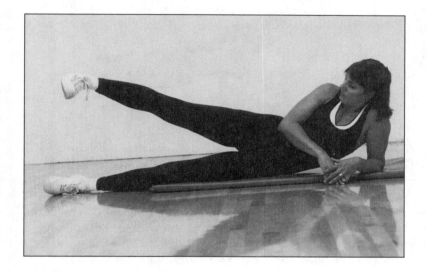

Leg lifts tone your gluteal muscles, but be sure to keep your back flat, not arched.

(Photo: Anne W. Krause)

To work your inner thigh, lie on your right side with your hips stacked. Cross your left leg over your right and place your left foot on the floor. This moves it out of the way of the right leg, which will be your working leg for this exercise. Lift and lower your right leg. When you are strong enough, finish with small pulses and then contract your muscles to hold your working leg at the highest part of the lift for a count of eight and then release. Switch legs. (The movements of these exercises are the same as for the outer-thigh leg lifts and inner-thigh leg lifts described in Chapter 7, but here, you are using just the weight of your own legs to provide resistance.)

Fitness Fact

The outer-thigh exercise is known as **abduction,** and the inner-thigh exercise is known as **adduction.**

This is another form of leg lift to tone your glutes and quads; be sure to keep your elbows on the mat to protect your back.

(Photo: Anne W. Krause)

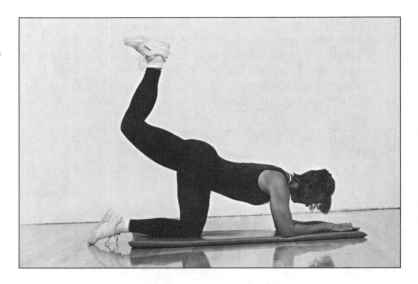

Rear Leg Lifts

To work your hamstrings and gluteals, get down on all fours on a mat or on the floor. Then, to protect your back, lower your elbows so that your forearms are resting on the floor. Raise and lower your right leg, keeping it straight behind you and elevating it no higher than the level of your hips. Then, bend your right knee, and raise and lower your leg with your foot flexed and the sole pointing to the ceiling. You can add a set of pulses in each position, and then, when you are stronger, you can finish by holding your leg up for a count of eight to 15 seconds. Another variation is to raise your leg with your knee straight, then bend it so that the sole of your foot points at the ceiling, straighten it again, and then lower it. Repeat with the left leg.

Gluteal Squeeze

To tone your buns, lie on your back on a mat or on the floor with your feet shoulder-width apart. Keep your lower back pressed to the floor and raise your hips, and then alternately squeeze and release your gluteal muscles. This is a very small motion. By keeping your feet in place but bringing your knees together, or by moving your feet a few inches farther apart or closer together, you will vary the exercise slightly and work a slightly different area. Finish the exercise by contracting the muscles as hard as you can and holding for eight to 15 seconds.

Squats

A tried-and-true lower-body exercise for anyone without knee problems is the squat, which helps strengthen and tone the quadriceps, hamstrings, calves, and glutes. Stand with your toes pointing straight ahead and your feet hip-width apart. Keep a natural posture with your back straight but arched out or hunched over. Keep your knees pointing straight ahead and press your hips forward without bending at the waist and keeping your back straight. You can steady yourself on a chair back, a barre, or another support if you need to, or you can rest your hands on your thighs or keep them out in front of you for balance.

Keeping your feet firmly on the floor and your heels pressed down, squat slowly and no deeper than 90 degrees (that is, no lower than a position in which your thighs are parallel to the floor). Rise up at the same tempo, pushing your body back to a standing position. When you get stronger, you can add extra weight in the form of dumbbells at your sides or, eventually, a barbell across your shoulders. To stretch, balance on the left foot, bring the right foot up behind you toward your butt, grab the forefoot with your hand, and stretch gently. Switch sides. Then stand on your left foot again and slide your right leg behind you, pressing the right leg toward the floor until you feel the stretch along the back of that leg. Switch sides.

Lunges

Lunges are wonderful for toning the whole leg, but they are not recommended if you have knee problems. In each of the versions described, you lunge by stepping with one leg and sinking down, which causes the knee of the stationary leg to bend. Switch sides to work both legs. (Some people prefer to alternate legs, while others prefer to do one set per leg and then change.) All lunges start from a standing position, and when you have done each one, return to a standing position:

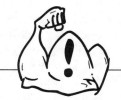

Fit Tip

You can ease into squats, but in the beginning, you may be more comfortable turning your feet out slightly for stability. This makes the exercise a cross between a squat and a plié.

➤ For the standing lunge, move your right leg straight back behind your body, flexing the right foot, and sink down. This causes your left knee to bend.

➤ For the diagonal lunge, move your right leg out at a 45-degree angle and sink down. This again causes the left knee to bend.

➤ For the lateral lunge, step the right knee out to the side and sink down, once again causing the left knee to bend. The important thing is to keep the left knee over the ankle.

Calf Raises

For a more shapely lower leg, stand with your feet slightly less than shoulder-width apart and hold on to a chair back or door frame for balance. Rise up on your toes and come down again, stopping just short of your heels touching the floor. Repeat the motion with your heels together and toes pointing outward. To add challenge, you can alternate raising your heels and toes, or you can stand firmly on an aerobic step or on a stair in your home, letting your heel drop below the edge each time you come down. In the most challenging version, place one foot behind the ankle of your other leg, and rise and come down on one leg at a time.

Trimmers and Toners from TV to You

Cable television is awash with infomercials for specialty items to help you trim or tone this body part or that. Such devices have been around for years, but seductive television infomercials, often with celebrity endorsements, imbue them with an in-your-face presence that makes them hard to ignore. Many of the products hawked on television also are available at discount stores, sporting goods retailers, and perhaps even supermarkets. Some products are sturdy and decently built; others are flimsy and marginally effective at best. It's hard to tell on the TV screen, and most people just shove purchasing mistakes away rather than take advantage of the money-back guarantees that usually are part of the offers. If a product seduces you, try to take a good look at a real sample and evaluate its quality in relation to its price. You can always go home and order it, or you can buy it locally, perhaps even on sale. If you buy from a local retailer, you won't have to pay the dreaded shipping and handling add-on, and if you are unhappy with the product or it doesn't live up to its claims, you're more likely to return it to a local retailer than mail it back to a distant company. You will also find that such items are often available at garage sales, because many people order them but never use them.

Over the years, the fitness marketplace has probably seen more types of abdominal exercisers than any other category. One early low-tech (and low-cost) product consisted of a system of cords and pulleys with five loops, one to go over a doorknob and four for the wrists and ankles. You just needed to lie on your back on the floor and alternately move the left leg/right arm and right leg/left arm. More recent abdominal exercisers have been tubular devices twisted into a cagelike form. You rest your head on a pad, and your hands grasp the side supports as you work your abdominals by doing caged crunches. Brands designed for abdominal exercising include Ab Rocker, Ab Sculptor, Ab Trainer, Ab Blaster, EZ Crunch, and Perfect ABs. At the peak of their popularity, they cost up to about $100, but prices quickly dropped dramatically.

Lower-body toning devices also abound. The ThighMaster, with its celebrity infomercial endorsement, enjoyed a high profile during its heyday. To use it, you put this resistance device between your thighs and squeeze your legs together. Other lower-body toners include Better Buns, Bun and Thigh Sculptor, BunTrainer, Fit Thighs, IsoBun, and UltraBurner.

In addition to these products that target specific body parts, multistation exercise machines and aerobic machines for home use are marketed on television. Some are sturdy, quality devices that really enhance your workout. These will be discussed in the section about setting up a home gym in Chapter 16, "Where to Work Out." Others are low-quality devices that mainly enhance the marketers' pocketbooks. Whatever the device, if it requires you to move your body or to work your muscles against resistance of some sort, it probably won't do any harm. If you're willing to make the investment in a product that appeals to you, you can add it to your home fitness arsenal and use it to spice up your routine or to supplement longer strength-training and aerobic workouts. Always remember that none of these fad devices will do anything for you that mainstream gear or traditional exercising won't do. And like all other fitness equipment and programs, such apparatus are only good if you truly use them.

Buyer Beware

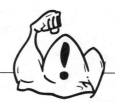

Do not believe exaggerated claims of calorie burning or conditioning in just a few minutes of exercising a day. In short, if a product or program sounds too good to be true, it probably is. The American Council on Exercise has specifically sited the example of Time Works, which markets an exercise machine that it claims helps achieve "full-body fitness in just four minutes a day." The device combines upper-body twisting and lower-body stepping. The manufacturer asserts that users can achieve a total aerobic workout, a total resistance workout, and a dynamic flexibility workout—all of which is equal to more than 60 minutes of traditional exercise.

Fit Tip

You can compare prices for products promoted on television infomercials (as well as obtain phone numbers and company addresses) at www.magickeys. com/infomercials/catl.html/.

The ACE commissioned Dr. David C. Nieman of Appalachian State University to test this $600 device. Not surprisingly, the study concluded that the manufacturer's fantastic claims are simply not true. The company asserts that people will "burn nearly three times the calories of a treadmill, rider, or strider!" In fact, study participants (12 men and 16 women of college age and average weight) burned eight calories per minute, and their metabolism returned to normal 15 minutes after they stopped exercising. Their total energy expenditure was about 40 calories, which is trivial in a fat-loss program. The subjects did gain some cardiorespiratory and lower-body strength benefits, but there was no gain in upper-body strength or joint flexibility. Harmful? No. Worth $600? Not really. The ACE also reported that from this product's release in early 1998 until early 1999 when the study was completed, Time Works racked up more than $60 million in sales. With profits like these, you can hardly expect infomercials for fitness products to go away.

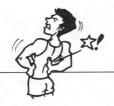

Strike Up the Bands (and Tubes)

You can do practically a full-body workout using *stretchercisers*—various styles of oversized elastic bands, cords, or tubes with or without loops or handles. These are portable, easy to use, inexpensive, and effective strength-training aids. Bands are flat pieces of elastic rubber with various resistance levels. Some come premade into loops; others need to be knotted for exercises that require loops. Exertubes are elastic tubes, usually with handles, that also come in various strengths. Less elasticity requires more strength and vice versa. Both types are color-coded so that their relative resistance is easy to identify. Just as you use different weights for different exercises, you may find yourself using different elasticities. You also can increase the amount of force required for an exercise by shortening a band.

> **Achtung!**
>
> Red–flag products include creams, pills, supplements, and other chemicals that you rub on or swallow. Although exercise gadgets at best can be beneficial and at worst can be a waste of money, lotions and potions often are useless even if you do use them, and some might carry hidden dangers to your health.

Bands and tubes are extremely versatile because you can do versions of various curls, presses, leg lifts, leg raises, and other stretchercises. They work the muscles when both stretching and releasing the tension—which, if you recall, is one of the benefits touted of expensive, gym-quality pneumatic and hydraulic strength-training apparatus. Exercising with bands or tubes mimics weight training, because they come in varying degrees of stretchability and require commensurate amounts of effort. Unlike iron weights, however, you can't precisely define how much resistance you are using when you are working with elastic. In other words, a 10-pound weight weighs 10 pounds, but a band offers relatively easy, moderate, or challenging resistance, and it can change as the band begins to wear. Before you begin working with any kind of "stretcherciser," check the band or tube for wear, especially in a gym, where it may get a lot of use.

SPRI Products sells several styles of stretchercisers: Xertube, Xercise Band, Can-Do Xercise Band, the Door Strap, the Xercuff, the Xering, and even the Step Tube, which is designed for use with a step routine. Most sell for less than $10. For information, call 1-800-222-7774.

Isometrics: Icing for the Fitness Cake

Charles Atlas was America's first fitness god. Before "beefcake" was a word and workouts were a way of life, his story was known all over the land. "I Changed Myself from a Puny 97-Pound Weakling into the World's Most Perfectly Developed Man," screamed magazine ads in the 1930s, '40s, and '50s. The Atlas approach to muscular training and body-building went by the trademarked name of Dynamic Tension—in other words, it was built on a strong isometric foundation. It is still around, and while it is a quicker fix than most fitness professionals now prefer, his system certainly has withstood the test of time. With a holistic approach to strength and health, Charles Atlas was way ahead of his time.

Fitness Fact

Atlas passed on some years ago, but Charles Atlas Ltd. is still around marketing its low-cost fitness program which promises fitness in "only 15 minutes a day." Contact the company at 888–MR–ATLAS or www.charlesatlas.com.

What worked for Charles Atlas and his 30 million reported students throughout the world can help you strengthen and tone, too. Think of isometrics as equipment-free strength training. Isometrics, which often are used as rehabilitation, are muscle contractions. Most people do not consider them to be their main workout routine, but they are good to have in your fitness repertoire because you can do them anytime and with no equipment. Isometrics use minimal movement to build muscles. Instead, the force of muscle contraction, muscle-against-muscle resistance, or muscle-against-stationary-object resistance builds strength. This concept is easy to understand as soon as you try it. Hold your hands out in front of you with your left palm up and your right palm down. Press your hands together as hard as you can. You can feel your pectoral, shoulder, and arm muscles working. This is an example of isometric exercise. (In fact, you can add this to a list of isometric exercises.)

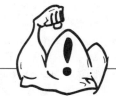

Fit Tip

Get into the habit of contracting and releasing muscles—abdominals, glutes, shoulders, even your chin—when you are stuck in traffic, standing in line, sitting in a theater waiting for the show to start, or anytime you think about it.

You most likely have been doing isometrics without even realizing it. When you suck in your gut, you're doing an isometric contraction. Runners automatically use isometric contractions to stabilize their torsos. Another example is the Kegel exercise, a contraction of the vaginal muscle, which women are counseled to do during pregnancy to counteract the pressure of the fetus on the bladder and afterward to tone the muscles stretched by childbirth.

Here are some isometric exercises that you can do virtually anywhere, anytime. Begin by holding each contraction for five seconds. Two sets of 10 repetitions is a good start. You can work up to 10 and then 15 seconds per contraction and then three or more sets.

➤ Stand in a doorway, hold your hands at thigh level, and then press the backs of your hands outward against the door jambs. This works the deltoids and supraspinatus.

➤ Stand in a doorway, raise your right arm above your head, and push your arm against the door frame. Change sides. This works the pectorals, obliques, and arms.

➤ Stand in a doorway, bend your elbows, and press the palms of your hands—at chest level—outward against the door jambs. This works the pectorals and biceps.

➤ Stand facing a wall about two feet away from it. Raise your hands to shoulder level and place your palms against the wall. Contract your abdominal muscles, straighten your elbows, lean your body weight toward the wall, and push against it. This works your arms and shoulders.

➤ Stand with your back against a wall. Tighten your abs so your back is firmly against the wall. Walk your feet forward, a few inches at a time, until your thighs are at least at a 45-degree angle but no more than a 90-degree angle from the floor. (At 90 degrees, your thighs are parallel to the floor, at a right angle to both your upper body and your shins.) Hold this position for as long as you can and then walk your feet back to stand up and relax. Repeat. This exercise also is known as the "wall-sit." It works the quadriceps and is an especially effective exercise for preseason ski conditioning.

➤ Sitting in a firm chair, place your hands on your thighs and press down hard, leaning forward slightly. This works your abdominals.

➤ Still sitting, place your hands palms down on the front of the chair seat and press down. This works your biceps and shoulders.

➤ Still sitting, press your legs tightly together or place a rubber ball between your knees and squeeze. This works your inner thighs.

➤ While sitting or standing, place your hands in front of you at chest level with your palms together, as if praying. Press your hands toward each other. This works the pectorals.

➤ Sitting in a chair, hook your feet under the edge of a desk (pad the tops of your feet with a folded towel or something else soft), the front of a sofa, or another large piece of furniture. Press your feet upward. This works the quadriceps. A variation for the quads that does not require hooking your feet under a piece of furniture is to raise one leg at a time and hold it parallel to the floor with the toes flexed.

➤ Standing beside a wall, door frame, or piece of heavy furniture, push your right ankle against the stationary object. Switch sides. This works the outer thigh of your right leg and inner thigh of your left leg.

➤ While seated in a straight chair, hold on to the front of the seat and pull your shoulders up and back, squeezing shoulder blades together. This works the rhomboids and trapeziuses.

➤ While seated at a table, press your palms against the underside of the table with your elbows bent at a 90-degree angle. This works the forearms.

Ball Game

Fitness can be a whole new ball game with a big, inflated, rubber orb called a fit ball or Swiss ball. Developed by Swiss physical therapists to help patients regain strength, balance, and flexibility, the fit ball makes a workout both productive and fun. Several dozen exercises have been developed to take advantage of this workout tool that looks like a great big toy. Here are several:

➤ **Abdominal strengthener.** Sit squarely on the ball. Slowly walk your feet out and simultaneously roll down onto your spine until your torso is parallel to the floor. Slowly roll back up, contracting your abdominal muscles to help regain the sitting position.

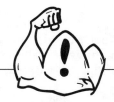

Fit Tip

To work your calves, not isometrically but still with minimal motion, stand with the front half of your feet on the bottom step of a staircase. Hold on for balance. Rise up on the balls of your feet and then let your heels drop below the level of the step.

➤ **Back strengthener.** Kneel behind the ball and drape your body forward over it with your hands flat on the floor in front of the ball. Slowly walk your hands forward so that the ball rolls down the length of your body past your hips. If you can, keep moving until your thighs are resting on the ball, maintaining a straight line from your head to your knees. Walk your hands back to return to the starting position. (Eventually, you might be strong enough to walk your hands so far forward and in such refined control that only the front of your ankles and tops of your feet are resting on the ball.) This exercise is sometimes called the "plank," and in addition to toning your back, it helps refine your balance and body alignment.

111

➤ **Push-ups.** Kneel behind the ball and drape your body forward over it with your hands flat on the floor in front of the ball. Move forward on the ball in the plank position as in the preceding exercise. When you are comfortably balanced, bend your elbows to lower your chest toward the floor. Straighten them to come up again. This push-up is easiest when the ball is under your hips, it is harder when the ball is under your thighs, and it is more challenging still when the ball is under your lower leg. These push-ups tone the pectorals, deltoids, and triceps. They also work your obliques and abdominals more effectively than conventional push-ups because you have to use these muscles to stabilize yourself from rolling off the ball.

➤ **Quadriceps strengthener.** Stand with the ball between your lower back and the wall. Squat down until your legs are at a 90-degree angle, keeping the ball against the wall. The ball will roll upward to about shoulder-blade level. Straighten your legs, and the ball will roll down.

When you first use a fit ball, you might feel wobbly and out of control, and you might even end up on the floor. The small, quick-reflex adjustments you make to stay on the ball will help your balance and tone the muscles of your torso.

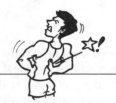

Achtung!

If you are just beginning to work out, are seriously overweight, and perhaps have problems balancing, start your fit-ball workout under a trainer's tutelage—or at least with a friend as a spotter—just in case the ball rolls out from under you.

Play the Roller Derby

Jyl Steinback, a personal fitness trainer who worked at the Elizabeth Arden day spa in Beverly Hills and at Arden's Maine Chance in Scottsdale, developed a stretching and toning program called "Roll Yourself Thin in 12 Minutes." This medley of 14 side-to-side rolling exercises, done sitting or lying on the floor, is pleasant and can help muscle tone and flexibility. Thinness—if it comes—is more the result of the fat-free diet Steinback also espouses.

The exercises are fun and easy, and with no equipment required, they offer do-anywhere convenience, so they are a useful adjunct to a more comprehensive fitness program. One example is Steinback's Love Handle Roll. Lying on your back, stretch your arms out to your sides with your palms up and your elbows bent slightly. Raise your feet over your hips with your knees together. Keeping your shoulders and arms on the floor, roll both knees alternately to the left and to the right. This and the other 13 exercises, which should be coupled with warming up before and stretching afterward, are described in a pocket-size book available by calling 888-FAT-FREE (888-328-3731).

Liquid Resistance

Aquatic exercise is one of the most effective ways to add resistance training to your program without compromising your joints. It is especially effective for obese people, pregnant women, arthritis sufferers, and anyone getting back to a workout routine after a back or knee injury. Water all but eliminates the effects of gravity on the body and cushions weight-bearing joints, making aqua exercises the lowest of low-impact workouts. At the same time, water provides resistance to force, which makes it an effective strength-training aid.

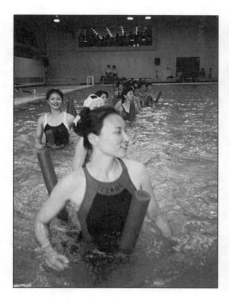

Hop into the pool for resistance training that won't stress your joints.

(Photo: Aquatic Exercise Association)

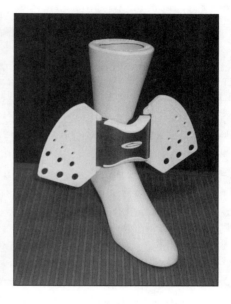

Fins add resistance to an aquatic workout.

(Photo: Claire Walter)

You can join a fitness class or buy special aquatic exercise equipment such as buoyancy devices that suspend your body with your shoulders, neck, and head above water. Other products designed for water exercises include webbed gloves, aquajogging belts, underwater runners, and paddlelike dumbbells that use an oversize surface area rather than weight to increase resistance. You also can increase your workload with a minimal investment. Commandeer a child's kickboard and push or pull it underwater to enhance arm, shoulder, and back muscles.

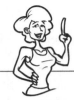

Fitness Fact

Water can be four to 42 times more resistant than air, depending on the speed of movement against it and the surface area being moved against it.

Here are some aquatic exercise tips from the manufacturer of AquaJogger (a buoyancy belt), AquaJogger Webbed Pro Gloves, DeltaBells (paddle-shaped dumbbells that use surface area rather than weight to increase resistance), and AquaRunners (underwater exercise footwear):

➤ Consciously work with resistance by finding the path of most resistance.

➤ Keep all moves below the water line.

➤ To make moves easier, bend the limbs and move more slowly.

➤ To increase resistance, straighten the limbs and increase speed.

➤ Push and pull the water to work forces equally in both directions to achieve balanced muscularity.

➤ Avoid being a "bobber" (a person who bounces up and down in the water), and try to keep your torso calm.

➤ Avoid using buoyancy-assisted moves.

➤ Because you are working with resistance, be sure to pay attention to any injuries. If a particular movement causes pain, eliminate it from your routine.

The Least You Need to Know

➤ More is not necessarily better. Slow, controlled movements are more effective than many repetitions with poor form.

➤ Fitness devices can be useful or useless, but most are harmless; check them out at stores and remember that most have a money-back guarantee.

➤ Exercise bands and tubes create resistance, because stretching them requires muscular strength.

➤ Water exercises are the kindest on the joints, because they are non–weight-bearing activities.

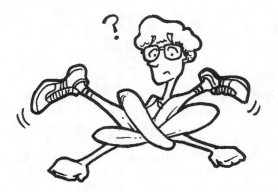

Chapter 9

Other Paths to Stretching and Toning

> **In This Chapter**
>
> ➤ Yoga enhances flexibility and emotional well-being
>
> ➤ Tai chi keeps elderly Chinese strong and supple
>
> ➤ Dancing is a fine way to shape up and have fun
>
> ➤ Pilates strengthens, lengthens, and tones the body

Some of the oldest paths to fitness are new again, and more people are embracing forms of holistic fitness that have long been understood in non-European cultures. Such approaches often are described in contemporary parlance as mind/body or mind/body/spirit philosophies. Many people are drawn to ancient Eastern practices such as yoga and tai chi to tone up and calm down at the same time. In addition to focused, somewhat introspective movements and postures, relaxation and meditation often are part of the appeal. These practices have been around for a long time but only recently have begun going mainstream. Their names often are derived from nature, which indicates the mind/body connection that has endured through the ages.

Another basic approach to fitness draws more from European and American practices such as Pilates, Feldenkrais, and the Alexander Technique. Their focus is on body balance and alignment as a way to enhance strength and fitness. They all adhere to concepts such as lengthening the muscles, stretching, and balancing the musculoskeletal system to be limber and free of pain. Many people—trainers and other fitness professionals as well as the general public—are now more aware of alternative paths and the mind/body relationship that is useful in embarking on and maintaining a healthy lifestyle. Such programs, developed by creative thinkers in fitness, stem from a Western tradition but often lead to the same results as older Eastern philosophies.

Yoga? Yes!

Yoga, a ritualized discipline, is as spiritual as it is physical. It is a versatile discipline that strengthens and tones the body, calms the mind, increases flexibility, and enhances introspection. It has even been called the world's oldest stress-management system. This ancient holistic philosophy from India now has as many branches as a cottonwood tree. Some are ancient traditions; others were founded more recently by modern masters. Although yoga is the foundation of a total lifestyle for some people, it is part of a fitness program for millions of others. In fact, many stretches now commonly used by athletes are yoga poses.

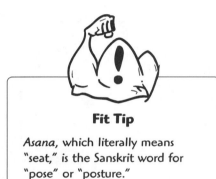

Fit Tip

Asana, which literally means "seat," is the Sanskrit word for "pose" or "posture."

Expert practitioners have flexible bodies that they can contort into a stunning repertoire of postures and movements that can be slow and deliberate or fast and flowing. Beginner yoga classes, available at health clubs, adult-education programs, and specialized yoga centers, focus on breathing and basic postures, and some of yoga's principles have been incorporated into the flexibility and relaxation portions of all sorts of fitness classes. Some clubs offer yoga-derived classes directed toward enhancing a sport, such as weight-lifting, swimming, or cycling. Whether you practice yoga as an end unto itself or as part of a whole fitness package, you might be happy with an elementary level, refined as skill and strength improve, or you might be drawn to a specific branch. At that point, you might seek out a yoga center or yoga studio, where more advanced programs are available. The most dedicated practitioners eventually work with a yoga master, either in India or in the West.

In addition to offering introductory classes, each yoga center tends to specialize in one or two branches of yoga, allowing you to go into yoga in great depth if you so choose. Health clubs and recreation centers might offer just one basic style at several levels. Here are some of the most common systems of yoga found in the United States, along with some clues as to how they might fit your needs:

➤ **Ananda.** Developed by an American student of an Indian swami, this system couples gentle physical movements and poses with affirmation and meditation. Enhanced self-awareness is one of its goals.

➤ **Ashtanga.** This system refers to the ancient body-mind discipline founded by the sage Patanjali, and it includes classical *asanas, pranayarsa* (breath practices), and meditation. A modern teacher named PataGhi Jo also refers to his style of teaching as Ashtanga yoga. This latter style is based on a series of challenging poses repeated over and over, with emphasis on a particular type of heating breath as the movement flows from one pose to another. It is easy to get comfortable with this style because you keep repeating and working to perfection the same poses. Once your poses are perfected, you can go on to a higher series. Each series takes about 90 minutes.

➤ **Bikram.** This is *asana* in a furnace. The poses are similar, but the setting is different. Bikram practitioners do 26 specific yoga poses in a very hot room. This helps warm and loosen your muscles, but some people find it uncomfortable.

➤ **Hatha.** This term usually is applied to classical body yoga. If it is meant to evoke anything, the sense is of meditative and deliberate poses and counterposes that integrate the body, breath, and mind. It is designed to move subtle energies in specific patterns and to balance and harmonize endocrine functions. If you sign up for a nonspecific yoga class, this is probably what you'll get. It's a good introduction.

➤ **Integral.** This is fusion yoga. It incorporates elements from various yoga systems into a 90-minute class that follows a prescribed progression. It includes poses, relaxation, and meditation.

➤ **Iyengar.** A modern movement, this is the Pilates of yoga emphasizing body alignment and precise movements and poses. In its purest form, this strenuous style requires practitioners to hold poses for up to two minutes, which can seem like an eternity. It is excellent for conditioning because of its challenge, but many beginning exercisers find it way *too* challenging. It also can employ blocks, belts, ropes, and other props to help less flexible or injured people reach the poses.

Fit Tip

Some clubs offer sport-specific yoga classes with positions and movements geared toward weightlifters, swimmers, cyclists, or participants in other activities.

➤ **Kripalu.** This three-part system begins with the understanding and practice of various postures, breathing, and movement. At the second stage, postures are held longer, and class members are encouraged to understand their feelings about what they are doing with their bodies.

➤ **Kundalini.** This refers to an ancient style of yoga in which the spiritual energy of the body is deliberately activated to attain higher consciousness. A modern teacher, Yogi Bhajan, also uses this term to refer to a style of *asana* that uses a rapid-breathing technique in each posture while that posture is being held. This is an excellent selection if you are stressed and want to harness Eastern philosophy to learn to relax, but like Iyengar, it requires you to hold each pose for a long time and is therefore very demanding.

➤ **Sivanda.** During 90-minute classes, students gently practice the postures in the Sun Salutation (see the next section), meditation, and deep relaxation, all of which are combined with chanting.

➤ **Viniyoga.** Mantras, chanting, meditation, and twisting postures that work deep into the musculature, organs, and glands are combined in this branch of yoga. It can be physically gentle but is complex and layered.

In basic classes, yoga often is presented as a one-style-fits-all discipline, but after you get beyond the introduction, its complexities unfold. You might have to shop around a bit to find the type that suits you best. "Picking the right style for each individual is crucial," says Dr. Sarasvati Buhrman of the Rocky Mountain Institute of Yoga and Aryuveda in Boulder, Colorado. "From a classical perspective, different poses and different styles of yoga *asana* affect basic *dohsas* or bioenergies in different ways. People differ from one another physically, physiologically, mentally, and emotionally, so it is important to match the practice with the person. Physiologically, *asanas* balance and stimulate the endocrine system, which is why yoga is effective for fitness and weight management."

Quote, Unquote

"There are two kinds of people in the U.S. right now: the seven million people actually doing yoga and the several hundred million who wish they were—even if they don't yet know it."

—Phyllis Berg, Eastern Athletic Clubs, New York

Salute to the Sun

This series of flowing movements and postures is one of the fundamentals of yoga. The Salute to the Sun also can serve as a warm-up for other activities, as a self-contained exercise, or simply as a good start to the day. Doing it for 10 minutes every day or two is a fast way to get the blood flowing and to enhance your well-being.

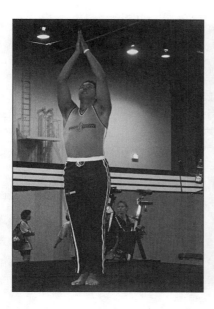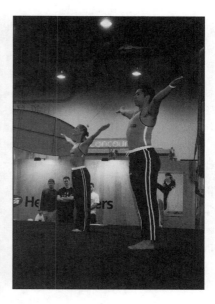

The Salute to the Sun is a flowing series of yoga postures to greet the day—or to stretch and energize anytime.

(Photos: Claire Walter)

The following postures (with Sanskrit names) are done one after another, and each one is a single continuous motion:

➤ **The Mountain (*tadasana*).** Stand with your feet together or parallel four to six inches apart. Contract your quads slightly and lower your hands to your sides.

➤ **The Lightning Bolt (*uktassana*).** Inhale deeply while raising your arms over your head. Exhale and lower your hands to chest level, palm to palm as if in prayer, and look toward the sky or ceiling. Inhale and raise your arms overhead again.

➤ **The Forward Bend (*uttassana*).** Exhale and, with a straight back, bend your upper torso toward the floor. Then, keeping your legs straight and your butt up, continue bending your torso until your head is down at your knees. Place your palms flat on the floor in front of you, if you can, or reach for your ankles with your hands.

➤ **The Plank (*chataranga dandassana*).** Inhaling, raise your upper torso until it is parallel to the floor, keeping your back flat and your arms parallel to your legs. Place your hands on the floor, and exhaling, walk your feet back and lower your body to the floor until you are in a push-up position.

➤ **The Cobra (*bhujangasana*).** Exhale and lower your body to the floor with your arms bent at your sides, the tops of your feet on the floor, and your toes pointed straight back. Straighten your elbows to push your upper body up while inhaling, and raise your head, tilt it back, and look at the sky or ceiling.

➤ **Downward Facing Dog (*adho mukha svanassana*).** Exhaling, keep your arms straight, and lower your head and shoulders toward the floor. Then straighten your legs, and rise up on the balls of your feet with your butt toward the ceiling. This posture resembles an upside-down V.

The Downward Facing Dog is another classic part of the Salute to the Sun.

(Photo: Claire Walter)

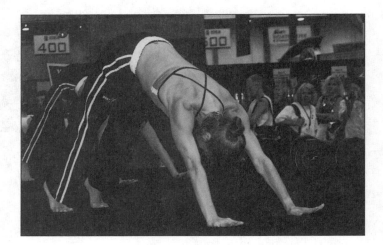

➤ **The Warrior (*virabadrasana*).** Inhaling, bring your right knee forward while keeping your left leg back in a powerful lunge. Bring your arms over your head, pressing the palms together. To do the warrior on the other side, repeat the Cobra, Downward Facing Dog, and Warrior with the left knee forward and the right foot back. Return to the Downward Facing Dog position.

➤ **The Forward Bend (*uttassana*).** Keeping your hands flat on the floor and maintaining the forward bend of Downward Facing Dog, step one foot at a time between your hands. Exhaling, move your body weight onto the balls of your feet.

➤ **The Lightning Bolt (*uktassana*).** Inhaling, raise your torso until your back is flat and parallel to the floor, look up, and reach your arms overhead, palm to palm. Exhaling, bend your knees slightly, tuck your head toward your knees, and reach your hands to the floor or to your ankles.

➤ **The Mountain (*tadasana*).** Inhale and straighten your legs to stand up tall with your feet flat on the floor, raise your arms overhead, and look toward the sky or ceiling. Exhale and lower your hands, bringing your palms together in a prayer position in front of your chin. Lower your hands to your sides and raise your head to look up at the sky or ceiling.

The Breath Factor

Although not all styles of yoga *asana* immediately emphasize the role of breath, most do. In fact, breathing is key to the whole philosophy. Breathing is viewed as the connection between the mind and the body and as the act that separates life from death. The one reason yoga develops the ability to achieve deep relaxation and flexibility is its controlled, deep, and focused breathing.

Some styles of yoga encourage you to breathe audibly, which serves as feedback that you are breathing correctly. Deep inhalation—filling the upper, middle, and bottom of the lungs—elevates the body's core temperature and helps make the muscles flexible. Interestingly, it also conditions your lungs just as exercise conditions the muscles. Yoga practitioners actually have increased lung volume, and their bodies have an enhanced ability to deliver oxygen to their muscles and organs.

Inversion Positions

Inverted yoga positions are those in which the head is lower than the torso. Suitable inverted positions for beginners include the Shoulder Stand, Downward Dog, and Forward Bend. Advanced practitioners can do handstands and headstands. For some people, inverted poses are truly invigorating and energizing, but they are not recommended for anyone with high blood pressure. Here are some useful tips, pithy observations, and benefits of the practice, compiled by the Om Yoga Center in New York:

➤ When your world turns upside down, turn yourself upside down with it and breathe.

➤ Inversions are rejuvenating and invigorating. At the same time, they give increased mental clarity and stimulate the hormones that aid sleep.

➤ Turning your body upside down reverses gravity's pull and improves the circulation of blood in the body. The facial muscles get to relax, and wrinkles tend to get fluffed.

➤ Inversions improve health and vitality. They aid in digestion, which helps with weight loss. They also let the legs rest from weight-bearing activity, which helps with varicose veins.

➤ Turning upside down allows your brain and other organs to bathe in the reversed blood flow.

➤ An inversion works like an organic facial, bringing fresh blood to the face to give it a rosy glow. This retards the aging process; it's like a natural face-lift.

If even the most basic inverted poses make you uneasy, you can get some benefits by lying across a bed on your back and allowing the head, neck, and upper body to hang over the edge. You also can lie on your back on the floor, raise your legs perpendicular to the floor, and rest them against a wall.

121

Quote, Unquote

"Inverted yoga positions allow you to see the world from another viewpoint."

—Cyndi Lee, Om Yoga Center, New York

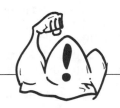

Fit Tip

To locate specific yoga classes, studios, and teachers in the United States, check www. chesco.com/yogafinder.

Nouvelle Yoga

America is nothing if not a fertile field for sowing hybrid and mutated versions of practices from abroad. Restorative Yoga (various locations), Phoenix Rising Yoga (1-800-288-9642, www.yogasite.com), Kali Ray TriYoga (310-589-0600), and Power Yoga (www. poweryoga.com) are among the made-in-the-U.S.A. yoga styles you will find. Most are available in just a few yoga studios, in a book, or perhaps on video. These are an early wave of the adaptations that might emerge with Americans' increased interest in yoga.

Tai Chi Touches Many Lives

The ancient study of tai chi chuan (usually abbreviated in the United States as tai chi) is a series of slow-motion movements ideally done outdoors to reduce stress, to keep the mind sharp, and to maintain the body's suppleness and muscular strength by moving the *chi,* or energy, through the body. Visualization is the key to success with tai chi. Its origins are in the martial-arts realm, but it is now thought of more as a way for people to remain fit and flexible. In China, the morning ritual of tai chi and a related discipline called *chi gong* is credited with helping create positive attitudes, emotions, and a sense of well-being. It also is said to help elderly people maintain their mobility, agility, and physical fitness.

Here is a sampling of some of tai chi's basic moves. The lyrical names mask the strength and control you will obtain if you practice them:

➤ **Sinking the Chi.** The image is one of gathering the energy surrounding you, bringing it into your body, and letting it flow through you to the center of the earth. Standing straight, slowly lift your arms out to your sides with your palms down. When they are at shoulder level, bend your elbows to bring your hands over your head with your palms still down. Exhale and let your palms float toward the ground or floor.

➤ **Supporting the Sky Like a Pillar.** The image is one of gathering energy and propelling it skyward with your hands. Raise your left foot, and turn it outward at about the level of your left shoulder, if you can. Keeping your shoulders relaxed, lift your arms in front of you with your palms facing each other. When your hands are at chest level, turn them so the palms face outward. Exhale and allow your hands to float down, inhale and raise them up, and exhale and let them float down again.

➤ **Penetrating Heaven and Earth.** The image is one of propelling energy both down to earth and up to heaven. With your arms extended to your sides at chest level, bend your elbows to bring your hands in front of you. Rotate your hands so that the right palm is up and the left palm is down. Exhale and raise your right palm toward the sky and lower your left palm toward the earth. Exhale and bring your hands closer to your body. Inhale and reverse.

Introspective Dance Plus

Neuromuscular Integrative Action is an effective, low-impact, cardiovascular program combining elements from tai chi, yoga, and dance forms such as jazz, ethnic, and even ballet to condition the body and calm the emotions. The elements of music come from dance, and the fact that it is done in bare feet relates to modern dance and yoga. Also from yoga is the emphasis on breathing. Power and strength moves are drawn from tai chi and other martial arts. Instructors use a great deal of imagery, which participants can interpret as they want and can. Although movements are suggested to the class, participants can tailor them to their own level of ability and agility. Adherents say that this program allows the emotions to flow even as the body moves.

Quote, Unquote

"If we move with tension, the intrinsic energy does not flow freely. When we move softly, the energy can flow. In life, we often learn that softness is stronger than firmness. It is like the oak versus the bamboo. The oak breaks and the bamboo bends. Or like the tongue versus the teeth. The tongue outlasts the teeth. Or water versus rock. The water wears away the rock."

—Justin Stone, "Tai Chi: Joy Through Movement," Public Broadcasting System

Pilates Pilots the Body to Fitness

The Pilates Method is a system of movement best known for its emphasis on balance, body alignment, flexibility, and building core strength. Joseph Hubertus Pilates (pronounced *pih-LAHT-ees*) was born in Germany in 1880 and lived in England. Because he was a diver, a gymnast, a skier, a boxer, and a physical therapist for circus performers, he learned about physiology and biomechanics before these fields really had names. During World War I, he used his knowledge to help rehabilitate wounded British soldiers, using hospital bed frames and springs as exercise equipment. In the 1920s, he extended it into a full range of complex yet effective exercises to strengthen, elongate, stretch, firm, and tone the body.

Dancers were the first to gravitate to The Method, as Joseph Pilates's system is widely known. More recently, Madonna, Uma Thurman, Sharon Stone, Vanessa Williams, and other actors and models who want tone without bulk have embraced it. "In 10 sessions, you'll feel the difference. In 20, you'll see the difference. In 30, you'll have a new body," is the way Joseph Pilates described his innovative system, and adherents over the decades would agree.

Pilates has two components: mat exercises and apparatus exercises. Between them, they include 500 exercises that require concentration rather than perspiration. Pilates involves low reps focused on strengthening the core, elongating the limbs, and rebalancing the body. At first glance, mat classes resemble other exercises done on the floor, but in fact they are more complex. The odd-looking devices associated with the Pilates Method are distinctive, even at first glance. To the untutored eye, Pilates apparatus—wooden contraptions outfitted with ropes, pulleys, springs, and padded footboards plus various padded boxes, platforms, and other paraphernalia—look like the brainchild of a mad scientist. They go by such fanciful names as The Reformer, The Cadillac, The Barrel, Ped-O-Pull, The Wunda Chair, and Magic Circles.

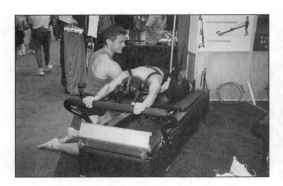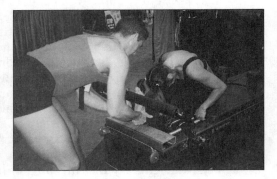

Two classic Pilates moves using The Reformer to limber, tone, and lengthen the muscles.

(Photos: Claire Walter)

Typically, you start Pilates with an evaluation and perhaps a few private sessions to familiarize yourself with the movements, the apparatus, and the approach. Many people then switch to Pilates classes, and some studios now offer group Pilates classes, inspired by the growing popularity of studio cycling and other group activities. The Method is useful for people of various ages and degrees of fitness. It often helps people with chronic back problems, hip and shoulder injuries, post-polio syndrome, and other conditions. In fact, in addition to serving as part of a fitness regime, it is used in hospitals and rehabilitation centers—truly going back to its origins.

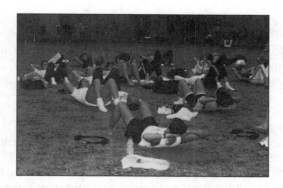

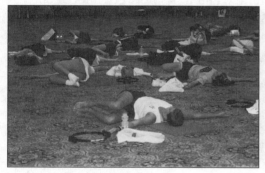

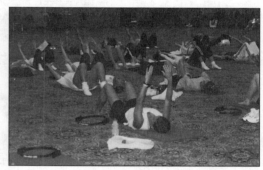

A series of positions in a Pilates mat class.

(Photos: Claire Walter)

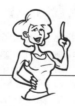

Fitness Fact

In 1976, there were just five Pilates studios in the world. Now it is taught in 500 studios, health clubs, and rehab centers in the United States alone.

Pilates on a Different Plane

Gyrotonics takes Pilates to a different plane. Like Pilates, Gyrotonics aims at elongating, realigning, stretching, toning, and conditioning the body. It has two components: with apparatus and without apparatus. Gyrotonic Expansion System exercises are done on a mat, and Spinal Dynamics exercises are gentle, repetitive torso rotations that are done seated, standing, kneeling, and prone on a mat. The Gyrotonics apparatus resembles a bench with a towerlike structure at one end and with straps, handles, and pulleys plus weight plates for added resistance. Breathing plays an important role in the program, as it does in Pilates and yoga. Pilates facilities have now grown to the hundreds, but Gyrotonics is still fairly exclusive. The apparatus is expensive, few trainers have been schooled in it, and it has not yet achieved popular status. Many who have tried it, however, tend to think of it as Pilates-plus.

The Methods of Moshe and Matthias

Dr. Moshe Feldenkrais (1904–1984) was a scientist, engineer, judo instructor, and an associate of Frederic Joliot-Curie at the Curie Institute in Paris. F. Matthias Alexander (1869–1955) was an actor who lost his voice and experimented with and developed methods to help him regain it so that he could return to the stage. The Feldenkrais (pronounced *FELL-den-krise*) Method and the Alexander Technique both aim to re-balance and realign the body for pain management, flexibility, coordination, and conduct of everyday activities. Both systems, which are practiced one-on-one with trained teachers and practitioners, gained favor with musicians and others who have to do repetitive movements in unnatural body positions.

Quote, Unquote

"Movement is life. Life is a process. Improve the quality of the process, and you improve the quality of life itself."

—Moshe Feldenkrais

Life in Balance

The goals of both ancient mind-body regimes and newer philosophies with mind-body orientation aim at improving balance, alignment, and flexibility. You don't hear much about strength or cardiovascular fitness in the mind-body world. If you don't feel comfortable with the old-tradition/New Age approaches to enhancing flexibility and balance, however, there are other ways to achieve this portion of a fitness goal.

Fit balls (or Swiss balls) are excellent tools for enhancing flexibility and balance (see Chapter 8, "Iron-Free Resistance Training"). Bongo Boards, balance boards, and balance disks are examples of balance-training devices. They feature a solid platform that is on, but not attached to, a cylindrical or round support. You climb on the platform and must subtly shift your weight to keep the board balanced on the moving support.

SRF is a company that makes the concept more technical with two disks, one fixed to a solid support on the floor and one sliding on an adjustable track, so you can do arm or leg stabilization and strengthening exercises. This device is especially useful for someone with limited strength or for rehab. For details, contact 1-800-FITTER-1 or www.fitter1.com.

Old Philosophies, New Programs

Although some of the powerful disciplines mentioned in this chapter have been around for centuries, they are not necessarily ends unto themselves in the modern fitness world. Just as Billy Blanks took traditional martial arts and combined them with modern elements to create Tae-Bo, which is discussed in Chapter 17, "Fight Your Way to Fitness" other innovators have taken their inspiration from various lands and times and have used that inspiration as a foundation for contemporary routines. Here are some examples:

➤ **Power Moves.** This is a choreographed melange of movements derived from several Eastern traditions. The class warms up with tai chi to "awaken the power." It proceeds with postures and movements from Ashanti yoga to "concentrate the power." Next, elements of kickboxing "release the power." Finally, the cool-down is inspired by Ch'i Kung, and it "calms the power." The instructor should emphasize the mind-body connection and proper breathing. For information, call 1-800-509-3607 or 805-646-0108.

➤ **JoSand.** A workout pioneer who goes by the name of Johnny G is credited with inventing Spinning. More recently, he developed a balancing act that he calls JoSand. The workout centers around a six-foot wooden stick, known in Japan as a *jo*. With the stick balanced on the fingers, participants do a series of moves, such as short runs, jumps, squats, and turns. Johnny G claims a connection between the participant and nature. In southern California, where this workout was created, it's done on wet beach sand at low tide. Stay tuned to see whether it will show up at your local health club.

➤ **Aqua Yoga.** Water or aqua aerobics and water or aqua jogging have been around for a while, but more recently, water or aqua yoga and water or aqua tai chi have appeared on the scene. The benefits of body buoyancy, the resistance of water, and the impact-free aquatic environment are added to ancient Eastern arts.

➤ **YogaFit.** This fast-moving hybrid combines the energy of aerobics with the flow and flexibility of yoga. Like aerobics programs, YogaFit is choreographed to music, but that choreography uses yoga movements and postures. (See Chapter 12, "Your Heart Will Love Aerobic Exercise.")

The Least You Need to Know

➤ Yoga comes in many forms, so it is possible to select the yoga discipline that suits your style.

➤ Breathing is an important part of all yoga schools, because it is viewed as the link between the mind and the body.

➤ Pilates lengthens the muscles and tones the body with movements that strengthen and stretch the body.

➤ Tai chi, an ancient ritual of full-body exercises performed daily, is credited with keeping older people fit.

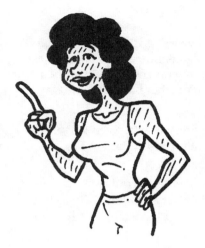

Chapter 10

Trainers' Tips and Tricks

In This Chapter

➤ Trainers' tips for an effective workout program

➤ Combine activities to benefit from cross–training

➤ A short workout beats no workout at all

➤ Keep tabs on your heart rate to monitor fitness

Personal trainers are hot. Exercisers from newcomers to fitness veterans see the benefit in spending time with a professional who helps them focus on their fitness goals, monitors their progress, and readjusts their program as they become stronger and fitter. Many of the benefits of hiring a personal trainer were discussed in Chapter 4, "Using All the Help You Can Get."

Personal trainers are to fitness what chefs are to haute cuisine. Just as these masters of the kitchen have tried-and-true tricks and techniques for producing culinary masterpieces, trainers have tips and suggestions that can help you perform wonders in the gym. This chapter includes some of the techniques trainers have for helping clients enhance their workout programs.

A Way of Life

If you talk to several personal trainers, each will have a slightly different philosophy on fitness and different training style. Trainers all agree, however, that a fitness program needs to be a way of life in order for you to gain the benefits of being fit. Here are a few other general tips that trainers agree can help make "fitness as a way of life" a reality:

➤ **Start smart.** Start your program easy and progress slowly. Even seasoned athletes must do this if they take a break from their training or are recovering from an injury.

➤ **Stay hydrated.** You can never drink too much water. Avoid caffeine and alcoholic beverages, especially before, during, and after a workout. These liquid refreshments will dehydrate you. Sports drinks can be okay as a supplement for hydration, but they do not replace water.

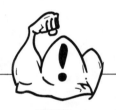

Fit Tip

If you are doing biceps curls and can lift 20 pounds but cannot manage 25 pounds, enlist a workout partner to help you get over your plateau. Have your partner help you curl 25 pounds, and then return to the starting position by yourself. A trainer will describe this as getting help on the concentric contraction (shortening the muscle) and doing the eccentric contraction (lengthening the muscle) by yourself.

➤ **Eat well.** Instead of a faddish diet promoted for rapid weight loss, weave a healthy, well-balanced diet into your life. Food fuels your body when you are working out.

➤ **Make working out convenient.** Join a gym or take a class near your home or workplace. Get home workout equipment. Pick a time of day for your workout that fits into your schedule. You won't work out if it is inconvenient.

➤ **Work out with a friend.** Find a training buddy if you can. A buddy with a similar goal—to get fit—provides camaraderie and motivation.

➤ **Keep a training log.** Use a training log or notebook to keep track of your workouts and your food intake. This can help you figure out when you have the most energy and when you are tired.

➤ **Mix things up.** If you do the exact same workout every day, you might get bored and in a rut. Variety is good for building up different muscles and helps prevent injuries.

➤ **Reward yourself.** Treat yourself to something special when you reach your goals. Set incremental goals so your ultimate goal does not seem unreachable.

➤ **Vary your lifting.** If you reach a plateau in your strength training, work with an eccentric-contraction routine, also called "negative repetitions," see the accompanying Fit Tip sidebar for a suggestion.

➤ **Have fun.** Last but by far not least, make working out fun! Being fit makes you feel better physically and mentally. When it is fun, you will do it more readily.

Targeting Problem Parts

If you go to a trainer and seek advice for dealing with specific problem areas, he or she probably will get you started on a general program to improve your overall fitness and shed fat. Once you're on that track, you can again seek help in targeting those touchy spots. Here are some of the most problematic areas that many people want to target. If you have one (or more) of them, here's what you'll probably be counseled to do (read on for more details on how a trainer might counsel you to tackle specific problems):

➤ **Flapping underarms.** Solution: Triceps exercises with weights, triceps dips, triceps extensions, and triceps push-downs on a weight machine.

➤ **Hollow chest or rounded shoulders.** Solution: Lat and pectoral exercises with weights; push-ups; chest press, chest fly, lat pull-down, and seated rows on a weight machine.

➤ **Love handles.** Solution: Aerobic exercise is the most important activity to rid yourself of love handles. In addition, do side stretches, oblique crunches, and back extensions.

➤ **Gut bulge or beer belly.** Solution: Crunches, crunches, crunches.

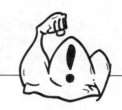

Fit Tip

If you are doing biceps curls and can lift 20 pounds but cannot manage 25 pounds, enlist a workout partner to help you get over your plateau. Have your partner help you curl 25 pounds, and then return to the starting position by yourself. A trainer will describe this as getting help on the concentric contraction (shortening the muscle) and doing the eccentric contraction (lengthening the muscle) by yourself.

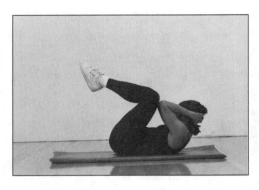 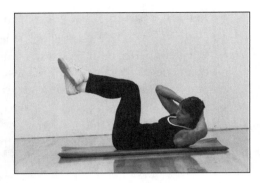

Crunches using your lower torso as well as your upper torso work all of your abdominal muscles.

➤ **Flabby thighs.** Solution: Side-leg lifts, inner-thigh lifts, abduction and adduction stations on a weight machine.

➤ **Flabby underarms.** Solution: Triceps exercises.

Remember that you can spot-strengthen, but you cannot spot-reduce. Spot-reduction will only show up when you lose the fat on top of the *problem part* that you have toned. That takes cardiovascular exercise and a sensible diet.

Quote, Unquote

"If spot reducing worked, people who chew gum would have skinny faces."

—Covert Bailey, author, motivational speaker, and founder of Covert Bailey Fitness

Amazing Abdominal Exercises

Most trainers and physiologists now recommend crunches rather than sit-ups as a tummy-toning exercise. Using the correct technique is more important than how many you can do. Lie on your back on a mat with your hands lightly supporting either the back of your head or your neck. Begin contracting your abdominal muscles to lift your upper torso while keeping your lower back on the mat. Use slow, controlled movements and be sure to work all parts of the abdominals—upper, lower, transverse, and oblique. For extra conditioning, hold at the top of each contraction for a few seconds. With each crunch, press your bellybutton to the floor as if concaving or sucking in your stomach. If you do abdominal exercises correctly and without momentum, 12 repetitions of each exercise will be sufficient to feel a burn and exhaustion. If you can do 100 or more reps of anything, you are not doing the exercise in the most efficient way. For more on crunches, see Chapter 8, "Iron-Free Resistance Training."

Build Your Chest and Arms

Chances are, when you began doing push-ups, you learned one hand position in relation to your body and have used it all along. This means you've been working your pectorals in exactly the same way. To make your push-ups build different parts of these muscles, you need to vary the position of your hands. When you move your hands closer together, you work the triceps and the inner or medial part of the pectorals. When you move your hands farther apart, you work the lateral part of the outer pectorals. As a push-up veteran, you will feel the difference as you experiment with different positions. Well-defined biceps are a sign of strength. If you have been doing biceps curls and push-ups, you have already been strengthening the upper arms.

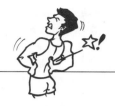

Achtung!

It is important not to arch your back and not to pull on or stress the neck when you are doing abdominal work. If you pull on your neck, you can stress the ligaments at the vulnerable cervical vertebrae and disks. If you arch your back, you stress the lumbar vertebrae or disks. Either can cause chronic neck or back problems.

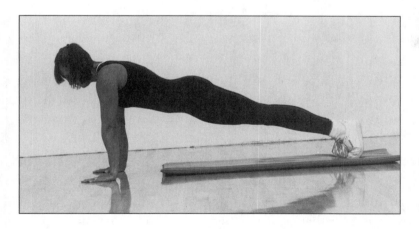

Push-ups with your legs straight add to the difficulty of the exercise.

Photo: Anne W. Krause

In the beginning, you can keep your knees on the ground as you perform the push-up. When you've aced this form of push-up, you can add to the challenge rather than increase repetitions. An effective way is to keep your legs straight with your feet on the ground. Next you can elevate your feet by putting them up on a step or bench, which is the most challenging form of a push-up and will build and strengthen your pectorals, arms, and even your abdomen—because you need to tighten it in order to maintain a horizontal body position.

Push-ups using handle grips ease the stress on your wrists.

(Photo: Anne W. Krause)

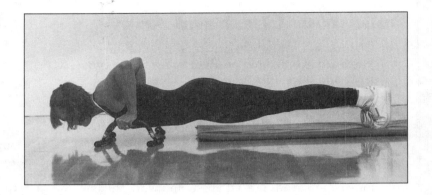

Using push-up handle grips to do push-ups is easier on your wrists and allows for a greater stretch of the pectorals as you move toward the floor.

A step used to lift your feet off the ground adds additional challenge to your push-up routine.

(Photo: Anne W. Krause)

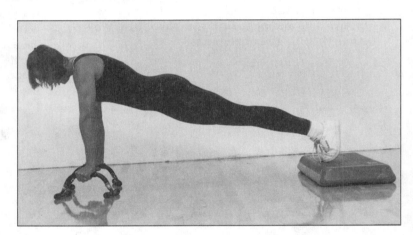

Triceps Training

Extra flesh on the back of the arms is a very common complaint among women, and older women or ones who have lost a great deal of weight are especially susceptible to it. You need to tone your triceps, either using free weights or a weight machine—or with this more advanced triceps exercise. Sit on a bench or a chair with your feet out in front of you. Slide off the seat, supporting yourself on your arms, until your butt and your back can clear the seat when you do your triceps dips. Start with straight arms and dip down, lowering your body so your elbows are bent to 90 degrees—or as far as you can bend them while still being able to pull yourself back up. Keep your torso erect so you are really using your triceps muscles, not your shoulders. To increase triceps dip difficulty, progress from dips with your knees bent to dips with (1) your knees straight, (2) your feet on another bench, and (3) a weight on your lap while your feet are on another bench.

To vary your triceps workout, use dumbbells for the three following exercises, starting with light weights, around three to five pounds each. In the first version, stand up and lean forward slightly with your left arm on a bench or a steady object, keeping your back straight, with a dumbbell in your right hand. Raise your right arm behind you so that your upper arm is parallel to the floor. Now extend your forearm straight back and then return it to the starting position. Repeat 10 to 15 times, and then switch arms. A second triceps exercise is to stand up straight and hold one dumbbell, or two lighter ones, behind your head. Keeping your elbows as close to your head as possible, bend and extend your elbows. Alternately bend and straighten. Do three sets of 10. As a final variation, you can do this exercise on a mat or on the floor. Lie on your back, and hold the dumbbells in your hands above your head with your elbows bent. Straighten your arms to raise the weights toward the ceiling, and then bend them to return to the starting position. You can mix and match these exercises to make up three sets, and you can increase the weight of the dumbbells as you get stronger.

Beef Up Your Biceps

Use dumbbells, again starting with lighter weights and increasing as you get stronger. Hold one dumbbell in each hand with your arms at your sides. Bend your elbow and contract your biceps, one at a time or both together. Don't use your back and shoulders or momentum to force the weight up. If you need to do this, the weight you are using is too heavy. Do three sets of 12 for each arm. There are many options for biceps training. In addition to the preceding basic exercise, you can use a single exercise bar or barbells instead of dumbbells. There is even a specialized curl bar, with grips at specific places, to work different areas of the inner and outer attachments of the biceps. Cable machines have positions for biceps curls. Push-ups also strengthen the biceps, and if you are really feeling strong, you can begin adding pull-ups or chin-ups to your strength workout.

Getting a Grip on Glutes and Thighs

If you want to tone the muscles in the buttocks area, here are a few exercises to firm up those sagging glutes. These exercises are great for new moms who gained weight in their gluts, hips, and thighs during pregnancy.

Fit Tip

No matter what you do, never sacrifice proper form in order to lift heavier weight.

➤ **Walking lunges.** Position yourself in a hallway or somewhere that you can take about 10 big steps. Standing with your feet about shoulder-width apart and your hands on your hips or by your side, step out with your right leg and bend your knee about 90 degrees to a comfortable position. Your knee should not bend out over your foot. Raise up and repeat the exercise with your left leg. Do three sets of 10 steps per leg. You can add to the challenge by holding dumbbells of 3 to 15 pounds in your hands while you lunge.

➤ **Side lunges.** Alternate taking steps to the right and then to the left. Return to the start position after each step. Do three sets of 10 per leg.

➤ **Squats.** Stand with your feet shoulder-width apart and your hands on your hips. Bend your knees, squatting until your knees are straight over your feet. Use your leg and butt muscles to push yourself back to a standing position. Repeat 25 times.

➤ **Leg lifts.** Get down on the floor on all fours with your thighs and arms perpendicular to the floor and your arms and knees about shoulder-width apart. Slowly lift one leg toward the ceiling. Visualize that you are pressing the bottom of your foot up toward the ceiling. Repeat 10 times with each leg for three sets. You can add challenge to this exercise by strapping leg weights around your ankles or above your knees.

Do these exercises three to four times a week. If you do cardio and strength workouts on the same day, the weight work should follow the cardio, because you will be warmed up. Otherwise, you can stretch lightly before strength training. However, remember always to take about 10 minutes to stretch when you're done so your muscles avoid soreness. If you have any pain in your knees while doing these exercises, consult a fitness trainer or your physician.

Putting It All Together: Cross-Training

Trainers helpkeep clients out of a rut, and the way they do that is by emphasizing cross-training. Think of it as mix-and-match exercising of various types: aerobic and strength training, indoor exercises and outdoor sports, strength training using weight machines and free weights, working in the gym and running, workouts, aquatic and dryland exercises, running and bicycling, or any other pair or combination of complementary activities. Cross-training combats boredom, prevents injury from repetitive motions, and enhances your overall fitness. Trainers are *very* big on cross-training.

Quick Tips for the Time-Impaired

Getting fit and losing weight require a time commitment. There are times, however, when you literally don't have more than a few minutes, even though your motivation remains high and your avoidance-and-procrastination mechanism has been shut off. So what do you do? Program a minimum of 30 to 40 minutes of activity into your day. Here is the bare minimum that the average, healthy adult needs to maintain overall fitness:

1. To warm up, five to 10 minutes of slow jogging, walking, or low-intensity movements

2. For muscular strength, at least two 20-minute strength-training sessions per week, which include all the major muscle groups

3. For muscular endurance, at least three 30-minute sessions each week that include activities such as calisthenics, push-ups, sit-ups, and weight training for all major muscle groups

4. For cardiovascular endurance, at least three 20-minute sessions per week of continuous aerobic activity, such as fitness walking, jogging, swimming, cycling, rope jumping, rowing, cross-country skiing, or using aerobic exercise machines in the gym

5. For flexibility, 10 to 12 minutes daily of slow stretching

6. To cool down, five to 10 minutes of low-level exercise (similar to the warm-up) at the end of each workout

These tips also apply after you have reached your goals and simply want to stay where you are fitnesswise. Keep in mind that, when you get into reasonable physical condition and have reached an attainable goal, you probably will want to continue getting fitter. At the point when you are satisfied, however, it doesn't take all that much effort to maintain your level of fitness.

Monitoring Your Heart Rate

Taking your pulse manually on your wrist or the carotid artery of your neck is the most basic way to monitor your heart rate. Trainers like more sophisticated methods for checking how closely their clients are working within their target heart rate range and how quickly they recover after an aerobic session, both of which are keys to general fitness and specifically to cardiorespiratory conditioning. For more details on these topics, see Chapter 12, "Your Heart Will Love Aerobic Exercise." Some high-end, gym-model aerobic apparatus, including treadmills and stationary bicycles, have heart-rate monitors built into the handrails or handlebars by reading through the palms of your hands, but these are far less accurate than personal heart-rate monitors.

Runners, cyclists, and others who are training to improve their cardio-conditioning are usually counseled to use a heart-rate monitor, and trainers increasingly recommend them to people trying to boost their cardio-conditioning. A number of designs from several manufacturers are on the market. You can compare features at running-equipment specialty stores, which usually carry the greatest variety. The most common design for personal heart-rate monitors is an adjustable band that straps around your chest, under your clothing, to monitor your heartbeat as you exercise. It transmits this information to a watchlike console on your wrist. The simplest models provide just real-time readouts at the push of a button, while more sophisticated models allow you to download your workout information onto your computer. Another option is the Heart Talker (1-800-639-5432), which accepts audio commands, calculates the workout program, and provides audio feedback by synthetic voice.

The Least You Need to Know

➤ A trainer can draw up a plan incorporating various elements of exercise and other lifestyle changes.

➤ You cannot spot-reduce, but you *can* sport-tone.

➤ Crunches really work when you want to firm and tone your abdominal muscles.

➤ As you get deeper into an exercise program, you will want to become more sophisticated in monitoring your heart rate.

➤ It is possible to do a quick, effective workout when you are pressed for time.

Part 3
Get Your Heart Pumping

Aerobic fitness, cardiovascular conditioning, and cardio-respiratory health all fall into the category of having a healthy heart, strong lungs, and a functioning circulatory system. These are the keystones to enjoying an active, productive life now and an investment in maintaining a high quality of life in the future.

No doubt about it: Aerobic exercise is the only way to gain and maintain cardiovascular health. It means you have to get moving and raise your heart rate to an aerobic level. You can do this by fitness walking, jogging, swimming, working out on a gym's cardio equipment, taking an aerobics class, or dashing up the stairs with a load of laundry to answer the call of a crying baby. You will recognize that you are in the aerobic zone when you become somewhat out of breath and feel your heart pumping fast. When you first embark on a fitness program, this might not take much—and it might feel uncomfortable or even scary. But as you become fitter and stronger, you will learn to love being in the aerobic zone, knowing that it is making you healthier and, yes, leaner too.

> *"Exercise is the best investment you can make in yourself."*
>
> *—Gabrielle Reece, professional volleyball star*

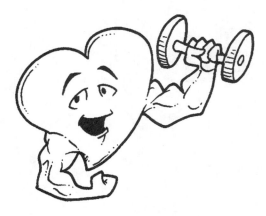

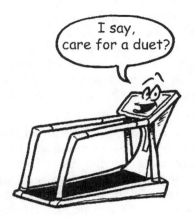

Chapter 11

I say, care for a duet?

Machines to Get Your Body Humming

In This Chapter

➤ Aerobic apparatus offered by modern gyms

➤ Indoor cycling, running, and rowing as workouts

➤ Using strength-training machines instead of pumping iron

➤ Beating boredom while using machines

Exercise machines can be divided into the same categories as exercises themselves—strength training, aerobic conditioning, and even flexibility enhancement. Fitness centers' gyms are equipped with an arsenal of apparatus, while a home gym (see Chapter 16, "Where to Work Out") usually just has one or two pieces—except perhaps in the home gyms of movie stars and millionaires. In most health clubs, the strength-training equipment is found in a weight room along with free weights, while the cardio equipment is grouped in another part of the facility. Home versions of many pieces are available, but they usually are not as heavy or as sturdy as gym models. Commercial gym models also have more sophisticated instrumentation and readouts than home models. Still, the purposes and functions of commercial and home equipment are similar.

Aerobic Apparatus

If you join a health club, you'll find yourself linked to an entire family of mechanized devices with which you can bond to enhance your aerobic fitness. Some of these cardio machines mimic some kind of natural or sports activity but in a climate-controlled environment. Stationary bikes, rowing machines, treadmills, and other apparatus allow you to use the same muscles as you would bicycling, rowing, running, or walking outdoors. Most can be programmed for a specific degree of challenge or can be operated in manual mode. Therefore, when you climb aboard, you can select the speed and/or resistance of these machines when you start and can readjust if necessary while you are exercising. In addition, elaborate display consoles on health-club models and even some high-end home models will help you monitor your workout. Where necessary, as on a stationary bicycle, these machines can be adjusted for users of various heights.

Typically, when you get on a cardio machine and begin walking, pedaling, or whatever movement the machine requires, the display prompts a series of questions. You answer by touching a keypad and pressing "Enter" after each response. Questions might include your weight, your age, the length of time you would like to work out, the degree of challenge on a scale of 1 to 10 (or 12 or 16), and the program you prefer. Most exercise bikes ask you to select the profile of the "ride" you are taking (random, interval, hills, and so on). A treadmill allows you to select the angle of the track from flat to a somewhat steep incline. When you've gone through the menu of questions, your exercise session automatically begins, and unless you chose "manual" mode, the apparatus determines your workout.

The machine's digital display tracks your progress throughout your workout and shows numbers such as elapsed time, distance, and estimated caloric burn. Some machines have handles with heart-rate monitors that you can grip to check whether you are in your target heart rate zone, as measured through your palms and fingers. Many experts are not impressed with the accuracy of this function (see Chapter 10, "Trainers' Tips and Tricks"). By contrast, time and distance readings are more reliable. Calories burned and heart rate are less-exact measures, but you can use them to monitor your progress—especially if you frequently use the same machine. Aerobic machines build warm-up and cool-down segments around your selected program.

This is a typical aerobic machine face that can be adjusted to suit all workouts and fitness levels.

(Photo: Claire Walter)

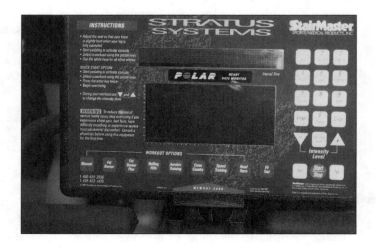

Assuming you are working at a comparable intensity, you will burn more calories using aerobic equipment on which you stand (such as treadmills, stairclimbers, and cross-country ski simulators) than equipment on which you sit (such as stationary bikes and rowing machines).

Stationary Bikes

This type of bicycle without wheels is a workhorse—and not just because it has a saddle. Health clubs' aerobic rooms usually have fleets of bikes, and if a small hotel, motor inn, or cruise ship has just a modest fitness facility, it is likely to offer at least a bike. Before you start riding, adjust the seat height so that your knees are slightly flexed when the pedal is at the bottom of its orbit. If the seat of an upright bike is too high, your hips and knees must go beyond their normal range of motion. If it is too low, you can stress your knees and tighten up your hip flexors because you aren't straightening your knees at any point during the exercise. Grasp the hand grips comfortably while you are riding but do not lean on the handlebars. You can often select the profile of your ride and the level of challenge, but your speed depends on how hard you pedal.

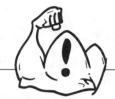

Fit Tip

Varying the intensity, duration, and type of aerobic-machine workouts lessens the chance of repetitive-motion injury.

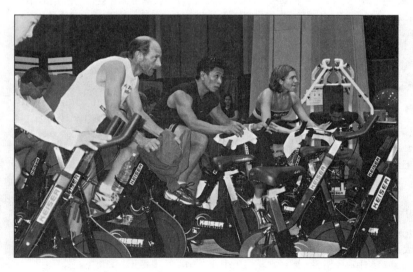

Pedaling on a stationary bike is a great cardiovascular workout.

(Photo: Claire Walter)

The mechanism of most bikes is encased in metal housing, but other types have a flywheel in the front. If you have lower-back problems, look for a *recumbent bike*. Instead of a relatively upright body position, you pedal with your feet extended in front of you, and you sit back in a bucket seat or a chair-type seat with a backrest rather than astride a saddle. Some stationary-bike designs feature movable handles that you can pump back and forth as you pedal in a synchronized motion for a bonus upper-body workout. You also might see a machine that resembles a bike, but with pedals that are handles at chest height in front of the seat. This is an upper-body exerciser.

Fitness Fact

In 1997, 19.5 million women and 15.3 million men rode stationary bikes as part of their exercise programs, according to the Fitness Products Council of the Sporting Goods Manufacturers Association.

Treadmills

The treadmill, another popular workhorse of the workout world, resembles a short, wide conveyor belt. There often is a support frame partway down the sides or a grip rail below the console. This machine conveys cardiovascular health to users. Its continuously looping treadbelt, which in commercial models is powered by an electric motor, travels over a cushioned deck that is about four to six feet long and 16 to 22 inches wide.

When you start the treadmill, you select the speed at which the belt moves so you can walk, jog, or run at the speed you selected. In addition to increasing or decreasing the speed of the belt, you also can adjust the incline of the deck from flat to an uphill "climb." Whatever speed and angle you select, you have to keep up with the treadmill's speed at the chosen angle. If it is going too fast, or if the incline is too steep, you have to slow the belt speed down or decrease the angle; otherwise, you will eventually be carried off the back end. Most treadmills also have a stop button—nicknamed the panic button—in case you have a problem and need to stop the treadbelt quickly. The machine will stop automatically if you catch your clothing and begin to fall or lose your balance.

Simpler models, including most designed for home use, are powered by the user. If you get on one of these, your pace determines the speed of the treadbelt. The faster you walk or run, the faster the treadbelt moves and the more intense the exercise. When you slow down, it slows down.

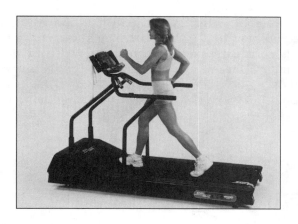

You can walk your way to fitness on the treadmill in your gym or in the comfort of your own home.

(Photo: Courtesy of Star Trac)

When using a treadmill, keep your posture and motions as natural as possible. This means lift your torso, let your arms swing, and keep your head up and looking forward as you walk or jog. Don't lean on the handrails, and don't press forward on the handlebar as if you were pushing a grocery cart. Walk or run in a full stride, hit the treadbelt with your heel, roll through the foot, and take off from the toe. If you find yourself moving toward the back of the treadmill, slow it down a notch so you don't slide off the back end. If you are not working hard enough, speed it up or select a steeper angle.

Retrograde Motion

One new fitness technique is called *retro walking*. Proponents assert that walking backward on a treadmill can strengthen the quadriceps, the calves, and even the abdominals, according to a report in the *Berkeley Wellness Letter*. Even a two-mile-per-hour *retro* pace can help your fitness. Experts suggest beginning with just a quarter-mile retro walk, even if you are in good shape, and gradually increasing your distance. You also can shift your workouts on a treadmill, a stairstepper, or an elliptical trainer, but not on a studio bike, because your feet can slip off the pedals and cause an injury. Retro walking also is not recommended for anyone with balance or back problems or for elderly exercisers. For anyone else, it is an interesting variation on cross-training.

Upper-Body Bonuses

In addition to using exercise bikes that allow for arm motion, you can use treadmills that offer ski-pole-type devices to add upper-body work to your exercise routine. Also, you can easily intensify the workout by pumping your arms as if you were power walking or running on the street or by using light hand weights. Specific treadmill accessories also are available for some brands. Precor's Smart Weights, for example, are a combination of hand weights and a remote-control device. Holding the one- or two-pound weights increases the aerobic benefit, and the weights also feature five small buttons so you can speed up, slow down, change the incline, or stop a Precor treadmill as you walk or run. ProForm equips one of its treadmills with an integrated unit that plays a special 30-minute CD featuring lively music and the encouraging words of a certified personal trainer who guides you through the workout. A PowerTread model has small built-in fans so you can stay cool during the workout.

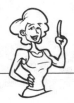

Fitness Fact

In 1987, 4.4 million Americans reported that they exercise on a treadmill. Ten years later, 36.1 million people do so, an increase of 720 percent, according to the Sporting Goods Manufacturers Association. Among people aged 35 to 54, the number grew from 1.5 million to 13.9 million, an increase of 827 percent.

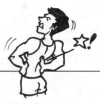

Achtung!

Do not support your body weight on your arms when you are using a stairstepper. Doing so decreases the amount of body weight you lift with each step and therefore erodes the aerobic benefit. It also can strain your elbows and wrists and can even cause forearm fatigue.

Stairsteppers

Stairsteppers, also called stairclimbers or steppers, consist of two footplates that resemble oversized pedals. As you stand on these pedals, you need to keep your body centered and upright without leaning on the rails. Your feet should be flat on the footplates throughout the motion. On some machines, pushing one plate down automatically raises the other. On other machines, the pedals operate independently of one another. The motion resembles climbing an endless flight of stairs to nowhere, and it results in an excellent lower-body workout. You can adjust the resistance, and you derive aerobic benefit from the level you select and the speed you use to push the pedals. Bigger steps work the butt muscles more; smaller steps work the legs and calves more. In addition to time and calories, the display usually will tell you the equivalent of how many flights and often how many vertical feet you have climbed. A Crossrobics machine resembles a stairclimber, but instead of standing on the footpads, you lean against a back support in a position similar to that of a recumbent bike.

StairMaster is a pioneering manufacturer of stairsteppers. The brand name has become virtually synonymous with this category of apparatus, even though many manufacturers now make this type of exercise equipment, and the StairMaster company now makes other types of apparatus.

Elliptical Exerciser

These hybrid machines combine many of the benefits of other aerobic equipment. You stand on footplates like those on a stairstepper, but these plates travel in an orbit around an axis like a stationary bicycle. Instead of a bike's round orbit, however, they travel in an elliptical pattern. The length of the stride often can be adjusted. The result is a no-impact, kind-to-the-joints motion that combines elements of a striding walk or run, pedaling a bike, and climbing stairs. One variation of these machines also has some kind of upper-body motion, usually upright ski-pole-style handles that you pump while moving your feet. This makes elliptical exercisers valuable cross-training tools, too.

Versaclimber

Some advanced exercisers like this apparatus for its cross-training and cardio benefits. This tall machine features pedals and arm levers of some kind attached to a center post. Your lower body climbs while your upper body pulls and pumps for a dynamite total-body workout. You have to be willing to look at the machine's center post, which puts some people off. Not surprisingly, rock climbers find it beneficial and don't mind the close-up view.

Row, Row, Row Your (Non-)Boat

A rowing machine, or rower, is a low-to-the-ground apparatus with a seat, footboards, and handles. Adjust the seat so your feet can brace comfortably against the footboard when you are leaning back at the apex of the rowing stroke. Most rowers' footboards have straps to secure your feet. The secret of effective rowing is to begin pushing back with your legs before you begin pulling on the handles. Although this is a good upper-body exercise, your legs should be doing 60 percent of the work. As you pull on the oars, allow your back to arch naturally but try to keep your elbows close to your sides. Return to the starting position in one fluid motion.

The machine's console tracks how many meters you have rowed, your time, your stroke output, and the approximate number of calories burned. Studio rowing classes and even competitions abound. There's even a computer interface that can simulate races with up to 10 boats at a time, and you can team rowers as singles, doubles, fours, or eights, as if they really are sculling on a lake or river.

If you prefer a kayak, Crossrobics makes a machine that simulates kayak paddling rather than rowing with oars. You sit astride the machine, brace your feet on the footblocks, and paddle with an alternate-arm movement. The bar angles across the body, and the end that is "out of the water" rises while the one "in the water" dips.

Ski Simulators

NordicTrack is the best known of the cross-country ski simulators. You won't have real skis on your feet or real ski poles in your hands, but otherwise, machines like this feel a lot like Nordic skiing. Just slip your feet into the stirrups mounted on the footboards, grab the handles affixed to cords that run through pulleys or vertical poles in front of your body, and begin the gliding stride of cross-country skiing. The ball of your foot will stay anchored, but your heel will rise with each stride. The motion is left arm/right leg and right arm/left leg, and this requires more concentration and coordination than many other kinds of equipment. As with stairsteppers, the footboards of some machines operate independently of each other. Some are more like stationary bikes or elliptical exercisers, because when one foot moves forward, the other automatically moves back.

Fitness Fact

Several Alpine skiing simulators also are on the market. They offer some aerobic benefit, but their main purpose is to get leg muscles in shape for skiing.

Spinning Your Heart into High Gear

You can literally ride your buns off with a fast-paced studio-cycling or group-cycling class, often referred to by the trademarked name Spinning. Spinning was created in 1987 by an endurance cyclist known as Johnny G as a training tool for the Race Across America. In 1993, Schwinn introduced a stationary bike specifically for such classes, and the concept really took off. The bike features a fixed gear and a heavy flywheel, the weight of which creates momentum that forces you to pedal continuously. Because resistance can be adjusted, however, each participant can custom-tailor the workout to his or her current fitness level—and in studio cycling, there are as many "hims" as "hers." The typical studio bike also has a racing saddle, contoured handlebars, pedals with toe clips, a tension knob that acts like a gear shift, a hand brake so you can stop the apparatus in an emergency, and a water-bottle holder for the hydration you will quickly need. Other manufacturers now also make special studio-cycling apparatus.

These indoor cycling classes are led by an instructor who participates in all the moves and also provides the motivation—all to a variety of musical beats. The instructor calls the shots on the program's pattern, which is designed to mimic the feeling of road cycling but without the traffic hazards, bumpy pavement, or weather issues. The instructor, on a bike facing the class, gives directions such as climbing out of the saddle, jumping (in and out of the saddle every two to eight strokes), sprinting, and pedaling with low resistance. He or she might ask participants to visualize the scenery on an imaginary bicycle trip. The whole routine is designed to be motivational and energizing. Studio cycling is an intense activity in which heart rates rev up fast and sweat-dripped shirts are a status symbol. A participant in a 40-minute studio cycling class can burn up to 500 calories.

Quote, Unquote

"Everyone can do this. In Spinning class, you can have a triathlete next to a deconditioned first-timer."

—Michael Potter, Schwinn spokesman

Since Schwinn's Spinning classes started the group studio-cycling craze, each manufacturer of studio bikes now has branded programs that go by such names as Cycle Reebok, FreeWheeling, Power Pacing, and Precision Cycling. Studio cycling has been such a success that it has spawned group classes for other kinds of studio apparatus. StairMaster, for example, has created a program called Stomp that uses stairclimbers, and Concept II has a program called Group Indoor Rowing.

You *Can* Fool Mother Machine

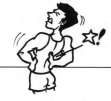

Achtung!

Leaning on the handlebars of a studio cycle can cause problems. When you lean too far forward, your shoulders hunch up, you could stress your knees, and you might even slip off the pedals. Only when you are standing up to *climb* is it all right to lean forward on the handlebars.

According to aUniversity of Tennessee study, the calorie calculators on many exercise machines are inaccurate. Even worse, they don't seem to be inaccurate in the user's favor. Stairsteppers, for example, often indicate the expenditure of 1 to six calories more per minute than are actually burned. This is a significant number if you are working out for 30 minutes or more, and other apparatus can be off even more. Suppose, for instance, that you spend half an hour on an aerobic machine that is off by six calories a minute. That's 180 calories—equal to a small bowl of breakfast cereal and skim milk or a container of low-fat or nonfat yogurt—each time you work out. In addition to some of the inherent miscounts, the machines also assume that you are not leaning on the support bar, which lessens your calorie use.

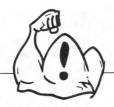

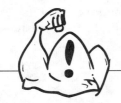

You can lie to the machine and outsmart it or extend
the time you spend on the device, but if you do, you
are only cheating yourself. If you do it right, you
won't have to work out as long to get the results you
want. When you are programming your workout profile, *Fitness* magazine suggests that you subtract about
20 percent off your body weight or stay on the
machine until it says you have burned about 25 percent more calories than your goal for that session.

Types of Strength-Training Apparatus

The kinds of equipment commonly found in a weight
room are multistation, variable-weight machines that
primarily use a weight-and-pulley system to provide
resistance. Other technologies also exist, which offer
refinements on the classic multistation principle.
Nautilus was the first brand to change the shape of the
pulley from round to spiral-shaped to provide more
consistent resistance throughout each lift. In addition,
Nautilus took inertia out of the equation by controlling resistance. The result is a timed movement that
takes two seconds on each lift or other resistance move
and four seconds on the return. Keiser machines operate with compressed air rather than iron and offer infi-
nitely adjustable resistance levels. Other brands of
weight machines include Body Masters, Cybex, Galileo,
Hammer, Magnum (Badger), and Universal. Gym rats
and gearheads may argue long about the physiological
benefits and user-friendliness of each technology or
specific brand, but basically, strength-training equipment is an invaluable fitness tool for anyone who gets
on and sticks to a program.

Flexibility Apparatus

Machines to make you stronger or aerobically fitter
are nothing new, but equipment to enhance flexibility
is now showing up in gyms. These passive devices
enable you to stretch without getting down on a mat
or finding a wall to lean against, a pillar or barre to
hang on to, or a vacant bench to put your leg up on.
Keiser's Stretch Zone and Stretch Corner feature posts,

bars, handles, and platforms suitable for doing various stretches. Precor's StretchTrainer is designed for eight seated stretches. The stretching apparatus that has been around the longest is The Reformer, which is used in Pilates workouts for strengthening and flexibility (see Chapter 9, "Other Paths to Stretching and Toning").

Beating Boredom

The most frequently cited disadvantage of cardio machines—treadmills, bikes, stairsteppers, and the like—is the tedium of moving without motion—of being in the same spot in the gym or studio. (Of course, some people find the ability to zone out while working out a relaxing aspect to machines.) Gyms make all sorts of efforts to keep things lively. Stationary bikes are equipped with racks so you can read a book or a magazine while you pedal. Music is a staple at many health clubs, but many people prefer their own music and use players and headsets. Virtual-reality bikes (nicknamed VR bikes) are like a cross between a video game and a cardio machine. They feature a video screen and speakers that replicate a town, a bucolic setting, or even a fantasy underwater bike ride past sharks, whales, and a shipwreck. Hop aboard a VR bike, start pedaling, and you'll "see" and "hear" attractions along the "route" of your "ride."

Many health clubs arrange rows of stationary bikes or treadmills facing television sets. At the Fitness Theater in Dallas, every bike has its own television. The Decathlon Club in Santa Clara, California, and ClubSport in Freeport, California, were among the first to equip stairsteppers and stationary bikes with Netpulse personal terminals that include a TV, a CD player, and even Internet access. Clients, it seems, like to check stock quotes and sports scores while working out. In other clubs, like the Aspen Club in Aspen, Colorado, machines are arranged in a circle, so exercisers can watch each other. The treadmills and bikes at the health club in the Shangri-La Hotel in Bangkok overlook the Chao Phraya River, which bustles with river traffic day and night. If you like to take your inspiration from other exercisers or simply gaze at the scenery, look for such features when you check out gyms that you might like to join.

The Least You Need to Know

➤ You can program most gym-quality aerobics apparatus for varying degrees of challenge, and each machine's console will display what you've accomplished.

➤ The stationary bicycle and treadmill are considered workhorses among cardio machines.

➤ If you have a bad back or other biomechanical problems, try a recumbent bike instead of a conventional stationary bike.

➤ Cardio machine readouts are not always reliable, but if you "cheat" when programming the machine, you exacerbate the problem and only cheat yourself in attaining your fitness goals.

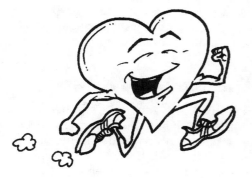

Your Heart Will Love Aerobic Exercise

Aerobics was the first wave of the big late-twentieth-century boom in intensive exercise. The word *aerobic* is such a part of the English language that it's hard to believe it has been around only since the 1960s. That's when Dr. Kenneth Cooper, the creator of a new and energetic style of exercise and the founder of the Cooper Institute for Aerobics Research in Dallas, coined the word to describe activities intense enough to get the heart and lungs pumping. These encompass a range of sports that involve running, pedaling, swimming, or ascending a steep hill, as well as gym activities, such as aerobics or energetic dance classes and the use of cardio apparatus.

In other words, aerobics encompasses all activities in which the body requires additional oxygen to enable the muscles to continue working, thereby strengthening the lungs and the heart. Dr. Cooper gave a name to the types of activities that get the heart pumping and the lungs working hard, and he created an indoor fitness activity designed to make that happen. Dr. Cooper's aerobics and its derivatives as we know them today are among the workouts discussed in Chapter 15, "Specialized Aerobics Programs."

Today, the definition has been expanded. Aerobic, as an adjective, describes any steady and repetitive activity that challenges the cardiorespiratory system and that makes the heart and lungs stronger. Aerobics, as a noun, has come to describe fitness routines based on dance and performed to music. These routines are done intensely enough to elevate the heart rate and thereby condition the cardiorespiratory system.

Cardiorespiratory Health: The Key to Fitness

You've probably heard a million times that heart disease is America's number-one killer. It also is the most preventable killer. Modern medicine can perform miracles in repairing congenital heart problems, mending damaged hearts, and reaming out clotted blood vessels. If you were born with a heart defect, it's wonderful that doctors can now repair the problem. If you started out with a healthy heart, however, it's unfortunate if you put yourself in line for major surgical procedures or rely on medications when you can be proactive in keeping your ticker ticking.

Quote, Unquote

"A man who does not care to exercise falls into ill health."

—Aristotle

There is a chicken-and-egg aspect to the relationship between cardiorespiratory health and fitness. If your heart and lungs are in good shape, you have a giant leg up on getting fit because your cardiorespiratory heart and lungs can handle a real workout. If you have been getting aerobic exercise and are fit, these organs are healthy. If you are sedentary, you have to work up to a hard workout. In other words, you have to build both strength and endurance. Building your heart's efficiency in pumping blood and your lungs' capabilities through aerobic exercise is crucial to maintaining (or restoring) your heart's health.

Experts differ in what they consider to be the bare minimum of aerobic exercise that is effective. Many trainers believe that cardiovascular benefits begin with 30 minutes of aerobic activity three times a week. Others say you need at least 20 minutes each day. To make sure that "at least 20 minutes" doesn't become a flat "20 minutes" or even less in many people's minds, the American College of Sports Medicine recommends 20 to 60 minutes of continuous aerobic exercise each day at 60 to 90 percent of your maximum heart rate. The ACSM defines aerobic exercise as rhythmic exercise that uses the large muscles, such as the thighs, calves, and glutes—walking, running, biking, swimming, or participating in organized aerobic exercise.

Allow one or two days of rest per week from aerobic activity. This does not mean sitting in the recliner and watching television. It can be "active rest," which refers to a lower level of activity than your aerobic exercise, such as a leisurely walk, a bike ride, a gentle swim, or simply doing chores that require physical activity.

Fitness Fact

According to the National Center for Health Sciences, the 10 leading causes of death in America in 1997 were heart disease (2,314,729), cancer (725,790), stroke (537,390), chronic obstructive lung diseases and allied conditions (110,637), accidents (92,121), pneumonia and influenza (88,383), diabetes mellitus (62,332), suicide (29,725), kidney disease (25,570), and chronic liver disease and cirrhosis (24,765).

Heart disease and stroke are the number-one and number-three causes of death for both men and women, and extra weight makes the problem worse. Studies have shown that overweight individuals have triple the normal risk of these diseases. Exercise is the best way to lower the risks. Even without weight loss, exercise alone decreases harmful cholesterol levels in the blood, improves circulation, and therefore reduces the risk of heart disease and stroke. More specifically, aerobic exercise increases the amount of blood your heart can pump with each heartbeat, improves circulation by making your blood vessels healthier, and increases the production of oxygen-metabolizing enzymes that allow you to use oxygen more efficiently and to eliminate waste products from your system. It also burns calories, resulting in weight loss. The result is a reduction of specific risk factors—and probably weight loss as well. In short, you can't afford *not* to do aerobic exercise.

What's a Target Heart Rate Anyway?

"Heart rate" is the fitness world's term for "pulse." In other words, it's the number of heartbeats per minute. It has become the accepted way of measuring the intensity of aerobic exercise. Your target heart rate is the level you need to maintain for at least 20 minutes to impact your cardiovascular fitness. It is not one number. Rather, it's a certain zone or percentage range of the maximum heart rate (that is, the most beats per minute that the heart can possibly pump).

Further, physiologists have come up with very precise numbers relating percentages to the exerciser's age. The heart rate zone numbers decrease with age, because as a person gets older, the heart muscle, like other muscles, diminishes. With the loss of heart muscle, the maximum heart rate also declines, even in very fit people. This explains why elite athletes generally peak in their 20s and 30s. If they continue training into their 40s, 50s, and beyond, their aim usually is to minimize the erosion of their peak capacity.

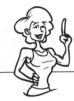

Fitness Fact

Older athletes predominate in endurance sports, not in sprints, because they can maintain a high degree of fitness for long distances but no longer produce the quick bursts of energy required for short distances.

In addition to a person's chronological age, his or her fitness level also affects the target heart rate zone. Endurance athletes concentrate their training on adding to their cardiorespiratory system's lifespan instead of focusing on strength training. They work hard on their cardio conditioning to stretch their competitive life for additional years. When older people get into competition, they also tend to look to distance events. Look at the increasing number of people competing in "masters" categories in running, swimming, and even the grueling triathlon.

Put another way, the fitness dividend shows up throughout life. A person of any age who is out of shape doesn't need to work very hard to elevate the heart rate, but to achieve cardiovascular benefits, the level of activity is relatively low. (In other words, an unfit person gets out of breath easily, and his or her heart starts pumping hard even after mild exertion.) By contrast, a very fit person, regardless of age, must run or cycle faster, swim harder, use a higher step, or ratchet up intensity in other ways to reach the appropriate target heart rate for his or her age.

Finding Your Target Heart Rate

You can check your cardiovascular fitness level by taking your resting heart rate (RHR). Ideally, take your pulse for 60 seconds before you even get out of bed in the morning. The target heart rate (THR, or target zone for short) is your aerobic workout aim. It is the range in which you need to work for better health and greater endurance.

The following formula establishes your target heart rate (THR) based on your age, your resting heart rate (RHR) and the maximum heart rate (HRH) for your age:

THR = 220 – your age – RHR × .6 or .8 + HRH

When you begin a fitness program, you probably want to stay at about 60 percent of your maximum heart rate (HRH); hence the .6 in the preceding formula. As you get fitter, you can increase your intensity to 80 percent of your maximum heart rate (hence the .8 in the preceding formula). Luckily, we don't have to keep doing and redoing the math. These calculations, which are used in THR charts posted in health clubs across the land, appear in the following table.

Target Heart Rate Zone

Age	Maximum Heart Rate	Aerobic Zone
20	200	140–160
25	195	137–156
30	190	133–152
35	185	130–148
40	180	126–144
45	175	123–140
50	170	119–136
55	165	116–132
60	160	112–128
65	155	108–123

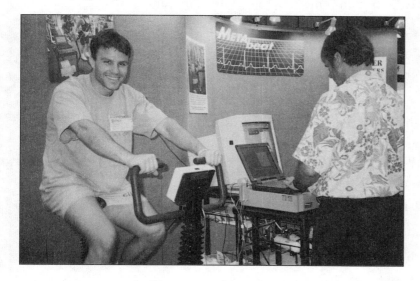

A trainer can determine your target heart rate zone for maximum benefit during aerobic exercise.

(Photo: Claire Walter)

A simpler way to evaluate how hard you've worked is Borg's Rating of Perceived Exertion (RPE). This is a 1-to-10 scale reflecting your assessment of how hard you think you worked. (Some RPE scales range from 1 to 20.) "Perceived exertion" relates to the ability to talk while exercising or the difference between breathing hard and panting while working out aerobically. Studies have shown a strong correlation between objective target heart rate zones and the subjective rating of perceived exertion.

Rating of Perceived Exertion

Rate	Subjective Rating
0	Doing nothing physical at all
1	Very light
2	Light
3	Light
4	Light to moderate
5	Moderate
6	Moderately hard
7	Hard
8	Very hard
9	Very hard
10	Extremely hard

Yet another method, developed by the Laboratoire du Travail et du Sport in France, is a 20-point logarithmic scale that measures the Estimated Time Limit (ETL) of how long a person estimates that he or she can continue an aerobic activity before exhaustion. In truth, the ETL corresponds more closely to heart rate and Borg's RPE at the lower levels (higher numbers) than at the higher levels (lower numbers) that new exercisers come up with. They are

ETL	Time Until Exhaustion
20	Less than 2 minutes
19	2 minutes
17	4 minutes
15	8 minutes
13	15 minutes
11	30 minutes
9	1 hour
7	2 hours
5	4 hours
3	8 hours
1	More than 16 hours

Fitness Fact

As you get fitter, you also will find that your resting heart rate begins to drop, which is desirable. This is because working out strengthens your heart and makes it more efficient.

Now That You've Found It, What Do You Do with It?

You only work out at 50 to 60 percent of your maximum heart rate three or four times a week to see improvement in your cardiovascular condition and endurance. If your main goal is weight loss, experts advise exercising five or six times a week at 60 to 70 percent (also called the fat-burning zone). If your only goal is to enhance your cardiovascular health, it doesn't take even that much effort.

Serious recreational athletes and fitness buffs generally set a target heart rate of 70 to 80 percent, which also is known as the aerobic zone. If 80 percent is good, you might wonder, isn't 100 percent better? Not at all. One hundred percent is all-out effort—the maximum anyone's cardiovascular system can pump. It is the point at which the body cannot process enough oxygen to sustain any more physical effort. This is called the anaerobic zone, and it's not someplace you want to be. Only competitive athletes routinely train above 80 percent, and only occasionally do they push to their limit. Wearing a heart-rate monitor and under the watchful eye of a trainer or physiologist, they can push to 100 percent of their maximum heart rate and can cross the anaerobic threshold, but they do so just for short bursts of only about a minute.

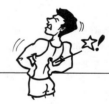

Achtung!

If you are obese, it might be prudent to keep your intensity below 60 percent to prevent joint injuries, but to compensate by exercising longer. The heavier you are, the more you might want to concentrate on non-weight–bearing exercises, such as water aerobics or a stationary bicycle.

Monitoring Your Heart Rate

When you begin working out, check your heart rate periodically to make sure you are working at the appropriate level of intensity for your goals. Aerobic instructors usually build into the fabric of the class a time for everyone to check his or her heart rate. To measure your heart rate, press your middle and second (or fourth) finger gently against your carotid artery on the side of your neck just below the jaw hinge or on the inside of your wrist, medical-style. Although the pulse feels the strongest on the carotid artery, some people get a little woozy from affecting blood flow to the brain. If this happens to you, the wrist is the best place to check your heart rate. You don't have to check your heart rate for a full minute. Starting at zero, count for six seconds and then multiply by 10 or do it for 10 seconds and then multiply by six. The result will be the same.

One of the interesting phenomena about sports participation and fitness conditioning is that veterans often have a good sense of where they are aerobically and can tell, from the way their bodies are reacting, where in the aerobic zone they are working. Ironically, these committed, long-time exercisers are also often the ones who want confirmation of exactly where they are. They can tell how hard they are breathing, sense how quickly their hearts are beating, and know whether they can still talk while working out. For such types, heart-rate monitors are the devices of choice. They monitor your heart rate throughout your cardio workout. For more on heart-rate monitors, see Chapter 10, "Trainers' Tips and Tricks."

A heart-rate monitor worn around the chest easily enables you to monitor your heart's beats per minute while you exercise.

(Photo: Claire Walter)

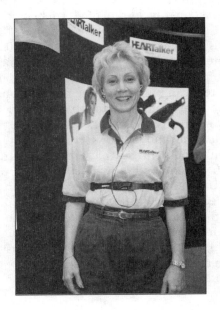

Let the Sweat Begin

Your individual preferences, and to an extent your body type, determine which forms of aerobic exercise suit you best. As long as you work in your target heart rate zone for the required time, your heart doesn't really care whether you are taking an aerobics class, working on an aerobic machine, running, cycling, or swimming. Find an activity—or two or three—that you really enjoy and use it to get your heart pumping.

One thing to remember is that, although it ought to be fun, a workout also is *work*. You won't do the best job for yourself or for your health without expending real effort—the kind of effort that not only gets your heart and lungs going but that brings sweat to your brow and perhaps an occasional grimace to your face. The best part is that, once you get into the workout habit, you will come to really enjoy it.

How Often? How Much?

The astonishing thing you will find when changing from being a nonexerciser to an exerciser is just how little time it takes to achieve some palpable results. No matter what options you prefer, your program will improve your whole body's strength and endurance—as long as you stick to it. Conscientious exercisers often work out for hours every day, but it's not really necessary, especially when starting a program. You should do at least 20 to 30 minutes of aerobic exercise five or six times a week and weight- or strength-train every other day. (Some experts now believe that you don't even need to do that half-hour of cardio all at once. Some believe that 10 minutes of aerobic exercise three times a day will give you the same results.)

If a major goal is weight loss, and if you are including aerobic exercise to help accomplish it, be aware that it is possible to work *too* hard to do the trick. Especially if you are overweight, when you exercise at the top of your target heart-rate zone, you might be

Quote, Unquote

"Don't worry so much about your heart rate when you exercise. Use common sense and exercise so that you could talk to me. If you get out of breath when you exercise, you're going too fast. If you don't feel a little breathless when you exercise, you're going too slow."

—Covert Bailey, author, motivational speaker, and founder of Covert Bailey Fitness

Quote, Unquote

"If you are unable to carry on a normal conversation when working out aerobically, you are working too hard. The proper level of exercise should not leave you tired, breathless, or in pain."

—Dr. Robert Bauer, medical director, Florida Pritikin Longevity Center and Spa lowering the glucose level in your blood instead of burning fat, which causes hunger and often causes the intake of more calories than exercising consumed. To exercise efficiently, do it right. Each of those 20- to 30-minute sessions should be within your target heart-rate zone, preceded by a warm-up and followed by a cool-down of 5 to 10 minutes each. That's less than an hour a day. Once you get hooked on exercise, however, your body will probably want more.

Putting Aerobics into Place

No matter what level of fitness you want to achieve, remember that a well-rounded program should incorporate the following principles, which makes it interesting as well as effective:

➤ **Weight-train to target specific muscle groups.** Include exercises that will affect particular muscle groups. Beyond general fitness, you also can train your muscles for other activities that interest you. If you are into swimming, for example, put extra emphasis on the upper body. If you want to improve your cycling, focus on the lower body.

➤ **Build progress into your program.** Increase the intensity, frequency, and duration of the activity to improve. This is true for both strength training and cardio conditioning.

➤ **Exercise regularly.** Plan to exercise five or six days a week to build and maintain your desired level of fitness. (In Chapter 10, you can find some ways to fit a workout into your schedule if you are pressed for time. You should consider three good weight workouts and at least five aerobic activities a week to be your ideal.)

➤ **Challenge yourself.** To bring about improvement in your fitness level, work out hard enough to overload your body above its resting level. This means challenging both your strength and endurance.

In short, cardio conditioning is part of a fitness program. It is not the entire program.

Heart Rate–Based Training

Heart rates are "in" with many people, especially those who train at a high level. In fact, more and more people are training according to their heart rate

Quote, Unquote

"[The minimum I work out is] an hour every day, and I have to do it in the morning. I know there are people out there [who are] a lot smarter than I am and have prettier bodies than mine, and they tell you they can do 30 minutes a day—10 minutes in the morning and maybe during lunch do 10 and then 10 minutes before they go to bed."

—Richard Simmons, television and video exercise host

zone rather than for a specific length of time or distance. People who really get into it purchase a heart-rate monitor, which is an excellent way to make sure you are training within your THR zone. There are two common kinds of heart-rate monitors. One looks like a watch and reads the pulse at the wrist; the other has sensors on a chest strap and reads the heart beats at the chest. (See Chapter 10, "Trainers' Tips and Tricks," and Chapter 23, "Shape-Up Shopping List.")

Even if you never get to the point of high-tech training for high-level competition, you will hear people talking about heart rate–based training. This practice started with hardcore athletes, but it has filtered down into the fitness community. It alternates between high- and low-intensity cardio workouts in a very specific pattern to improve speed, increase pace, and become race-ready. The idea is to train to your peak, avoiding both overtraining and undertraining.

This is not a do-it-yourself process. It is complicated and should only be undertaken with a trainer or kinesiologist. Athletes who embark on this type of high/low training are measured accurately for heart rate, oxygen consumption, and more. (In fact, one phrase you might hear often is *VO2max,* which is shorthand for "oxygen consumption.") The three stages in this type of gonzo training program include conditioning and *over-distance* work to increase both endurance and maximum oxygen utilization, specific training to increase the heart rate alternating with low-intensity maintenance workouts, and alternating low-intensity and brief anaerobic bursts. Heart rate–based training is not for the casual exerciser, but some of what has been learned from it has filtered down through the gym hierarchy.

The Least You Need to Know

➤ Heart disease and stroke are among the leading causes of death in America, and exercise is the best way to lower the risk of these diseases.

➤ Your target heart rate is the intensity of exercise for which you need to aim.

➤ The best aerobic exercise is the one you will do regularly.

➤ People who train at a high level use heart monitors and high–intensity techniques to further increase their fitness.

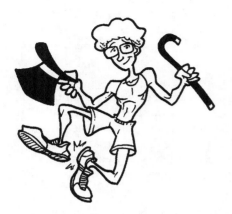

Chapter 13

Footwork Plain and Fancy

In This Chapter

➤ Walking for better health

➤ Increasing speed, distance, or challenge

➤ Starting a running program

➤ The do's and don'ts of running

➤ Walking versus running

Sometimes it seems as if we are a nation populated by people with stomachs but no feet. As a people, we spend millions on exercise equipment and diet plans to help us shape up and lose weight, but success can be much simpler and cheaper. If we simply put our little-used feet into action, step outside the door, and start walking, we're embarking on one of the best, simplest methods of shaping up. So lace up, step out, and start walking regularly. Once fitness walking is a habit, it might even be such an ingrained part of your life that you cannot imagine a week without it.

Simple footwork falls into a natural continuum of activity. From short, leisurely walks, most new exercisers progress quickly to longer, faster ones. Aggressive walkers get into PowerWalking (also called fitness walking), which is a real calorie hog and hip-slimmer. Some hardcore walkers eventually become race walkers, participating in a demanding sport that is generally eclipsed by running. Other people start walking, but first break into a jog and then often begin running. Remember Forest Gump? He was a fictitious character, but he symbolized what real people have experienced. Joggers-turned-runners who have seen their pace and endurance pick up begin looking at races. Before you know it, the casual exerciser has a real goal.

Walking Is Wonderful

Your initial walks don't have to be mega-marches. Fitness success stories abound in which extremely sedentary people simply begin walking around the block and eventually become well-conditioned runners. A block might be all some people can handle at first, but most people can start walking 20 minutes a day. No matter where you start, make your walking time count. Take comfortable strides with your arms swinging naturally at your sides—left arm/right leg and right arm/left leg. Then, as you make walking a routine, start to do it more energetically.

Fitness walking is the next step up. It is no place for twinkle-toes or flat-footed plodding. As you rev up your walking, remember that you are turning casual exercise into a more athletic activity. Like other athletes who nurture their body awareness, become conscious of what your foot is doing through each strike. You should be able to feel the entire cycle moving smoothly—heel strike, forward roll of the weight, and push off from the toe. Move your arms aggressively through the stride, consciously bending your elbows, swinging them back, and letting your hands come up to chest level. This upper-body motion will add aerobic benefit and burn more calories.

Walk tall—that is, with your back straight and your abdominal muscles tight—when you are going at a moderate pace. Any forward lean should originate at the ankles. You may start modestly, but chances are that you will soon be tooling along at a smart pace. To maintain a good cadence for a fitness walk, keep that pace at a steady 100 to 120 steps per minute if you can. You can also add disciplined breathing to your fitness walk by inhaling for three or four steps and then exhaling for three or four steps.

When you increase your pace, it might feel natural to add some forward lean from your hips—not enough to fall forward but enough to reinforce the feeling of motion. Sherry Borman, author of *Walk Yourself Thin,* asserts that you should also rotate your upper body with each step you take so that your right shoulder comes forward when you step forward with your left leg and vice versa. The arm should continue moving forward even as the shoulder rotates. Her contention is that a rotation helps tone the abdominal and gluteal muscles and even helps stabilize the back.

As you become more comfortable with going a certain speed and a certain distance, add up to five minutes at a time to your walk as your endurance increases. When you can easily walk the length of time you have available, begin picking up your pace to increase your intensity. Again, you can be modest in this increase, just taking a few extra minutes or going a block or two more in your allotted time.

You can use a Walkman or another personal cassette player to listen to energetic, upbeat music that you love, a tape specifically recorded for walking, or even an audio book. The miles will fly by, and you'll be entertained or enriched while you exercise.

several names. Fitness walking relates to all the good things it does for you. "Health-walking" is a word coined in 1982 by Jake Jacobson, the walking coach (who has worked with Olympic athletes) and motivational speaker who began promoting walking for fitness in the late 1970s. Race walking is a specific athletic technique distinguished by the aggressive hip movement required to maintain foot contact with the ground at all times and to straighten the knee with each step while at maximum speed. Another race-walking characteristic is the powerful elbows-up arm pump. Race walking takes training and practice to perfect, and many people don't even want to do it because it looks so ungainly.

Fitness Fact

In the 1996 Summer Olympics, Ecuador's Jefferson Perez won the men's 20-kilometer race walk by covering the 12.4-mile course in a sizzling 1 hour, 20 minutes, and 7 seconds. Russia's Elena Nicolayeva, the women's 10-kilometer gold medalist, sped through the 6.2-mile course in 41 minutes, 49 seconds.

Even without the refinements of race walking, you can increase the challenge of your walking program by stepping up your pace, adding hills, adding distance, or extending your time. Another way to intensify your workout is to carry hand weights. One-pounders, or two at the most, can do wonders in revving up your intensity. Never use ankle weights for walking, because they can stress your ankle and knee joints. One popular, balanced, walking-based routine alternates one day of walking for 60 minutes with one day of walking for 30 minutes and then doing moderate strength training for 30 minutes.

The American Volkssport Association conducts some 2,000 recreational walking events annually and has developed about 1,000 routes in major cities, interesting towns, parks, and historic sites that you can follow on your own. Most walks are roughly 10 kilometers (6.2 miles) and take about two hours. For more information, contact the AVA at 1-800-830-WALK or www.ava.org.

A walk in the park is a wonderful way to get your daily exercise.

(Photo: Telluride Visitor Services)

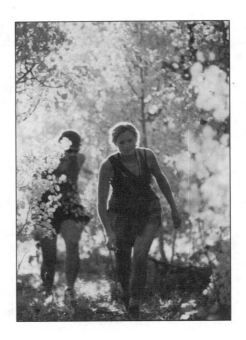

Quote, Unquote

"If you want to become the best runner you can be, start now. Don't spend the rest of your life wondering if you can do it."

—Priscilla Welch, U.S. Masters Champion

Revving Up for Running

Walking is enough for many people, but others—perhaps even you—begin to feel like a horse that longs to break into a trot. Go ahead. Put a little spring in your step, let your rear foot leave the ground before the front foot lands, and let your arms swing in rhythm with your stride. The aerobic benefits of a slow jog and a fitness walk are similar, but you might find yourself getting winded sooner because your feet are not in constant contact with the ground. You don't have to give up walking completely. When you start running, walking can still serve as your warm-up and your cool-down. If you get serious about running and go for more speed and distance, a slow jog can serve as your warm-up and your cool-down.

Once you decide you want to begin running, a good way to gently move into it is by jogging, which is a slow, recreational form of running. In the beginning, you can alternate walking and jogging either by time or by distance. If you have access to a track, try this: You can begin by alternately walking half a lap and jogging half a lap. Gradually increase your jogging time in relation to your walking time. Jog three-quarters of a lap and walk the rest. Then alternate running a lap and walking fractions of laps. Finally, eliminate the walk (except for the warm-up and cool-down periods) until you can jog for about 45 minutes.

If you use park paths, streets, or sidewalks instead of a track, you can start your shift to becoming a runner by alternating one to three minutes of walking with two or three minutes of jogging, or you can jog a block and then walk a block. In the beginning, you might find that such a "sprint" is all you can do, but pretty soon, the jogging segments will come more easily. That's when it's time to lengthen the jog and shorten the walk. Follow the same pattern as you would on the track until you can jog for about 45 minutes, which might mean a three- to four-mile jog. When you are comfortable and are able to carry on a conversation as you jog, you might find yourself naturally lengthening your stride and quickening your pace until you are running. The changeover should be gradual, taking anywhere from several weeks to several months.

Running, of course, is not for everyone. It is a high-impact activity that is not always suitable for overweight or older people, whose joints just can't take the constant pounding. Each time a runner's heel strikes the ground, the flexed ankle and knee act like shock absorbers. The vibration from the heel strike is like a shock wave that travels up the leg at 200 miles per hour. By the time it reaches the hip, it has been reduced to one sixth of its original intensity. By the time it reaches the head, this vibration is one tenth of its initial intensity, which means your brain may be serene, but your ankles, knees, and hips feel the jolt with each footfall.

The good news, however, is that running does not cause bone or joint degeneration. In fact, like other weight-bearing exercise, it helps build bone density. According to a nine-year Stanford Arthritis Center study of 28 long-time runners age 58 and older, the runners, who ran an average of just two hours a week, had more bone mass than the 27 nonrunners also tested.

That alternate walking and running that experts here recommend as a transition stage between walking and running takes the form of recreation in Scandinavia. The word "fartlek" sounds indecent, but this Swedish word means "speed play," and it is a way to vary your program. It combines walking strides and jogging for various lengths of time or running different short segments—say, from light pole to light pole—at different speeds. You can create your own pattern. You might walk at a warm-up pace for three minutes, for example, jog for 30 seconds, walk fast for five minutes, jog for one minute, race-walk for two minutes, walk for five minutes, jog for three minutes, walk for 10 minutes, and so on until your adventure is over. The variations are limited only by your imagination.

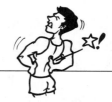

Achtung!

If you are a new exerciser, are 40 years of age or older, have a heart condition or knee problems, or are 20 percent overweight or more, it is crucial to consult with a physician before you begin running.

The following is a list of running do's:

➤ Walk or jog for three to five minutes to warm up before running and for the same amount of time at the end of your run to cool down.

➤ Stretch lightly at the beginning of your run and more specifically at the end when your muscles are warm.

Try this stretch for your outer thighs after a jog or a brisk walk.

(Photo: Anne W. Krause)

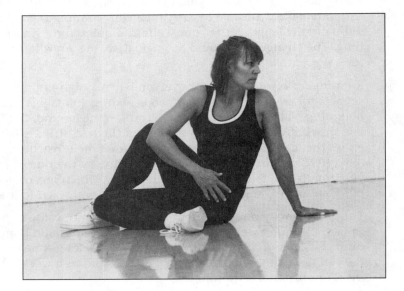

➤ As you run, keep your body erect, your head balanced on your neck, and your eyes looking forward and down just slightly. Keep your shoulders down and relaxed.

➤ Bend your elbows so your arms form a 90-degree angle. Use a natural, efficient motion with your arms close to your body and your palms relaxed.

➤ Try to land lightly on your heels and roll through your entire foot, from your heels to your toes, with each stride. (Some people naturally land midfoot or even on their toes. If you tend to do this, consult a trainer or a running coach for an evaluation.)

➤ Use your arms more when running up a steep hill.

The following is a list of running don'ts:

➤ Don't start up at full pace without warming up and don't pull up to a stop at the end of your run without cooling down.

➤ Don't skip a light stretch or stretch too strongly at the beginning of your run, and don't forget to stretch at the end.

➤ Don't lunge forward, hunch your shoulders up to your ears, or look down at your feet as you run.

➤ Don't clench your fists, press your arms against your body, or let your arms flail wildly.

➤ Don't overstride or land on the balls of your feet.

➤ Don't pick up your knees like a drum major or majorette (except when sprinting, which you'll rarely, if ever, do as a beginning runner).

Ready, Set, Race

If you set a goal of racing, you will want to improve your running. The most sensible way is to first increase your distance and then gradually try to pick up your speed. You can further vary your routine by adding sprint intervals. For example, you can walk faster or jog for two to three minutes several times during a fitness walk; or if you run, you can pick up the pace and sprint for short distances. You can add hills or go off-road, running cross-country or on hiking trails. The soft-dirt surface will be kinder to your joints than concrete or asphalt. You also can join a local running club that provides camaraderie, coaching, companionship, and support for recreational runners and racers.

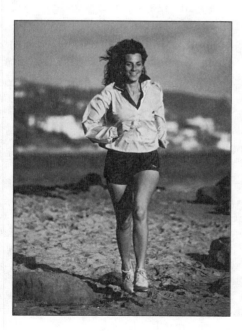

You can jog just about anywhere. A dirt trail is softer than asphalt and is easier on your joints.

(Photo: Anne W. Krause)

173

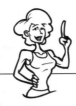

Fitness Fact

A runner's pace is stated as "running an X-minute mile," not as "running X miles per hour." A novice runner will jog about a 10- to 15-minute mile. A recreational runner with some experience can run an 8- to 10-minute mile. A serious, well-trained runner might run a 6-minute mile. A world-class male runner can sustain a 4½- to 5-minute-mile pace in a 10-kilometer race.

Colleen Cannon, a former triathlon competitor and director of Women's Quest fitness camps, has the following tips for starting and maintaining a running or general-fitness program:

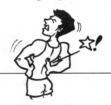

Achtung!

Runner's knee (technically, chondromalacia of the patella) is the degeneration of the underside of the kneecap. It causes pain when running downhill, when walking down stairs, or even when standing after prolonged sitting. In many cases, this biomechanical misalignment can be prevented by proper footwear or orthotics. It can be remedied in various ways, including physical therapy; strengthening of the thigh, hip, and/or ankle muscles; or body-realignment techniques.

➤ Keep training fun by making a game of it. Say "I'll love running 30 minutes today" instead of "I have to run 30 minutes today."

➤ Get with a group. It is hard to go on long runs alone. Going with others makes it more enjoyable.

➤ Be moderate in the beginning. Some people start exercising too hard and too soon, and they get injured or lose their motivation.

➤ Be disciplined. The root word of "discipline" is "disciple." Be your own disciple. Exercise for yourself, not for anyone else.

If walking or jogging is your preferred aerobic exercise but lousy weather keeps you in the gym, walking or jogging on a treadmill or riding a stationary bike can be a good substitute. Experts say that five miles on a bike equals one mile of walking on a treadmill at comparable settings. You can play videotapes of trails in Hawaii, the Swiss Alps, the Grand Canyon, and other places to visualize walking or running there while on a treadmill.

Rules of the Road for Runners (and Walkers)

Unless you do loops on a track, you have to run or walk in harmony with playing children, pedestrians, cyclists, in-line skaters, motor vehicles, or a combination of these. If you can, run or walk on a sidewalk or a recreational path, where at least you won't have to contend with motor vehicles. On a recreational path where motorized vehicles are prohibited, keep to the right so that cyclists and skaters can pass you safely. If you run on the road, run facing traffic but try to pick routes with little traffic. Avoid deserted or poorly lit areas if you are out after dark, and heed the following safety tips:

➤ Run during daylight hours if you can. If you can't, wear light-colored clothing with reflectors. Also make sure your footwear has reflectors built into the heel and sides.

➤ Always run or walk against traffic.

➤ If you are in a group or with another person, run single file and stay on the shoulder or at the very edge of the road.

➤ Anticipate vehicles and cyclists at intersections—not just other streets but also alleys and driveways—especially if there are hedges, fences, or other obstructions. You can hear them coming, but they can't hear you.

➤ Remember that, although a personal tape or CD player can be a diversion or motivation for running or walking, headphones also block out many street sounds. You need to be alert to what's going on around you. When wearing a headset, you might not hear cars, bicycles, or other potential threats. If you need to use one, don't crank up the volume so high that it blocks out all street sounds.

➤ Always carry identification with you. Money for a pay phone or a cell phone also can be useful in case of an emergency.

➤ If a belligerent driver approaches you without making room, don't challenge the car. Move off the road.

Comparisons and Contrasts

As you now know, walking is excellent exercise to tone your body and burn calories, but you might want to break into a jog or begin running seriously. Your caloric burn will vary according to your body weight, the activity, your intensity, the duration of your walk or run, and whether you follow a hilly or flat route.

All other things being equal, runners use energy faster than walkers, although a fast walk does burn more calories and elevate your heart rate more than a leisurely trot. Walking is easier on your joints than running. A walker exerts one to one-and-a-half times his or her body weight with each footfall, while a runner exerts the force of three to four times his or her body weight. Light jogging is in between, exerting more force than walking but less than full-out running. Because walkers straighten their knees with each stride and maintain constant contact with the ground, their backs, knees, and other joints are better protected.

The following chart has been adapted from Fitness Partner's Activity Calendar and is computed on the basis of 45 minutes of walking or running. It's simply a guideline, not gospel. As they say in car commercials, "Your mileage may vary." You can calculate your calorie consumption by logging on to www.primusweb.com/fitnesspartners/jumpsite/.

Walking and Running

Activity	110 lbs	150 lbs	180 lbs
Walking (17-minute-mile pace)	158	216	259
Walking (15-minute-mile pace)	178	243	292
Walking (13-minute-mile pace)	198	270	324
Jogging (<10-minute-mile pace)	238	324	389
Race walking	257	351	421
Running (5-minute-mile pace)	317	432	518
Cross-country running	356	486	583
Running (10-minute-mile pace)	396	540	648
Running (8-minute-mile pace)	495	675	810
Running (6-minute-mile pace)	653	891	1,069

Shoes and More

Footwear can make or break your walking or running program. Properly fitting shoes that are broken in but not broken down and cushioning socks are crucial, especially if you use hard surfaces. Hitting the road with a companion is excellent motivation, but if you are going solo, a small tape player that you can carry in your hand or on a belt is good company. Some just play tapes; others include radios so you can walk with the news or your favorite program. Other accessories include sports watches and heart-rate monitors. For more information about such products, see Chapter 23, "Shape-Up Shopping List."

Ready to Race?

Foot races lure millions of competitors from the casual to the serious, and you don't have to be a marathoner to participate. Recreational races take place in many cities, suburbs, small towns, and resorts across the country. Many races donate the proceeds to charity. (The Race for the Cure series benefiting breast cancer research is probably the most famous.) Five- and 10-kilometer and 5-mile lengths are common. These are reasonable distances to shoot for after you've begun walking regularly or have escalated your walking to a running pace. A specific race at a specific time gives you a training goal.

Competitors can be subdivided into several different categories. Common ones include men's and women's divisions, wheelchair racers, recreational and elite racers, runners and walkers, and age-group categories. Some races also have a short course, perhaps a kilometer or a mile or two, that is designated as a "fun run" or a "family race," and novices and even small children can compete. On the other end of the spectrum, many races also attract a field of professional-name runners who race for prize money. Most entrants are in it to test themselves, perhaps trying for a "personal best" over a certain distance or a specific course—or just to have fun.

The sports or outdoors section of your local newspaper might publish articles containing race-training tips in the weeks leading up to a big local event. Generally, it is possible to sign up for these races in advance or on race day. You just fill out an entry form, pay a fee, and you're in. Major races in big cities might limit the field, but the limit is in the tens of thousands. Your race fee gets you a bib with a number; a T-shirt, a water bottle, or another prize; and perhaps lunch or at least a snack.

In some communities that host foot races, you can find tune-up classes to help you prepare for your first competition. If you later get really serious about competing, running and race-walking coaches can help you get the best results. Even in casual classes, it is fun and beneficial to train with a group, and you'll also learn how to pace yourself, what to eat before the race, how much to hydrate, and how to handle race-day weather that is

Quote, Unquote

"I used to think I had to run at least three miles a day, [but] I can always walk fast if I want to break into a sweat. Now I love to hike with my dog up in the hills where it's just beautiful. No pressure. It feels good. I've gone out more since I got my dog."

—Daphne Zuniga, actress

Quote, Unquote

"The only difference between a runner and a jogger is an entry blank."

—Dr. George Sheehan, recreational running guru and author

very hot, humid, cold, or rainy. For committed competitors, the race must go on—no matter what the weather. The energy and enthusiasm generated by the crowd on race day will help you go the distance and might even give you the incentive to better your time next year.

Here are some races open to runners and walkers:

➤ **Squaw Valley Mountain Run and Fitness Walk.** This ski resort in California's Sierra Nevada near Lake Tahoe has hosted this uphill race since 1980. The 3.6-mile course climbs 2,000 feet from the resort's base to the High Camp Bath & Tennis Club at 8,000 feet. The race takes place in late July. Contact 530-550-0885 or www.jps.net/sagamtn/public_html/mtnrun.html.

➤ **Bolder Boulder.** This 10-kilometer running and walking race attracts more than 35,000 participants who run through the streets of this scenic city at the foothills of the Rockies. The race finishes with a big party for all participants at the University of Colorado football stadium. It takes place every Memorial Day. Contact 303-444-7223.

➤ **Mackinac Island 8-mile.** This 8-mile race offers stunning views of Lake Huron as it follows the very flat perimeter trail of the historic and beautiful Mackinac Island in Michigan. No cars are allowed on the island; you must take a ferry or a plane to get there. The race is held annually in September and is open to runners and walkers. Contact P.O. Box 233, Flushing, MI, 48433.

➤ **George Sheehan Classic.** This 5-mile run and 2-mile health and fitness walk is held in Red Bank, New Jersey, each August. Dr. George Sheehan played a big role in the running boom that started in the late 1970s, and his memorial classic is noted as one of the country's top 100 races by *Runners World* magazine. Contact 732-988-7725 or go to the Web site at www.sheehanclassic.org.

➤ **PRA Seafood Festival 5K Run.** This 5-kilometer flat course loops through the historic downtown of Pensacola, Florida, and the race is open to runners and walkers alike. It is held annually in September in conjunction with the Pensacola Seafood Festival. Contact 850-433-6512 or e-mail fiesta@fiestafiveflags.org.

If you decide to up your mileage to prepare for a race, don't overdo it. To reduce the risk of injury, increase your mileage and your pace gradually, run on soft surfaces or a treadmill whenever you can, stretch faithfully before and after each run, and take a day off between runs. Biking, swimming, cross-country skiing, and snowshoeing are good cross-training activities for runners.

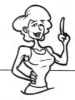

Fitness Fact

Off-road running on dirt trails and unpaved roads can be beneficial in two ways. Because the earth gives, some runners believe that muscles actually become stronger than when running on unyielding pavement. Second, and perhaps more important, the dirt has a cushioning effect that is easier on the joints, ligaments, and tendons.

The Least You Need to Know

➤ Walking is a great way for sedentary people to start a fitness program.

➤ Start a running program by alternating walking and jogging segments.

➤ Proper footwear prevents injuries and increases comfort.

➤ Instead of concrete or asphalt, try to run on dirt trails to lessen the impact on your joints.

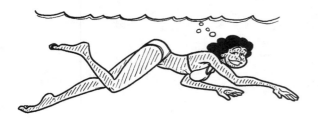

Chapter 14

More Great Moves

> ### In This Chapter
>
> ➤ Swimming is an effective, no-impact exercise
>
> ➤ Jumping rope provides intense cardio conditioning
>
> ➤ In-line and ice skating are topnotch muscle-toners
>
> ➤ Cross-country skiing and snowshoeing are great winter activities

Some people get into shape, or stay in shape, to participate in sports. Others partici-pate in sports to get or stay in shape. Some people do both, exercising specifically to train for a particular sport—or several—and in the process, becoming fitter. Sports, like gym exercises, use and therefore strengthen different muscle groups, require various amounts of agility and speed, and call for different levels of coordination. This chap-ter deals with individual recreational sports and activities, while Chapter 18, "Playing Your Way to Fitness," focuses on organized individual and team sports that have rules.

With an increased number of apparatus mimicking particular sports, training for a specific one is getting easier and easier. Chapter 11, "Machines to Get Your Body Humming," explored stationary bikes, treadmills, rowing machines, versaclimbers, and ski simulators. These machines can be an end unto themselves or can provide training specifically for cycling, running/walking, rowing, and rock-climbing. Still, for many people, nothing surpasses the "real thing"—the thrill of being on a bike, on a trail, in a kayak, or on a cliff.

Swimming into Shape

Swimming is a powerful and effective shape-up tool. It strengthens the heart and lungs, builds a strong upper body, and burns calories, all while being a no-impact activity that is gentle on the joints. The strokes, from the most energetic stroke to the least, are

➤ Butterfly

➤ Crawl/Freestyle

➤ Breaststroke

➤ Backstroke

Treading water, which basically involves using your legs and arms in constant, coordinated motion to keep your head above water, is another calorie-burning activity to try in water.

Swimming laps is a great workout for the entire body.

(Photo: Anne W. Krause)

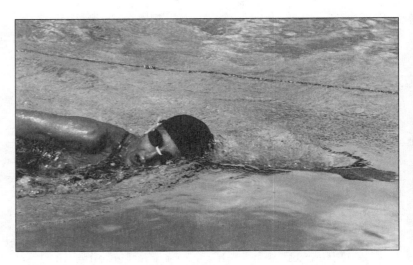

In warm weather, you can swim outdoors in a pool, a lake, or the sea, and you can swim year-round indoors. Perhaps you haven't been in a pool to swim for exercise since you were a kid. To find facilities where you can start again, check with your local recreation center, Y, or fitness club about adult swim lessons. The best time to swim for exercise is when the pool is only open for swimming laps. Most pools designate lanes for slow, medium, and fast swimmers. If you swim for fitness, mix various strokes to avoid tedium and injury, and also to tone your muscles in slightly different ways. When you've reestablished your strokes (or learned them properly for the first time), try a masters' swim workout, which is simply an adult swim workout under the direction of a coach. Swimming also is a great cross-training activity for other sport-specific training.

Jump Ropes: They're Not Just for Children Anymore

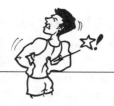

It's no coincidence that boxers, who are extremely attuned to training, have been jumping rope for conditioning since Joe Louis was a pup. Rope jumping is cardio training to the max, so a few minutes go a long way. Jumping or skipping rope combines high-impact aerobics with a constant heart-rate-raising arm motion. In addition, it helps tone your legs, arms, deltoids, and abs. If you play sports that require fast footwork, such as tennis or racquetball, you might even find that rope work can help improve your coordination for such sports.

As beneficial as jumping or skipping rope can be, the potential for overdoing it, or doing it wrong, is real. Be sure to select cushioning footwear, such as aerobics shoes, and only jump on a yielding surface. A wooden gym floor is the best; concrete is the worst. To minimize the impact on your ankles and knees, and to avoid pains that range from backaches to shin splints, don't overdo jumping. Land softly, using your feet and knees as shock absorbers. Your feet don't have to jump high off the floor to benefit from rope jumping.

Start out by alternating jumping for one minute and resting for one minute. You'll be surprised at how quickly your heart rate zooms after so short a time. Work up to two minutes of jumping with one minute of rest and then three minutes of jumping with one minute of rest. Even many pros don't jump rope for more than 10 minutes per session. Keep in mind that "rest" doesn't mean sitting down. It means walking around or moving to keep your blood flowing. (For more information about jump-rope routines, see Chapter 15, "Specialized Aerobics Programs.")

Be a Good Skate

Skating can be excellent for toning the legs, enhancing cardiovascular fitness, and burning calories—provided that you become skilled enough to skate quickly, fluidly, and aggressively.

Achtung!

Freestyle, also known as the American crawl works the front of the shoulders more than the back and increases the risk of shoulder tendonitis and rotator-cuff injuries. Alternate the crawl and the backstroke. If you swim for fitness regularly, mix various strokes to avoid repetitive-motion injuries.

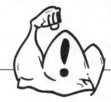

Fit Tip

An old hunk of clothesline isn't suitable for fitness rope jumping. It's too light and can snag under your feet. Sporting goods stores carry ropes with a little more heft to them. Even inexpensive ones have comfortable handles and are sized to fit the user's height. You can determine the correct length of the rope by measuring from one armpit to the other while standing on the middle of the rope. The best jump ropes are made of leather rope.

Line Up for In-Line Skating

If you thought the four-wheeled skates you strapped to your shoes as a kid were fun, you'll love the freedom that in-line skating provides. This new sport is based on a design in which four wheels are lined up one after another, which makes them easier to use and more maneuverable than old-time skates. First marketed in 1980, in-line skates have all but supplanted traditional roller skates. In-line skates have one row of wheels in a line (hence the name in-line skates). Go fast, feel balanced, and get a workout while rolling along on a recreation path, in the park, or in a big empty parking lot.

Today's skates are designed for comfort, balance, and ease of use. Made with high-performance materials, they provide support and are breathable to keep your feet cool. Skating works your quads, thighs, and glutes, among other muscles. Experts note that you can burn about 400 calories an hour by skating at a rather leisurely pace.

If you want to try skating, many bike and outdoor stores rent skates by the hour or by the day. Wrist sprains and fractures are among the most common skating injuries. It is important to wear a helmet, wristguards or special gloves, and kneepads and elbow pads when you are in-line skating. When you're just starting out, your feet might get tired within an hour, so don't have expectations of skating all day. A good place to try skating is on a smooth recreation path that is relatively flat or in a big parking lot without cars and traffic. There are brakes on the back of skates to help you slow down or stop. As you improve, you will find that you can maneuver up and down gentle grades, skate backward, and make quick turns. Rollerblade, the company that developed in-line skating, has divided the sport into three skill levels and even offers moderately priced classes and workshops in a program called Bladeschool. These levels are

➤ **Novice.** Stopping, striding, turning.

➤ **Intermediate.** Crossovers, transitions.

➤ **Advanced.** Backward skating, powder slides.

For information on where to find a Bladeschool program, contact 1-800-232-ROLL or www.rollerblade.com.

Skating can take you places. It is not unreasonable to go 10 to 15 miles per hour, so you can skate a considerable distance in a short amount of time. Some skates are available with a wheel base that can be removed to create a shoe. This enables you to use your skates to get some exercise while running your errands.

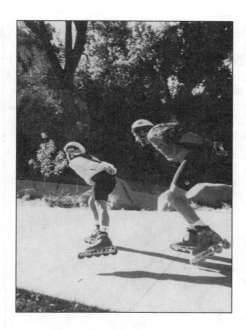

Roll along while enjoying a heart-strengthening workout.

(Photo: Anne W. Krause)

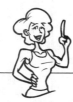

Fitness Fact

About two thirds of people injured in in-line skating accidents aren't wearing helmets, elbowpads and knee pads, or wristguards when they crash, according to the Consumer Product Safety Commission.

The Ice Is Nice

Almost everyone has watched figure skating on television, at least during the Olympic competitions. At its highest level, it is a graceful yet astonishingly athletic sport, but you don't have to be a pro to have fun on the ice. If you are intrigued by watching figure-skating competitions, you too can enjoy skating and reap the fitness benefits of this graceful exercise.

There are indoor ice rinks in many towns and cities throughout the country, and out-door rinks with natural or artificial ice abound in the North. If you're on a winter vacation, many resorts have maintained and lighted ponds or rinks along with rentals and instruction. Rinks offer many programs, from lessons to rentals to public skating sessions—even adult hockey leagues (see Chapter 18, "Playing Your Way to Fitness"). If you haven't skated since you were a youngster, and you don't want to jump onto the ice without some coaching and reassurance, sign up for some lessons. They will give you the confidence you need to chaperone your child's skating party during that Friday night public skate session—and perhaps they will get you motivated to skate for exercise yourself. Give one of your local rinks a call to see what programs it offers.

Warm up winter while gliding along to fitness.

(Photo: Anne W. Krause)

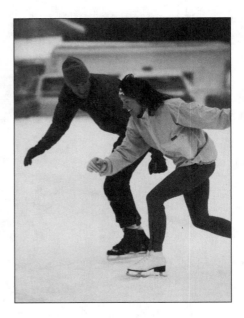

When renting skates, get a pair that is at least as small as your shoe size. Even if you are skating outdoors, wear thin socks, because thick ones will prevent the skates from providing proper ankle support. Lace the skates snugly and all the way to the top. If your toes become numb within minutes, you have laced your skates too tightly. If your ankles flop to the inside, your socks are probably too thick, you have laced the skates too loosely, or the skates are too big.

If you're ready to get right on the ice without a lesson, but you haven't skated in a while, start out by walking on the ice. Keep your back and head up straight, hold your arms out slightly to the side, and bend your knees and ankles. When you've got your balance, add the glide and have fun. In the winter, you can rent skates and go down to the local lake or pond after it is frozen solid. They can be treacherous if the ice is thin or water is moving beneath the surface, so be extra careful if you want to skate on a frozen lake or pond. Heed any warnings posted at natural lakes and ponds. Make sure any outdoor ice you want to skate on is thoroughly frozen. Do not venture out on thin ice.

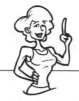

Fitness Fact

The primary reason for bicycle use among Americans is recreation, at 92 percent; followed by fitness, 26 percent; commuting, 10 percent; and racing, 1 percent, according to The Bicycle Council. The ratio of male to female riders is 54 to 46. Nearly 77 million adults, age 16 and older, ride bicycles, and 25 million say that they ride an average of at least once a week. Forty-three million youngsters age 16 and under ride bikes.

Pedal Power

Bicycling not only is great exercise, it also is a lot of fun. You don't get the joint impact of jogging or aerobics, and pedaling in the fresh air is invigorating and refreshing. You can turn it into excellent conditioning by adding hills or riding fast. Cycling is excellent aerobic conditioning and also strengthens the legs, especially the quadriceps.

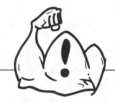

Fit Tip

If you're looking for a cool place to walk, run, bike, cross-country ski, or snowshoe, check out the Rails-to-Trails Conservancy's Web site at www.railstrails.org. At last count, the organization had converted some 700 trails nationwide to recreational use.

Here are several approaches to bicycling:

➤ **Commuting.** You can use your bicycle as an environmentally sound commuting vehicle to get to work, to go to the store, to visit a friend, or to get to the gym. A mountain bike is good for negotiating uneven pavement and potholes, but some commuters prefer a specially designed city or street bicycle.

➤ **Mountain-biking.** Developed more than two decades ago on Mt. Tamalpais in Marin County north of San Francisco, mountain-biking rapidly escalated from an oddity to a mainstream sport. The term has been extended to include any type of off-road cycling from unpaved roads to gonzo downhills and grinding uphills that revs up the heart rate, gets the lungs pumping, and gets the leg muscles working overtime.

➤ **Family cycling.** Cycling is a family activity that everyone can do on one level or another, and there are several ways to include small children. You can use your bicycle to tow a toddler or two in a sturdy Burley trailer, which features a top and side panels and a zip-up screen or plastic "windshield." You can use hook it onto an adult bicycle and tow a toddler or two behind you as you ride. Another option for preschoolers is a durable child's bicycle seat that mounts behind the saddle of your bike. Children old enough to "help" pedal can ride a bike extender, which consists of a wheel, pedals, and handlebars, that attaches to the back of your bicycle. However your youngster cycles with you, make sure he or she wears a helmet—and set a good example by wearing one, too.

➤ **Road-racing.** If the Tour de France is the stuff of your fantasies, you can get into serious cycling. Try setting a goal to train for an organized event, such as a vacation bicycle tour, a fund-raising ride, or even a citizens' bike race.

Cycling can be fun on your own as well as a great way to build camaraderie with a spouse or training partner. If you don't have a cycling partner, many cycling clubs throughout the country put together group rides and offer cycling and bike maintenance clinics. Check with your local bike shop, recreation center, Y, or health club.

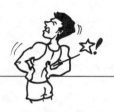

Achtung!

If you get into any sort of distance riding, be sure not to grip the handlebars too tightly or lean your weight on your forearms. Such habits can result in handlebar palsy, which has symptoms such as numbness, tingling, cramping, or weakness of the hands and perhaps the forearms.

Today, there are a number of different bicycle types to choose from. Mountain bikes have fat, knobby tires and pedal well over rough terrain and along dirt trails. Road bikes have skinny, smooth, high-pressure tires designed for going fast on the road. Both road and mountain bikes have many gears that can be adjusted for the terrain. Recently, bike manufacturers revitalized the "cruiser bike," which is a throwback from days gone by. Cruisers look cool and really are only good for easy commuting. The tires are smooth but not skinny, and these bikes generally have few if any gears. Cruiser bikes often have higher handlebars that enable you to sit up straighter. This often is appealing to older, overweight, or pregnant cyclists. There are also a number of *hybrid bikes* on the market that are a cross between a mountain bike and a road bike. Finding one of these may be your best bet if you plan to use your bike mainly for multiple tasks.

Before investing in a bicycle, set some cycling goals. Do you want to pedal short distances to do errands? Do you want to ride on dirt trails? Do you want to ride fast on the roads? Have you been intrigued by a bicycle tour or a fund-raising cycling event in your area? When you have determined the type of cycling you want to do, find a bike shop that will suit your needs and try a number of different bikes. Make sure the shop helps you find a bike that fits you properly. A bike that doesn't have the proper fit can lead to injury over time.

The Bicycle Council offers the following tips for selecting a bicycle:

➤ **Suitability.** Make sure the bike fits your lifestyle. Buy a bike for its intended use. Will it be for recreation, commuting on paved surfaces, dirt paths, or rough terrain?

➤ **Fit.** Get your bike properly fitted for your body. When you are comfortable, you are in better control, which means safer, more comfortable, and more enjoyable rides. To determine the proper fit from the ground to the seat, straddle the top tube of the bike. The clearance between the bike and the body should be between 2 and 4 inches. When seated with one foot on the pedal at its lowest extension, the knee should be slightly bent. The reach from the seat to the handlebars can mean the difference between a painful ride and an enjoyable one. Different brands vary in distance for the reach, so the best bet is to try several models to determine which is the most comfortable for you.

➤ **Quality.** Buy a properly assembled bike with quality components. A quality bike is a better value in the long run. Buying a poorly assembled bike often leads to a breakdown or poor riding performance and an unpleasant experience.

In addition to a properly fitted bike, you should invest in a few other things. You will need a helmet, a water-bottle bracket (also called a cage) and water bottle, a bicycle tire pump, a tire patch kit, a spare tire tube, and perhaps some bicycle shorts. Bicycle shorts are a must for long rides, because they have additional padding in the crotch area to alleviate soreness.

Quote, Unquote

"Many people want a bike just to ride on the weekends. Others use their bikes as a healthy form of transportation to and from work. Most people who cycle start out riding recreationally. Later, some slowly graduate to medium- and long-distance touring. Others eventually take their interest in cycling to racing. That was the case with me—I got my first bike because I enjoyed the outdoors; after a few months I was ready to start racing."

—Greg LeMond, three-time Tour de France winner

Paddle Power

You might have seen Meryl Streep's shapely arms in *The River Wild*. She did her own rowing and paddling in the film, which is how she built those arm muscles. There is no need to aspire to running a wild river to enjoy paddling and reap the benefits of an outdoor upper-body workout. The options for boating include canoeing, river kayaking, sea kayaking, rafting, and river rowing. If you live near a river or a lake, you probably will find boat rentals and tours nearby. If you're planning a vacation near a lake or a river, check with the local chamber of commerce or your hotel to find a place that provides rentals or guided tours for paddling adventures. A day on the river won't change your shape, but it will introduce you to the world of white water or flat water.

Hiking and Trekking

You don't have to be Sir Edmund Hillary and have aspirations to climb Mt. Everest to enjoy hiking and trekking. In fact, quite the opposite is true. Hiking provides the opportunity to enjoy nature and to get some healthy exercise. It is yet another outdoor activity that accommodates all ability levels. It really is just a form of walking, but it implies that you are on a scenic and somewhat uneven trail going through the woods, across a wildflower meadow, to a waterfall, or up a mountaintop—and it's a great way to spend quality time with family or friends.

Hiking takes you into nature, whether it's on a trail through the woods at a nearby state park, a hike to a scenic mountain vista, or a walk on the wild side in an exotic locale. For a sedentary city dweller, even a brisk walk to and around the local park can seem like a hike, and it does benefit your heart and muscle tone. While hiking, you can talk with your hiking companions or simply enjoy the environment in silence. Look around at the flowers and vegetation and learn more about where you are.

Enjoy friends and aerobic fitness pedaling along a scenic mountain road.

(Photo: Anne W. Krause)

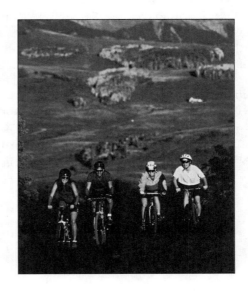

If you are planning to hike on dirt trails through uneven terrain, sturdy boots with good traction and thick, cushioned socks are important. If you plan to hike in an area where it rains or the ground is moist, invest in boots lined with Gore-Tex or other waterproof material. If you live in tick or mosquito country, clothing with long sleeves and long pants that you can tuck into your socks will prevent discomfort. Many outdoor stores sell lightweight and comfortable hiking boots that are not too expensive, and these shoes are just fine for day hikes when you are carrying only water, snacks, some extra warm or water-proof clothing in case the weather changes, and other basics. If you are going on a long hike, make sure someone knows your itinerary and when to expect you home.

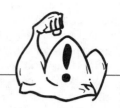

Fit Tip

If your feet tend to blister or you are breaking in new hiking boots, do some preventive maintenance by applying moleskin, Second Skin, Band-Aid's Blister Block, or another cushioning product as soon as you feel a hot spot develop.

Outdoor stores and bookstores often carry a variety of hiking guidebooks for various areas around the country. If you are planning a trip somewhere or you want to get to know the trails in your area, there probably is a guidebook to help you out. Most guidebooks provide trail distances, elevation gains, difficulty ratings, and what you can expect along the way. In addition, local state and county park systems, forest service offices, and other public agencies have trail information about the trails under their jurisdiction.

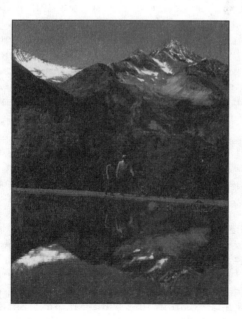

Hiking offers scenery, serenity, and a super workout.

(Photo: Telluride Visitor Services)

If you're looking for some camaraderie on the trail, contact a local hiking club, recreation center, or health club. These organizations are likely to put together group hikes and treks that offer companionship, expertise on places to go, and support for those tough spots on a hike. When you hike with a group, you also might earn the fitness dividend of picking up your pace to keep up with the pack. If you find you really enjoy hiking, you might want to extend your range. You might develop aspirations to climb a mountain or to go on an extended multiday trek to a foreign land—Peru, Nepal, Switzerland, and others come to mind. Regional hiking and mountaineering organizations such as the Appalachian Mountain Club, the Colorado Mountain Club, or the Sierra Club often put together trips led by experienced volunteers. Adventure travel outfitters also put together commercial hiking and trekking vacations to suit a variety of ability levels. Many of these are "supported" expeditions in which gear is carried by porters or pack animals, leaving clients free to enjoy the scenery while carrying only a lightweight day pack.

Quote, Unquote

"Ten minutes' drive from my apartment, there is a long, grassy ridge from which you can look out over park land and sprawling metropolis, over bay and ocean and distant mountains. I often walk along this ridge in order to think uncluttered thoughts or to feel with accuracy or to sweat away a hangover or to achieve some other worthy end, recognized or submerged."

—Colin Fletcher, *The Complete Walker III*

Winter Wonder Sports

If snow is the order of the winter day where you live, there is no need to hole up indoors by the fireplace. Skiing and snowboarding are high-profile winter sports, but the season's more low-key activities actually provide better exercise. NordicTrack provides an indoor simulation of cross-country skiing, which ranks as one of the best overall conditioning activities—as long as you do more than simply shuffle along a totally flat trail. Cross-country skiing, also called Nordic skiing, is the real thing. It works your legs and your arms as well as your heart and lungs. Snowshoeing, which has gained popularity in recent years, is like hiking with big floppy feet attached to your real feet so that you can stay on top of the snow.

Cross-Country Skiing

Cross-country skis are lightweight boards that let you glide along in a set of parallel troughs etched into the snow. Your toes are affixed to the skis, but your heels move freely. Classic cross-country skiing is a kick-and-glide motion that offers a good overall body workout that's easy on your joints. It requires use of your legs and arms, both pumping backward and forward (your arms using poles) as you glide along. Skating is done on a flat track using shorter, lighter skis and longer poles. Instead of gliding and striding, you push off aggressively with the inside edge of your free ski and add propulsion with a strong pole-plant. The motion is similar to an in-line skating motion. Skating is one of the most intense activities in the sporting world, summer or winter.

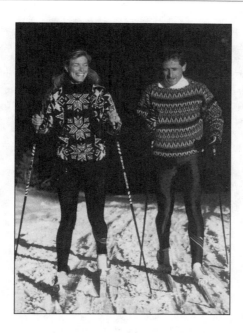

Cross-country skiing works your arms, your legs, and your heart.

(Photo: Anne W. Krause)

You can do both of these activities at a Nordic center (also called a cross-country center), which grooms its trails. The terrain can vary from virtually flat to very hilly. The trails might meander scenically through woods or be out in the open along golf-course land. The center will rate its trails from beginner to expert so you won't end up on a trail that's over your head. Ski rentals and lessons are available at most Nordic centers, and there generally is a fee to use the trails. Some Nordic centers also have added dedicated snowshoeing trails.

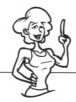

Fitness Fact

Ball State University and the University of Vermont conducted studies regarding the caloric benefit of various cross-country skiing activities. The hourly caloric expenditure is 420 calories at 2.4 miles per hour, 510 calories at 3 mph on packed snow and a flat trail, and 740 calories at 3.5 mph. When powder snow blankets the flat trail, the hourly energy expenditure is 744 calories for women and 984 calories for men at 3.5 mph. If the trail is hilly, the hourly burn is 774 calories for women and 1,046 for men at 2.9 mph.

Snowshoeing

Learning to snowshoe is simple. All you need to do is get used to walking with gear on your feet that flops up and down while you walk. Modern snowshoes consist of a lightweight metal frame with a platform made from a durable material such as neoprene or flexible plastic for flotation. There's a binding that enables you to affix almost any boot or shoe to it. It also lets the foot move in a natural free-heel stride. Most snowshoes have metal talons on the bottom for traction.

Romp through the powder on snowshoes for a heart-pumping experience.

(Photo: Anne W. Krause)

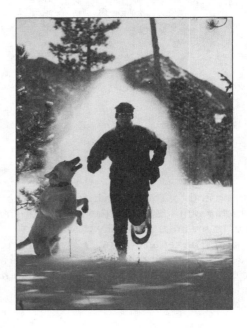

Snowshoeing offers the chance to go on a serene winter hike. You can get to your favorite summer spot that's snow covered for the winter. If you're headed on a winter vacation, chances are you'll find snow-covered hiking trails at your destination. Snowshoes are available for rental at many outdoor stores in locales that get lots of snow in the winter. Stores that rent snowshoes also can provide information about great snowshoeing trails.

Dressing for Winter Fitness

Dress in layers for both cross-country skiing and snowshoeing. The basic layers should include a synthetic underlayer, windproof pants, an insulating upper layer, such as fleece or a vest, and a wind- and waterproof jacket. You also will want warm synthetic socks for both sports. For cross-country skiing, boots are part of your rental package. For snowshoeing, you will want a pair of warm, waterproof boots and leg gaiters, which are waterproof "cuffs" with Velcro closures that are worn to keep the snow from coming into your boot tops. A hat and a pair of warm gloves complete the outfit. You might heat up or cool down, so be prepared to shed or add layers along the way.

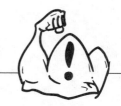

Fit Tip

Adjustable poles are gaining popularity with hikers and snow-shoers. Some experts believe that using poles while hiking and snowshoeing can help improve your balance. Poles also can take some pressure off your knees when going downhill.

The Least You Need to Know

➤ Swimming is a fantastic, no-impact sport for cardiovascular training.

➤ Jumping rope provides a high-intensity, high-impact aerobic workout.

➤ Skating, both in-line and on ice, is great exercise and fun, too.

➤ Bicycling is an aerobic sport you can participate in for fun with your family and friends, or for commuting, touring, or racing.

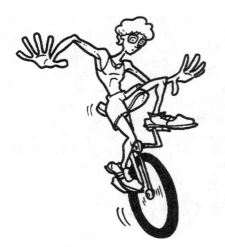

Chapter 15

Specialized Aerobics Programs

In This Chapter

➤ High, low, and high-low aerobics

➤ Rebounding using minitrampolines

➤ Dancing as exercise

➤ Aqua-aerobics: the ultimate in impact-free exercising

You know you have to get your heart rate up, but with so many choices, what should you do to get into shape? The obvious general answer, which this book espouses time and again, is to select activities that you enjoy, that you have time to do, and that you can do where you live. You might adore swimming, but if there's not a lap pool within 50 miles, it's not a practical activity for you, and chances are you won't get into the water too often. If you live in a congested city with plenty of traffic and stoplights but with no park nearby, you might not do well on a running program.

Virtually everyone has access to a gym with a choice of aerobics classes of all sorts. If you join, consider the gym to be the home base for your aerobic workouts. There you'll find cardio machines (treadmills, stationary bikes, and so on, which are discussed in Chapter 11, "Machines to Get Your Body Humming") and an array of scheduled fitness classes. Many people feed off the contagious energy of a good instructor and an enthusiastic group. You can select the class or a handful of classes that suit you and build on those with walking, running, or other sports as your fitness increases and your desire for exercise grows. You also can sample classes of various types as your schedule and mood dictate. Two of the hottest trends in aerobic conditioning are group cycling and its offshoots (again, see Chapter 11) and martial arts–based classes (see Chapter 17, "Fight Your Way to Fitness").

People keep returning to the gym to participate in the classes it offers. In addition to the dynamics of a class and the motivation provided by the instructor, some of the appeal is the physical facility itself—a good studio with a great sound system, a resilient floor, and climate control for comfort. All these factors can help you get more out of your aerobics class than the same workout at home. Still, if there's a particular type of class that you enjoy, you usually can buy a tape by a national fitness figure and continue your routine at home as well.

The High and Low of Aerobics Classes

Fitness instructor Jackie Sorenson is widely credited as the mother of aerobic dance. She devised it as a way to relieve the boredom she saw in many people who had trouble sticking to such cardio activities as running, jogging, walking, or swimming. Aerobic dance classes done to upbeat music combined vigorous dance moves, jumping jacks, running in place, and power moves that often involved leaping into the air. The classes could be done indoors in a climate-controlled gym and therefore had the additional benefit of being weatherproof. Aerobic dance was energetic, youthful, and fun, and it helped fuel the fitness boom of the 1970s.

Quote, Unquote

"Walking, jogging, and bike riding are wonderful if you don't think about your problems. If you come to an aerobics class, there's not too much time to think about your problems because there's a lot of activity."

—Linda Kennoy, The Energy Center, Boulder, Colorado

Over the years, this evolved into what we now generally refer to by the broad name of "aerobics," with the original concept now referred to as "high-impact aerobics." High-impact aerobics have been in a decline as the population of original aerobics exercisers has grown older, people have become wary of the injury risks, and more types of cardio workouts have developed. More people now choose step aerobics and various forms of low-impact or no-impact workouts.

Whatever their style, aerobics classes typically last one hour, but they can run anywhere from 45 minutes during a lunchtime workout break to 90 minutes for a class that combines aerobics with a significant toning and stretching section. Some gyms include unlimited aerobics classes in their membership fees; others charge extra for each class taken. Typical fees range anywhere from $2.50 at a public gym to $10 at a private club, although $20 is not unheard of for a popular class at a swanky club in an expensive part of the country.

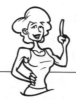

Fitness Fact

In 1988, 13,961,000 people in the United States participated in high-impact aerobics classes, 11,888,000 participated in low-impact classes, and step aerobics was not yet on the radar screen of the *Sporting Goods Manufacturers Association*. Ten years later, high-impact aerobics participation had dropped dramatically to 7,460,000, but 12,774,000 were taking low-impact classes, and 10,784,000 did step aerobics, showing a significant increase in this type of aerobics participation.

Most instructors stick to a favorite choreographed routine so that regular participants know what's coming, but a good instructor also gives clear directions in advance for new participants or for people who just haven't memorized the routine. You should be able to hear the instructor over the music. Directions should include specific moves, changes of direction, and add-on moves. If a combination is complicated, the instructor often will demonstrate it before inviting the class to join in.

Good aerobics classes start with a warm-up and end with a cool-down and a stretch. Many also include a short toning segment such as abdominal and upper- and lower-body exercises just before stretching. Many instructors also will have you check your heart rate at the end of the cardio session and compare it with a posted chart.

When you are looking at a health club's offerings, classes listed with catchy, capitalized names are trademarked routines that do not vary from gym to gym. Instructors are trained by the developer and are certified to teach those classes. Classes listed in lowercase type often are developed by local instructors. They might be knockoffs of popular brand-name workouts, but this does not mean they are bad. It just means they don't use the same music or exactly the same moves. Examples of various kinds of aerobics classes follow.

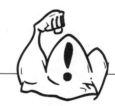

Fit Tip

To view literally hundreds of aerobic patterns and routines, log on to www.turnstep.com. The information is divided by category: step, high-low, aquatic, cycling, box-aerobics, and other categories. An aerobic dictionary on the site lists all the common moves and a few unusual ones, too.

High Impact: The Original

Music, motion, and energy are the enduring appeal of high-impact aerobics classes. To coordinate with the four-beat music that prevails in aerobics studios, most routines are based on eight repetitions (or multiples of eight) for each exercise, and exercises are usually grouped into sets. The instructor calls out each movement and demonstrates it if it is complicated or the class is populated by newcomers. The classes rely on a choreographed routine featuring heart-rate-revving moves such as hops, jumps, and jumping jacks. If the intensity gets to be too much, you can always back off and do low-impact variations of high-impact moves.

Low Impact: The Spin-Off

Some people don't like to jump, some (especially new or significantly overweight exercisers) cannot jump, and some have been injured and are now wary of jumping. With low-impact routines, one foot is always on the floor. The cardiovascular benefit, however, might be equivalent to high-impact aerobics because the pace often is faster. Low impact also is common for senior citizen and prenatal fitness classes.

Keep one foot on the floor for a low-impact workout.

(Photo: Claire Walter)

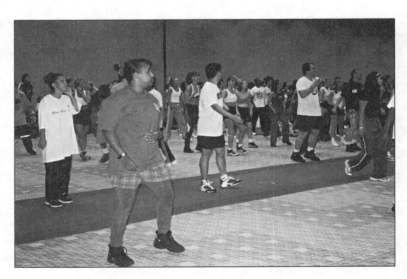

High-Low: The Combo

These classes alternate high-impact and low-impact patterns. They are good for people who want a little air time but don't want to jeopardize their joints by going full-out in a high-impact class. You often will be directed to jog or march in place as a holding pattern while the instructor provides new information on the next move.

Arms and the Exerciser

No matter what style of aerobics classes you take, your arms have a lot to do with your level of intensity. Even if your feet are making exactly the same moves, what you do with your arms affects the intensity of your aerobic workout. When your arms are at or above shoulder level, your workout is more intense than when they are between waist and shoulder height. If you need to bring down the intensity of your workout, simply let your arms hang loosely at your sides.

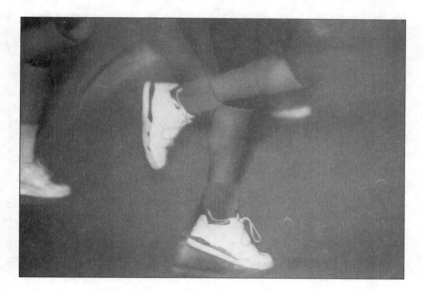

Running or marching in place is part of many aerobics classes.

(Photo: Anne W. Krause)

Step Up (and Down) for Fitness

Step aerobics (usually called just "step") uses a variable-height, heavy-duty, molded-plastic bench that you step up onto and down from. An original brand called The Step launched numerous imitators that have been using the word generically. The top platform of The Step, or other brand of bench, usually is 4 inches high, and the top surface is covered with a nonslip material. When you start doing this kind of exercise, you'll probably place the platform directly on the floor. As you become accustomed to the moves, get stronger, and improve your coordination, you can add 2- or 4-inch nonskid risers under the ends of the bench. Even a tall, well-conditioned step exerciser rarely adds more than three risers. If a person wants more intensity, he or she generally uses light hand weights during the routine. Another option is a new program, such as Super-Step, which uses two same-height benches set close together to add variety to the workout.

Step to the beat of the music for a great workout.

(Photo: Anne W. Krause)

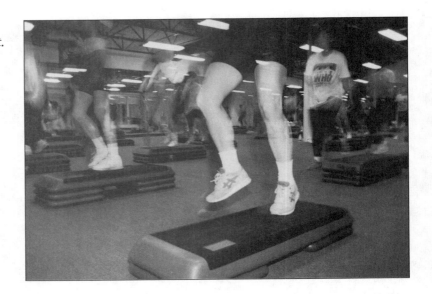

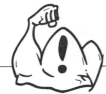

Fit Tip

Be sure you always step up onto the bench with your whole foot. In other words, do not let your heel hang off the edge of the bench, which could cause you to slip off.

Vocab-Aerobics

Aerobics routines are a choreographed progression of moves that come in a staggering assortment of combinations, but they all are assembled from building blocks of moves that have become standard. Instructors might combine them in unusual ways or match different arm movements to the common foot patterns. If you know the moves and the words, however, you can follow the instructor's directions no matter where you take a class.

Some of these moves are used only on the floor, some are used on a bench, and others are used in both contexts. For the sake of convenience, some of the most common moves are described here from a feet-together position (unless specified otherwise), beginning with the right foot leading. Obviously, these moves can be done in both directions.

➤ **A-step.** As a floor move, you step your right foot forward and to the right at a 45-degree angle, bring your left foot next to it, and then, with your right foot, step back to the right at a 45-degree angle. As a step move, you start behind the left corner of the bench, bring your right foot to the center of the bench, bring your left foot up next to it, and step down behind the other corner of the bench with your right foot and then your left foot. Whether on the floor or using the bench, the movement resembles the capital letter A, without the crossbar.

➤ **Across the top.** This energetic bench movement goes sideways across the length of the bench. Start on the floor, next to the left end of the step. Step your right foot to the middle of the bench, bring the left foot next to it, and then step off the right end with the right foot, bringing the left foot down next to it.

➤ **Around the world.** This move circumnavigates the bench. Start on the floor, perpendicular to the bench. Begin by stepping sideways onto the bench with your right foot. Bring the left foot up and make a one-quarter turn. Step off the end of the bench with the right and then the left foot. Repeat the move, stepping up with the lead foot, bringing the other foot up while turning, and then stepping down until you have worked your way all around the bench.

➤ **Basic.** In this fundamental step move, you stand behind the bench. Step up onto the bench with your right foot, bring your left foot next to it, and then step down to the floor first with your right and then with your left foot.

➤ **Change lead.** To change the lead in a step routine, return to the basic or other move and touch the toe of the nonlead foot to mark a beat. Then switch to lead with the opposite foot.

➤ **Circles.** You might be asked to circle your shoulders or your arms. This movement, done forward or backward, is a full rotation of the shoulder socket and is often used as part of the warm-up or cool-down.

➤ **Corner to corner.** In this move, you begin by stepping up diagonally onto the bench with your right foot and then lifting your left knee up. Step down with your left foot, and bring your right foot next to it on the floor behind the bench. Change sides.

➤ **Criss-cross.** This floor move begins with your feet shoulder-width apart. Flex your knees and step forward with your right foot, keeping most of your weight on your left foot. At the same time, raise your left arm in front of you above head-height and press your left arm down and behind you. Change sides.

➤ **Diagonal.** This move begins at the side of the bench near the end. Begin by stepping up to the middle with your right foot, bring your left foot up past your right foot, and step off the other corner with your right and then your left foot.

➤ **Flat back and roll up.** This is a common warm-up or cool-down move. Begin with your feet shoulder-width apart. Exhale and bend at the waist until your torso is parallel to the floor. Inhale as you roll up, one vertebra at a time, until you are upright.

➤ **Grapevine.** To begin this traveling floor move, take a long stride to the right with your right foot. Cross your left foot in front of or behind your right, and take another long stride to the right with your right foot. Then bring your left foot next to your right foot.

➤ **Half-jack.** This is a low-impact alternative to the jumping jack (described later in this list), in which you begin with your feet together and alternately move your right and left feet out to the side.

➤ **Hamstring curl.** Standing with your feet shoulder-width apart, bend your right knee as if to kick yourself. The motion is energetic and aggressive. It can be done on the floor as a high-impact move with a left-foot hop or as a low-impact move with a left-knee flex. It also can be done from the step.

➤ **Hop turn.** This advanced move is done from behind the bench. Step up onto the middle of the bench with your right foot, and hop on that foot while turning a half-rotation so you can step off facing in the opposite direction from your starting position.

➤ **Jumping jack.** This is a classic calisthenic move adopted by aerobics instructors. Stand with your feet together, jump out to the sides simultaneously with both feet, and raise your arms to waist or shoulder height (or, for maximum intensity, over your head). The half-jack (previously described) is a low-impact option.

➤ **Knee-up.** Standing with your feet shoulder-width apart, raise your right knee to hip level. The motion is energetic and aggressive. This move is done on the floor as a high-impact move with a left-foot hop or as a low-impact move with a left-knee flex. It also can be done stepping onto the bench. Some instructors do knee-ups to the front and to the side. In a variation, you can lower your left elbow to your right knee.

➤ **L-step.** This move starts at the left end of the bench. Step up with your right foot, lift your left knee, and immediately step down to the floor with your left foot. Step back with your right foot, and then bring your right foot next to your left foot. Step back onto the end of the step with your right foot, lift your left knee, place your left foot on the floor, and then bring your right foot down next to it.

➤ **Lunge.** This move can be done on the floor or on the bench. Stand with your feet together. First, flex the left knee and at the same time step back with the right leg, keeping your right foot flat on the floor. Change sides. The lunge often is done with a quarter-turn to the side. It can be a floor move with or without a hop, or it can be done from the step. In this case, the stationary foot remains on the step while the other foot steps back and down to the floor.

➤ **Over the top.** This move is similar to across the top (previously described), but it goes across the width rather than the length of the bench.

➤ **March in place.** This warm-up, cool-down, or mark-time sequence is done on the floor or on top of the step.

➤ **Plié.** This is a traditional ballet move. Stand with your feet shoulder-width apart and your knees and feet pointing outward. Bend your knees and sink down until your thighs are parallel to the floor. Rise to a full upright position.

➤ **Repeater.** A same-leg sequence (usually three or four repetitions) of a knee-up, a lunge, a hamstring curl, a side leg, or a similar move.

➤ **Side leg.** From a standing position, raise your right leg from the hip directly out to the side. This move is done on the floor as a high-impact move with a left-foot hop or as a low-impact move with a left-knee flex. It also can be done while stepping up onto the bench.

➤ **Side to side.** Often a warm-up, cool-down, or mark-time sequence, this move is done on the floor. Step your right foot out to the right side and bring your left foot to it; then step your left foot to the left and bring your right foot to it.

➤ **Squat.** Stand with your feet shoulder-width apart and facing forward. Sink down until your thighs are parallel to the floor. Your arms can come forward for balance if this is comfortable for you. This move can be done on the floor or with one foot on the bench.

➤ **Straddle.** This is an across-the-bench move. Begin by standing at a right angle to the side of the bench. Step up with your right foot and then your left. Step down with your right foot on the right side of the bench and your left foot the on the left side so that you are straddling the bench. Then, step back up with the right foot and then the left. Think "up, up, down, down" when doing this move.

➤ **T-step.** This move begins near the end of the bench. Step up onto the bench with your right foot, bring your left knee up, step back down off the end of the bench onto the floor along the side of the bench with your left foot, and bring your right foot down next to it.

➤ **Turnstep.** This step move begins at a right angle to the end of the bench. Begin by stepping up onto the near corner with your right leg, make a quarter-turn to step onto the other corner with your left leg, and step down with your right leg. You end at a right angle to the other end of the bench.

➤ **V-step.** This is the opposite of the A-step (previously described), and it can be done on the floor or by stepping onto the bench. Step your right foot forward to the right at a 45-degree angle and then your left foot to the left at a 45-degree angle. Return your right and then your left foot to the starting position.

These steps sound more complicated than they are once you have seen them demonstrated. You can practice them slowly at home, perhaps to a television show or tape, so that you are more comfortable putting them together faster in a class. You can also see these steps in sequence on the Web at www.turnstep.com.

No Impact: Slide and Glide

Speed skaters developed sliding as an off-ice training device for practice. The first slide boards were homemade, but now they are standardized. A board consists of a slick, flat, personal track that is 5, 6, or 7 feet long. It usually is made of polymer with a super-slick top surface and rubber bumpers on each end that can be adjusted in one-foot increments to customize the board's length. Inline and speed skaters and cross-country skiers who use special skating skis (see Chapter 14, "More Great Moves") use slide boards to increase their lateral strength and power as well as the balance, agility, and speed that their sports require.

Slide classes use the same type of board. You put nylon booties on over your footwear so you can slide easily across the board's smooth surface. Classes involve pushing off from one foot to another in power-skating strokes. You will get significant aerobic benefit from powering across the board to get from one bumper to the other, especially if you couple the move with arm swings. In addition to the cardio workout and increased endurance, you will find that slide classes tone your hips and both the inner and outer thighs.

For the smoothest, safest workout, wear flat-soled aerobics or dance shoes under the booties when you slide, not running shoes with heavy treads.

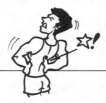

Achtung!

If you have ankle or back problems, the slide board might not be for you. The push–off can stress your ankles, and the Bonnie Blair–style speed skater's forward bend can compromise your back.

Plyometrics, Please

Plyometrics, the machine-gun routines of aerobics classes, include rapid-fire moves that contract and extend the muscles to enhance strength and power as well as your aerobic fitness and metabolic rate. These advanced moves can be front to back, back to front, or lateral. Visualize a leaping cat to get an idea of the principle behind plyometrics. You start a typical plyometric move by sinking down into a muscle contraction, launching into the move with a springing motion, landing, and then immediately sinking down into a shock-absorbing muscle contraction.

Plyometrics are not for beginners. You need to have quite a lot of strength before starting a "plyo" regimen, because it is easy to get injured if you start too soon in your exercise program. Because plyometric moves are so intense, often bringing people to the anaerobic threshold, they are done as interval exercises with recovery periods in-between. Some gyms offer short, intense plyometric classes, and many aerobics instructors now insert short, optional plyometric segments into their classes.

The old-fashioned medicine ball is another element of plyometric training. This weighted ball, which is larger than a basketball, can be used for a series of floor and mat exercises as well as for exercises such as throwing it back and forth with a friend, passing it from person to person in a circle, or throwing it for height or power.

City of Rope

Jump rope is more than just a kids' playground diversion. Done correctly, it is one of the most effective cardio workouts and an excellent plyometric component of cross-training. In fact, that's why hardcore athletes such as boxers and football players incorporate rope jumping into their training programs. This high-endurance activity is the choice of many professional athletes. (For more information about jumping rope, see Chapter 14.)

FreeStyle Roping is a branded class and video that combines rope jumping's aerobic benefits with a street-savvy, hip-hop attitude. Common moves include jumping, skipping, cross-hand turning, speed changes, and other tricks.

Louis Garcia, FreeStyle Roping's founder, helps beginners get the hang of the rope by working up to complex moves. First you practice the foot and arm moves with an imaginary rope to get the timing and coordination down. Then you practice the same steps while holding both handles in one hand and swinging the rope on one side of your body. Finally, you put it together with the jump rope twirling in two hands. Jumping rope is an intense and effective aerobic activity.

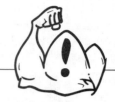

Fit Tip

The Strength Shoe is a frontal platform shoe that was developed to enhance plyometric training by taking the body weight off the heels. Because it moves the body weight and boosts the effective workload, it is an aerobics aid that also is an extension of strength training, because it works the calf muscles and stretches the Achilles's tendon. For more details, contact Strength Systems at 1–800–451–5867.

Many instructors also include a jumping segment in their cardio or general fitness classes, and a few studios even offer classes that center around jumping rope. For basic rope jumping, keep your hands at hip level with your palms facing forward. Stand erect with your head up, and keep your elbows bent at a comfortable distance from your body. Turn the rope with a motion of the wrists, push off from the balls of your feet, and land lightly. You can also adapt moves from aerobics classes, such as marching or running in place, while turning the rope alongside your body. These resting or neutral moves will help you stay in your target heart rate zone. Once you are comfortable, you won't have to jump more than an inch or two off the ground to derive aerobic benefit.

A good jump rope is not just a hunk of old clothesline, but even a good rope is an inexpensive fitness investment. Serviceable models found in gyms and sporting-goods stores are plastic or beaded-plastic in construction with comfortable, full-rotation handles. Most ropes weigh about half-a-pound and are sturdy enough to make a full loop without flopping and tangling under your feet. Ropes come in different lengths. Whether selecting a rope in the gym or buying your own, find the right length by holding the rope in one hand, stepping on the bottom of the loop, and pulling it up. The tips of the handles should reach your chest or armpits. For experienced exercisers who are not susceptible to wrist or elbow problems, weighted ropes (from one to six pounds) are available to boost the aerobic benefit even more. These are safest for short periods of exercise.

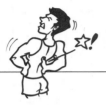

Achtung!

If you jump rope on your own, be sure to do so on a resilient surface such as wood. Jumping on asphalt and especially concrete can cause injury.

Bounce your way to fitness on a minitrampoline, now known in the fitness world as a rebounder.

(Photo: Claire Walter)

Fitness on the Rebound

Rebounding classes are aerobics with an overlay of childish joy. The playthings are 28- to 33-inch-diameter minitrampolines (the type that people once used for indoor jogging in place), which are now called rebounders. The games involve aerobics moves such as jumping, turning, twisting, kicking, kickboxing, running, and, not surprisingly, given the popularity of martial arts–themed workouts, punching. The trampoline adds a plyometric bonus to the moves. The workout also contains an abdominal segment, which involves crunches while sitting on the rebounder.

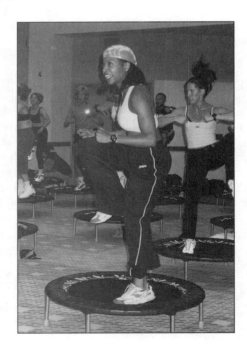

In addition to the cushioning effect of the trampoline being kind to the joints, fans assert that rebounding's cardio benefits and calorie consumption exceed that of the same moves done on a wood floor. The theory is that your body is heavier when it decelerates or comes down from the bounce, so you have to work harder to jump back up. In fact, the National Aeronautics and Space Administration determined trampolines provide a workout bonus because the additional gravitational pressure of bouncing briefly makes you two-and-a-half times your regular body weight. This in turn makes your muscles and cardiovascular system work harder than during other exercises. The first popular rebounding routine, called Urban Rebounding, was launched at Crunch Fitness Centers. For more information, call 212-734-6313.

Dance Yourself into Shape

From the time the Charleston and the jitterbug replaced more sedate dances to the disco days of the 1970s when *Saturday Night Fever* spirit permeated the land, young people have kept aerobically fit by dancing—and the young-at-heart have kept right up. Energetic dances and dance-based exercise programs are fast-moving and fun. Dance in all its forms is still a great way to get and stay in shape and to loosen up joints and muscles. Besides, dancing is *fun*. The following sections describe some of the classes you will find.

All That Jazzercise

Jazzercise, the forerunner of dance-based aerobics programs, was conceived in 1969 by a professional dancer named Judi Sheppard Missett. Like so many dance-based programs that have come along since then, it was launched in a dance studio rather than in a gym. In 1972, she was teaching it in a YMCA gym, and it spread quickly. It was the first program to franchise its instructors, and although it is now a multimillion-dollar corporation, Missett still leads classes and choreographs a new routine every 10 weeks to keep classes varied and lively. Classes use a musical medley of jazz, pop, country, funk, and classics as a backdrop for an ever-evolving routine.

The basic format is a warm-up, 30 minutes of aerobic exercise that's a blend of jazz dance and studio exercises, a strength segment using hand

Quote, Unquote

"People have an innate desire to jump up and down like little kids on Mom and Dad's bed. It helps bring the fun into fitness."

—JB Berns, Urban Rebounding creator

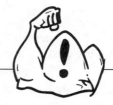

Fit Tip

If you took dance classes as a kid (or always wanted to), look for adults-only ballet, tap, modern dance, and jazz classes offered by many dance studios. Many studios even offer beginner classes.

weights, and a cool-down with stretching. Jazzercise formats now include Jazzercise Plus, which is similar to the original but in a 90-minute version; Simply Jazzercise, a toned-down program for beginners; Jazzercise Lite, which is for beginners, seniors, pregnant women, and significantly overweight exercisers; and even Musical Chairs Jazzercise, a seated exercise using light weights or resistance for people of all ages with limited mobility.

Jazzercise boasts of being the world's largest dance-fitness program, with 19,000 classes a week offered in all 50 states and 38 countries. More than 13 million participants have taken Jazzercise classes in its three decades, and some 450,000 people a week do now. The trend that Jazzercise set off continues to this day with styles of music and movement to suit various tastes.

You Gotta Dance!

Dance-based classes done to ethnic music of all kinds are especially appealing to young people who love to work out to strong, loud music and a prominent beat. In many locations, these classes attract a greater proportion of guys than the traditional aerobics sessions. The freeform street and dance-club scenes, such as hip-hop and funk, have morphed into full-on choreographed routines designed to provide a quality aerobics workout. These energetic classes are full of funky moves with a city-savvy attitude, and they are done to a strong rap or funk beat. Some instructors direct their classes to beginners, but many feature complicated choreography and can be very difficult to follow unless you've been doing it for a while.

Classes based on hip-hop, Latino, and swing sounds are less structured and often vary more from instructor to instructor. Other classes are based on African rhythms or traditional Latin dances, such as the merengue, rumba, cha-cha, and salsa. There are even cross-cultural fusion routines such as Hip-Hop Italiano, Latino Groove, and Afro-Brazilian Cardio! The music and the energy carry classes through high-intensity but usually low-impact workouts. Other classes are less intense and have more to do with suppleness and toning than heavy-duty cardio work. Examples include belly-dancing and hula, which not only help cardiovascular endurance but also help develop a strong and supple torso.

Inspiration for variety in aerobics routines never ends. Tinixing, developed by trainers Amy Roman and Lorie Lewis, is based on a Philippine pole dance called tinikling. Instead of bamboo poles placed on the ground, participants arrange pliable 42-inch poles called Tinix Stix on a gym floor in the forms of boxes, ladders, crosses, and stacks. In each choreographed routine, participants step over, jump over, weave through, and step around the poles in a variety of patterns to enhance cardio fitness, plyometric conditioning, and agility. It's a little like souped-up hopscotch with changing patterns rather than chalk boxes on the sidewalk. Offshoots include Tinix Stations, a circuit class; Interval Stix for advanced aerobic conditioning; Sport Stix, which was inspired by athletic drills; Stix for Kids; and Stix N Kix, a combination of Tinix Stix and kickboxing. For more information, contact TriEd Fitness at 703-455-1896 or www.TriEdFit.com.

The Classics

Some people who studied dance as youngsters stay with it to remain active and supple, while others find that returning to dance is satisfying both physically and aesthetically. Many studios offer adult ballet, jazz, modern, and tap classes for beginners and experienced dancers—although you won't find many adult beginner ballet dancers en pointe! Most studios stick to traditional dance forms, but in this mix-and-max era, dance-based hybrids are also available in some places.

And then there's the joy of social dancing, available in such places as dance studios, clubs, and singles' and couple's organizations. Cheek-to-cheek slow dancing is romantic, but you'll rev up your heartbeat with more energetic dances. Swing, tango and other Latin dances, the second running of disco dancing, square dancing, and anything else that gets you really moving is good exercise.

Watery Workouts

Aquatic exercise is booming. It provides year-round indoor exercise and is a fine way to stay cool in summer or at a tropical resort. More than the comfort of being underwater, however, aquatic exercise is the ultimate impact-free exercise that is kind to the joints and is good for cardio endurance as well as strengthening and toning (see Chapter 8, "Iron-Free Resistance Training"). It is popular among older exercisers and is a topnotch method of rehabilitation after an injury, because it minimizes the loss of both cardiovascular endurance and muscle strength even before the injury is healed.

Aquatic exercise is not swimming. Developed by physical therapists for rehabilitation, to help people with chronic physical conditions, and to speed injured athletes' postinjury recovery and training, it has grown into a family of pool-exercise programs. There are two basic body positions. In shallow water, exercises are done with the body in a vertical position and feet on the pool bottom, water at chest level. In deep water, participants use flotation equipment because they cannot touch the bottom. These exercises range from underwater jogging to aqua aerobics, underwater yoga, and others.

Quote, Unquote

"The whole process with my trainer led me back to ballet (which I studied for eight years). I love it so much. Now, instead of worrying what my muscles are doing, I'm worrying about how graceful I am and whether I can hold my positions."

—Portia de Rossi, actress

Keep cool and be kind to your joints with an aqua-aerobics class.

(Photo: Courtesy of Aquatic Exercise Association)

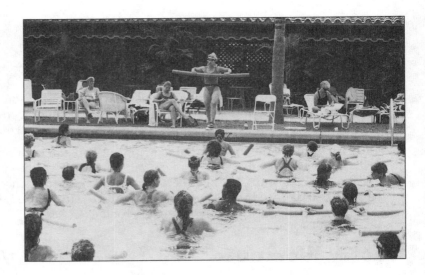

Because your body is buoyant in water, impact on the joints is far less than on land. At the same time, water is more resistant than air, so your muscles work harder just to move through the medium. Because the water's resistance is constant, you work opposing muscles in a balanced way as you move a limb through the water. Some exercisers like to work out until the perspiration drips from their brows. Some people hate it. Water cools more efficiently than air, so even in a comfortable 80- to 85-degree pool, you will not heat up as much. If you do heat up some, the water rinses the perspiration away.

Just as there are many versions of dry-land exercises, aquatic programs come in an assortment of styles to meet different goals. To increase your cardiovascular health and use underwater exercise for weight management, look for classes that focus primarily on using the legs, such as jogging underwater and aqua-aerobics classes. You'll need a flotation belt, and you also might want finlike resistance gloves for your hands and paddles for your ankles as you get stronger. Special shoes to provide traction on the bottom of the pool also are useful.

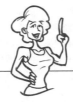

Fitness Fact

In 1995, 4.1 million Americans participated in pool exercise programs. By 1999, the figure had risen to 10 million, according to the Aquatic Fitness Association of America.

Put It All Together with Combo Workouts

The late 1970s saw the introduction of a workout called The Firm, which combined an aerobics circuit with light weight training. This two-in-one program that used hand weights for strength training and aerobic conditioning captured the public's imagination. Tens of thousands of tapes were sold. Now the concept of hybrid routines is so accepted that most gyms offer some kind of combination classes—often several. Generically called circuit training, cardio-strength training, cardio-sculpting, or something similar, these classes intertwine cardio and strength training. They usually are action-packed and lively, providing a two-for-one punch that experienced exercisers often crave.

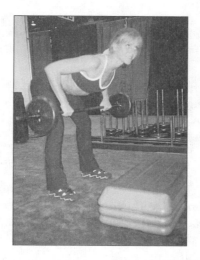

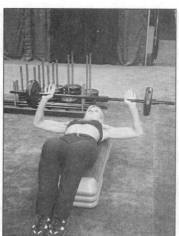 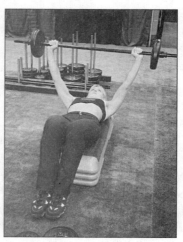

Weight-train to the music during Body Pump, a free-weight program originated in New Zealand.

(Photos: Claire Walter)

At their most basic level, many aerobics classes have at least some element of combination workouts, often ending with some ab exercises and perhaps pushups. Other popular combinations include aerobics or step-aerobics routines supplemented with segments using hand weights, stretch bands, fit balls, or other strength-training aids during some or most of the workout. More recent developments combine aerobic routines or even aquatic programs with yoga postures and moves. All of these inject an element of cross-training benefit into exercise classes.

The most common combo classes involve circuit training, but instructors are dreaming up other hybrids all the time. Classes can be quite intense, because they alternate aerobic and strength work in rapid-fire succession. Most routines include weight-training and aerobics apparatus—and often mats and the floor as well—for anywhere from 30 seconds to three to five minutes per exercise. When the instructor calls a command or blows a whistle, everyone shifts to the next exercise. Watching it is like looking at a mad-dash fire drill or a game of musical chairs. Participating makes the clock spin fast.

Such combination routines might make purists shudder, but some of these hybrids might capture your fancy and work for you. Your gym might offer the following trademarked combination workouts. When the programs are successful, local instructors sometimes develop knockoffs with different names and somewhat different moves. Tapes often are available so you can do these routines at home. Here is a sampling of the trademarked, franchised, and licensed hybrid programs you might find:

➤ BodyAttack, BodyFlow, BodyPump, and RPM comprise the BodyTraining family of programs promoted by The Step Company to bring club-to-club consistency to popular kinds of programs, sometimes with an interdisciplinary spin. BodyPump originated in New Zealand, where an instructor named Les Mills began choreographing a free-weight program, thereby adding the energy and motivational music of aerobics to the strength components of pumping iron. For more details, log on to www.bodypump.com.

➤ The Step Company added a choreographed kickboxing program called BodyAttack, a routine combining elements of yoga, Pilates, and mind-body training called BodyFlow, a retro-step class called BodyStep, and a studio cycling class called RPM. For more details, call 1-800-SAY-STEP.

➤ The Burst 'n' Boost circuit, developed by a Canadian trainer named Peggy Cleland, alternates high-intensity intervals (strength and speed, quickness, and good reaction time) and with lower-intensity intervals ("recovery intervals" and body sculpting). For more details, call 416-782-2456.

➤ Esprit de Danse was developed by Stephanie Herman. As a professional dancer, she performed ballet, modern dance, and jazz dance, and she also studied Pilates, the Alexander and Feldenkrais techniques, tai chi, yoga, and other disciplines. Building on a Pilates foundation but drawing from other fields, she calls her basic program Fitness Through Conscious Movement. It combines alignment, breathing, balance, and control into a vigorous but no-impact choreographed routine that challenges the body and the mind. Advanced routines include Heartbeat Ballet, Muscle Ballet, Muscle Ballet Weight Training, and Stretch and Feel It. For more details, call 1-800-775-1580 or log on to www.ijs.com/dance.

➤ Jazzercise has spawned the following hybrid programs: Body Sculpting Jazzercise with additional ab, arm, and leg muscle toning; Circuit Training Jazzercise, which adds strength training with weights, resistance tubes, and balls; and Step by Jazzercise, which adapts popular choreography to a step format. For more details and information about other Jazzercise formats, call 1-800-FIT-IS-IT or log on to www.jazzercise.com.

➤ YogaFit was developed by Beth Shaw, who is certified as an Integrative Yoga Therapist, a Cycle Reebok instructor, and a massage technician, to bridge the gap she felt existed between the mental discipline of yoga and the physical workout that many exercisers desire. It has been described as "an athletic approach to yoga." The routine features basic yoga postures put together in a sequence for cardio conditioning, and it is followed by a cool-down that stresses meditation. For more details, call 1-888-786-3111 or log on to www.yogafit.com.

➤ Dancer and instructor Jessica Sherwood developed Balletbootcamp, which combines stretching, warm-up, abdominal work, an upper-body aerobics segment inspired by military boot camp drills, traditional ballet exercises done at the barre, and a simple choreographed ballet routine into a fairly rigorous, total-body workout.

Whether they are done in a class setting or from a tape, such combinations of seemingly contrary disciplines provide cross-training opportunities and keep interest high.

The Least You Need to Know

➤ All aerobics workouts should start with a warm-up and end with a cool-down.

➤ Exercising to music keeps classes lively and interest high.

➤ Plyometrics are not suitable for most beginning exercisers, because they require strength and a high degree of cardiovascular fitness.

➤ Both trademarked and generic exercise programs are available at most gyms and health clubs. Trademarked programs are nationally franchised routines, while generic programs are designed by local instructors.

➤ Combination programs combine aerobics and strength training.

Part 4

Fitness Is More Than Just Working Out

Fitness for its own sake will help you to live longer and healthier, and that alone is worthwhile. But that's just part of the picture. Fitness is the means to an enhanced quality of life as long as you live. It will allow you to enjoy the physical aspects of life too. You may find a vacation to a health and fitness spa to be an effective way to jump-start a fitness program, which you can then continue at home. You can join a gym or health club, for these facilities are designed, equipped, and staffed to provide a variety of exercise opportunities, notably strength training and aerobic conditioning. You can also work out at home, while you are traveling, and even in some enlightened business settings.

Housework and yardwork, when done with energy, can enhance your quest for fitness. Once you get into a routine, you will find that outdoor activities, sports, and adventure travel that might have seemed impossible to keep up with are now within your capabilities. You'll be able to take a hike, play a game of tennis, or walk or cycle through exotic or beautiful vacation destinations. No matter what your starting point, you will be surprised at all of the things you can do when you add physical activity to your life.

Dieting without exercising or exercising without dieting is only a half-way measure to achieving good health. It takes changing your lifestyle to become trimmer, fitter, and more able to take on life's challenges and take advantage of its opportunities.

"Courage is very important. Like a muscle, it is strengthened by use."
—*actress Ruth Gordon*

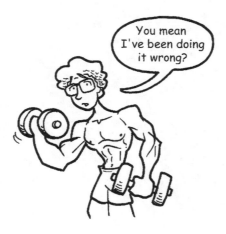

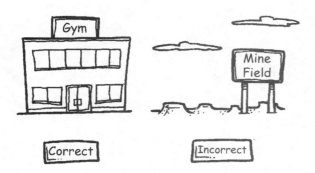

Where to Work Out

People who want to embark on a fitness program are confronted with an array of choices, not the least of which is where to exercise. You might prefer to exercise in the privacy of your own home, and if you have the space and the finances to outfit a home gym, you can work out any time you want. On the other hand, you might be the sociable type who craves the buzz and bodies of a health club or gym. Maybe you're a business traveler who's on the road more than you're at home. Or you might simply be one of the confused new exercisers who wants a routine but doesn't quite know how to go about launching a new lifestyle.

Jump-Starting Your Workout

The choices of where, when, and how to exercise can be so overwhelming, especially to a new exerciser, that it sometimes seems easier not to do anything at all. If you can get away for a fitness vacation, you will get a fitness assessment, a suitable exercise program, perhaps an eating plan, and most important, the positive reinforcement and encouragement of fitness pros who want you to start off right. The health and fitness experts at Arizona's Canyon Ranch say that you are a candidate for a spa vacation if you have made one or more of the following resolutions:

➤ To get your weight under control

➤ To improve your eating habits

➤ To quit smoking

➤ To learn to deal with stress

➤ To reduce your risk of heart disease

➤ To make a change in your life

➤ To learn to live a healthier lifestyle

➤ To make health a priority

➤ To have a fun and healthy vacation

➤ To relax, refresh, and renew

➤ To go hiking and biking

➤ To enjoy outdoor sports and activities

➤ To lose a few pounds

➤ To exercise and eat right

➤ To get away from it all

➤ To become aware of foods for healthy living

➤ To have an annual physical

Here are some examples of the range of fitness vacations now being offered:

➤ **Fit Camp.** Think of cruising as a weight-gaining vacation? Think again. Body-building champion Greta Blackburn directs shipboard fitness vacations that include all sorts of classes, motivational and informational seminars, and active shore excursions. For more information, call 1-800-727-2888 or log on to www.fitcamp.com.

➤ **Global Fitness Adventures.** Though headquartered shipboard in Aspen, Colorado, this is actually a moveable fitness feast, offering its hiking-oriented fitness vacations in venues from the Rockies to the Caribbean. There's no gym component to these outdoorsy itineraries that include anywhere from six to 18 miles of hiking a day, plus horseback riding, rafting, or other sports where available. Founder Kristina Hurrell also adds a good dose of yoga, meditation, group energy, and fine, low-fat fare into the mix. For more information, call 1-800-488-8748.

➤ **Mountain Trek Fitness Retreat & Health Spa.** A rustic 16-room lodge on Lake Kootenay in southeastern British Columbia is the setting for a holistic health and fitness retreat that specializes in jump-starting guests' introduction to healthy eating and exercise. Yoga with master Nateshvar Ken Scott, hiking, mountain biking, kayaking, a daily massage, and access to a nearby hot spring are featured activities. The fit who want to get fitter can sign up for Tesh Trek Challenge Boot Camp Week. This is a coed camp, but it does offer a women-only weight-loss retreat. For more information, call 1-800-661-5161 or log on to www.hiking.com.

➤ **Mountain Tune-Up Mini Spa.** Four-day summer programs at Keystone, Colorado, combine such outdoor activities as hiking and biking with low-fat cooking and relaxation techniques. Groups of beginning, intermediate, and advanced exercisers go at different paces and sometimes follow different itineraries. The program is directed by ex-Olympic cross-country ski racer Jana Hlavaty, now in her 50s and still a superlatively conditioned athlete. For more information, call 1-800-438-7251.

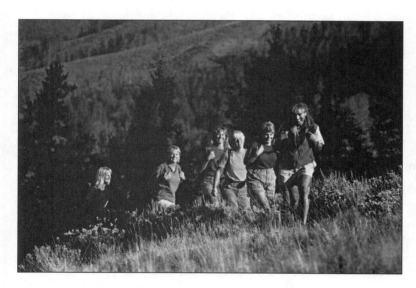

Fitness vacation programs such as the Mountain Tune-Up Mini Spa can build camaraderie while hiking in the mountains and are for women of all fitness levels.

(Photo: Courtesy of Keystone Resort)

➤ **Red Mountain.** This resort in southern Utah's spectacular canyon country specializes in fitness vacations. It combines medical and fitness evaluation capabilities with a choice of routes to start or enhance a fitness program: excellent gym facilities, an array of classes, holistic nutrition programs, outdoor activities such as guided hikes and power walks, and spa services. For more information, call 1-800-407-3002.

➤ **Sun Valley Mountain Wellness.** This Memorial Day weekend festival of good, healthful living and healing at last count featured more than 65 free fitness and wellness activities. These activities include a run/walk event, wilderness hiking, and fitness classes, as well as such newly rediscovered practices as Feng Shui, crystal healing, meditation, Reiki, and others. For more information, contact the Sun Valley-Ketchum (Idaho) Chamber of Commerce at 1-800-634-3347 or www.visitsunvalley.com.

➤ **The Ashram.** This long-running fitness spa in Calabasas, California, began offering New Age mind and body conditioning when the New Age was truly new. It still is a leader in the field. Simple accommodations, a vegetarian menu, 10 to 15 miles of mountain-hiking a day, and yoga form the framework for this spartan spa. The feel-good reward is a daily massage. For more information, call 818-222-6900.

➤ **Tone & Tan.** This one-day program at the National Hotel in Miami's trendy South Beach area includes a one-hour workout with a personal trainer, a one-hour outdoor massage in a private garden alcove, and unlimited use of the hotel's pool and beach. For more information, call 1-800-327-8370 or log on to www.nationalhotel.com.

➤ **Walking the World.** Ward Luthi offers more than two-dozen international trips a year for travelers over age 50. (He calls his clientele "50 and better.") The trips, led by local guides and accompanied by a company representative, appeal to people who want to hike in beautiful environments and also learn about other countries and cultures, step by step. Difficulty levels vary, but they range from easy to moderate trips for relatively new walkers to arduous, high-altitude treks for fit and experienced hikers. For more information, call 1-800-340-9255 or log on to www.walkingtheworld.com.

➤ **Women's Quest.** World-class triathlete Colleen Cannon runs this summer program at Winter Park, Colorado, for beginning to experienced female runners who want to become fit (or fitter). It combines physical and mental training for athletic endeavors with New Age nostrums. Running is at the core of the program, which also includes yoga and singing to help participants "follow their bliss." For more information, call 303-545-9295, or log on to www. womensquest.com.

If you are going on a fitness vacation—or are just hiking or mountain biking—at high elevations, be alert to altitude sickness. Mild symptoms include shortness of breath, sleeplessness, and headache. Nausea, loss of appetite, and insomnia are signs of more acute mountain sickness. Most symptoms disappear after a few days, especially if you avoid alcohol and caffeine and drink plenty of water. If that fails, the cure is retreating to a lower elevation. If you have difficulty breathing and develop a cough, however, see a doctor, because these are symptoms of pulmonary edema, a more serious condition.

Gym-Dandy Clubs

If you have no trouble getting yourself out of the house, gyms and health clubs are exemplary venues for working out. After all, that's why they're there. They are equipped and staffed to help you get into shape. For in-depth information about different kinds of clubs, see Chapter 21, "A Primer on Gyms."

Fresh Air and Sunshine

Going for a daily walk or run can become the core of your fitness regime, or you might want to stay in shape with such outdoor activities as bicycling, in-line skating, tennis, or heavy yard work. They all carry the image of clean air and sunshine, but the great outdoors isn't always so great. Polluted air, heavy traffic, and uncomfortable humidity are among the factors that can drive all but the most dedicated outdoor exercisers indoors, and overexposure to the sun has been established as a health hazard.

If you live in a city with bad air pollution, try to schedule outdoor activities such as walking, running, cycling, or in-line skating as early in the morning as possible. The *University of California at Berkeley Wellness Letter* also recommends breathing through your nose rather than your mouth to decrease the amount of pollutants that actually reach your lungs. Traffic is a major cause of the problem. The daily pollution index is therefore likely to be at its lowest at dawn. However, if you have allergies, exercising outdoors in the morning can be problematic because that's when the pollen count is the highest. Less vehicular traffic equals safer cycling and running as well. From an air-quality standpoint, the worst possible time to exercise outdoors is during rush hour, especially the afternoon rush.

Quote, Unquote

"Everybody is an athlete, and we just help them find it."

—Colleen Cannon, triathlete and director, Women's Quest fitness camps

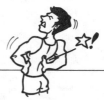

Achtung!

The air can be particularly bad in the summer. That's when sunlight and warm weather work on nitrogen oxide and organic compounds in the air to produce ozone, which can cause or exacerbate respiratory problems.

How can you deal with these problems and still exercise outdoors? You'll have to adapt your program. Instead of city streets, you can walk, run, or bike in a park, on a recreational path, or on a promenade along a river, lake, or seashore, because the plants partially counteract the pollutants in the air. If you live in a polluted city and also are allergic to pollen, your best solution might be to exercise indoors during the week and to escape to the country on weekends for outdoor activities.

Because all the exercise in the world won't ward off melanoma, use sunscreen when you are exercising outdoors. To be most effective, sunscreen should be put on at least 20 minutes before you go out into the sun. Experts say that if you are medium- to dark-skinned, use SPF 15; if you are fair-skinned, SPF 20 or higher is better. Apply it to your face, neck, ears, arms, hands, legs, and any exposed parts of your chest and back. Reapply every four hours for dry-land activities and every two hours if you are swimming. In the summer, 50 percent of the injurious ultraviolet rays hit between 10 A.M. and 2 P.M.

Setting Up a Home Gym

If you'd rather keep your workouts to yourself, creating a home gym is a feasible option. Today, you can find a myriad of fitness equipment designed for the home. "Two of the major pitfalls I see clients falling into are one, not spending enough money to get quality; and two, buying something new and different on impulse without trying it out first to see how well it works," cautions Angela Renee Settle, President, Settle for the Best, Inc., a fitness consulting firm.

Just like equipment that you can find at a gym, some machines are designed to improve cardiovascular fitness (stationary bikes, treadmills, rowing machines, NordicTracks, stairsteppers, or climbers) and others are used for strength training (free weights, weight machines, bands, and tubing). Before you buy anything, realistically assess your fitness goals so you can look for the equipment that will help you meet them. A piece of fitness apparatus will quickly become an eyesore in your bedroom if it remains unused.

Here are some tips for setting up your home gym:

Quote, Unquote

"In your home, every inch counts. Everybody wants equipment to be invisible."

—Richard Miller, president, The Gym Source, a large fitness retailer

➤ **Evaluate.** Before buying anything, evaluate the space you plan to use. Try to set up your workout space in a room that you truly want to spend time in. Measure the space available, write the measurements down, and take your tape measure with you when you go to look at equipment. Make sure the equipment you want fits into the space that you have. Remember to measure vertical space as well as floor space. Some equipment folds up, but if you have particularly low ceilings or hanging plants in the room that will be your gym, some apparatus may be a little too tall.

➤ **Test.** Wear workout gear or something loose and comfortable to the store and try out the apparatus you are interested in. Test not only the equipment you think you'll buy, but take a little time to try out other types of machines as well.

If the store carries several brands, check them all out, and have the salesperson go over the features of each so that you can evaluate the cost-benefit ratio of each model. Even if you don't think you'd want a particular machine, you might find that you like it when you try it.

➤ **Shop wisely.** Buy for value, not just price. Don't automatically go for the cheapest equipment, because a flimsy apparatus won't be as smooth or as enjoyable to use as a quality model. By the same token, don't be sucked into purchasing a high-end training apparatus that has features you'll never use. Think about what you need and make sure that your choice is going to work well and last for a long time. The old adage "You get what you pay for" also applies to gym equipment.

➤ **Find bargains.** Expertise, warranties, and the opportunity to comparison shop are good reasons to make such a high-ticket purchase as exercise apparatus from a reputable dealer. However, it may be beyond your budget to buy that way—even if the store is running a sale. New equipment is available at discount stores, but it generally is of lower quality than at dealers specializing in sports or workout products, and the sales staff at big-box chains can be spectacularly unknowledgeable about exercise equipment. You can find used equipment at garage sales; listed in your local newspaper's Classified section; and even in thrift stores such as the Salvation Army, Goodwill, or your local hospital auxiliary or other charity. The price will be right, and you might score the deal of a workout lifetime. Or the equipment might be abused, worn-out, or simply unsuitable for you. You can't comparison shop, there are no guarantees, and you won't have any recourse but to try to sell or donate the apparatus if it doesn't work for you.

➤ **Inquire.** Ask questions about warranties when you make a purchase. A reputable dealer often will give you a trial period during which you can use the equipment at home for, say, 30 days and then return it for a full refund or merchandise credit if it isn't right for you. Also ask about repair and maintenance policies. Again, the dealer should have a trained technician available to handle repairs and maintenance.

➤ **Set the tone.** Set up your equipment in an area you enjoy being in. Setting things up in a dark, cold, and uninviting basement is a formula for procrastination, excuses, and possibly failure to meet your goals. If your gym area is part of your regular living space, think of creative ways to make it look good when not in use. Decorating ideas include a plant on wheelers, a decorative Japanese shoji screen, or a folding screen that can partition the room and easily go in front of the machine when not in use.

➤ **Entertain yourself.** Make your TV, VCR, and stereo accessible in your workout area. You might want the TV on rollers so you can see it easily while you work out. If you have a VCR, you might want to work out to exercise tapes. Make sure

you have remote controls for all your media so you can change the station or adjust the volume without interrupting your workout.

➤ **Protect the floor.** Place some kind of rubber matting under your cardiovascular equipment so that sweat does not drip onto your floor or carpet.

➤ **See yourself.** A full-size mirror can be useful in your workout area so you can watch your form while you are lifting weights or doing aerobics or yoga. Many home exercisers enjoy working out in front of a mirror.

➤ **Make it social.** Invite a friend over to work out with you. It is good to have camaraderie; it can help both of you to be honest with your commitments and meet your goals.

The Fitness Products Council of the Sporting Goods Manufacturers Association publishes a booklet called "How to Buy Exercise Equipment for the Home." Request it by writing to Publications, Fitness Products Council, 200 Castlewood Drive, North Palm Beach, Florida 33408.

Fitness Fact

Forty-five percent of people with home offices surveyed by *Income Opportunities* magazine said that they exercise more often working at home than they did when they left the house for their jobs.

Looking at equipment that stands idle can be unmotivating in and of itself, so make the effort to create your home gym in a space you will want to spend time in and make sure you buy equipment you want to use. Then enjoy not having to go anywhere to get your workout. To get you going on the right track and to motivate you, you might want to invest in a few personal fitness trainer sessions as soon as you have set up your home gym. Some equipment dealers even offer a complimentary personal training session with your purchase, so be sure to inquire during the purchasing process.

In addition to the conventional manual, many companies that market home-exercise equipment also make videotapes to help people use their products. Some firms—especially those that market high-ticket items—will send a complimentary video in advance to show how it works; others send the tape along with the product.

Stairs, Chairs, and Other At-Home "Apparatus"

You actually don't need to invest a penny to work out at home. Chances are, your home already is equipped with the basics that can be adapted easily for important exercises. Stairs, furniture, and even a blank wall are useful, particularly for lower-body work.

A straight chair can provide a change of position when you want to work your abdominals. Lie on a mat or a carpeted floor on your back and in front of a straight chair. Place your thighs at a right angle to your upper body and your calves on the seat of the chair. If you are short-legged, you might want to rest the soles of your feet against the front of the chair seat. From this extended Z-shape, you can effectively do abdominal crunches. You can do both straight lifts to work the rectus abdominus and twisting lifts (shoulder toward opposite knee) to work the obliques.

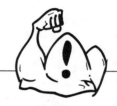

Fit Tip

As you would in a gym, start each exercise with 10 repetitions of each exercise (or on each side, for leg work). Try to do two or three sets of each exercise, resting for a minute between sets. Work up to 15 and then 20 reps per set.

Exercise instructors often have participants line up at the ballet barre to work their hamstrings. The back of a chair can serve the same function. Stand behind it and hold on to the back of the chair for balance while you do hamstring curls with or without ankle weights. To strengthen your quadriceps and tone your inner thighs, again stand behind the chair. Hold on to the back, turn your feet out as far as is comfortable (ballet's second position, if that reference is a useful image), and with your weight centered, sink down in a plié, keeping your back straight and making sure your knees do not extend beyond your ankles. Come up again.

Another way to work the quadriceps is a partial sit. Standing in front of the chair with your feet pointing forward and shoulder-width apart, hold your hands out in front of you and slowly sit down—but don't really sit down. Just as your backside grazes the seat, come up again slowly and in control. You can use an armless chair or a solid, low stool (not a high barstool) for some of the upper-body exercises you would do on a bench at the gym. Sit straight with your feet flat on the floor, as if at the end of a weight bench, to do seated exercises with hand weights to work the biceps, triceps, deltoids, and upper back.

You can even use a plain wall to strengthen your quads. See the example of the wall-sit in Chapter 8, "Iron-Free Resistance Training." Some exercise enthusiasts keep space available next to their wall-mounted telephones so they can do this effective exercise while chatting.

A staircase also can be an exercise tool. You can do laps on a flight of stairs, being careful to maintain your footing. This does not provide the constant climbing motion of a stairstepper, but alternating the ascent and the descent does work your leg muscles in different ways. Carry a set of weights if you want to increase the workload. Start with five to 10 minutes of going up and down the stairs. If you live in a high-rise apartment building, all the better, because you can go up and down many stairs.

You also can use the bottom step as if it were a bench or a step in a gym. Stand two to three feet in front of the bottom step. Step one foot forward onto the bottom step and lunge, rising on the toes of your back foot and taking care not to move your front knee farther forward than your ankle. Repeat using the other gastrocnemius leg. To strengthen your gastrocnemius, the big calf muscle, stand with the front half of your feet on the bottom step and your heels hanging off the step. Rise onto your toes and then slowly allow your heels to drop below the level of the step (keeping your legs straight but without locking the knees). Change foot positions—feet parallel, toes in, heels in—to work the different parts of the calf muscles.

Workplace Workouts

Enlightened companies that recognize the increased productivity and morale of employees who exercise often help make working out easier. Many find a side benefit to be a lower absentee rate, because fit employees call in sick less frequently. Some companies install workout rooms and showers in the building. Some subsidize employees' health-club memberships or at least arrange for group discounts at nearby gyms. Club Fit in White Plains, New York, offers classes to employees at the nearby headquarters of IBM, and across the country in Seattle, Microsoft employees are eligible for good rates at nearby health clubs. Not surprisingly, sports-oriented companies are most enlightened about the range of fitness perks they can offer employees:

➤ Based in Berkeley, California, Clif Bar, Inc., has an on-site gym featuring a 22-foot climbing wall. It also supplies personal trainers for every one of their 80 employees. When this manufacturer of energy bars became a sponsor of a series of long-distance bicycle rides to raise money for AIDS-HIV causes, it offered to pay the airfare and accommodations for any employee who participated, it did not count the race as vacation time, and it helped employees who didn't have suitable bikes get a good deal on them.

➤ Based in Aspen, Colorado, skiwear manufacturer Sport Obermeyer encourages employees to follow the example of its octogenarian founder, Klaus Obermeyer, who plays 90 minutes of tennis every day—taking some of his staff with him—and, in the winter, heads to nearby Aspen to make some turns. Obermeyer believes that people need time off during the day to work out, run, ski, or pursue other athletic activities, and he feels this makes for better employees. In the winter, Sport Obermeyer offers each worker four "Powder Days" per season. When it snows more than four inches the night before, employees can make arrangements with their supervisors to ski from lift opening until noon. The company also has a solar-heated lap pool on site (Obermeyer swims every day), and there is a hiking and biking trail nearby. Employees are encouraged to develop a workout plan that works for them, and to work with their supervisor to fit it into their schedule.

Businesses from accounting firms to zoning and planning consultation companies can offer their employees fitness facilities. Some companies put in their own workout rooms; others find buildings that are so equipped. Dallas-based Goodbody's Fitness Centers, for example, operate workout facilities with health club–quality equipment and classes in new high-rise office towers in several cities. Developers and building managers view such centers as worthwhile amenities that attract commercial tenants willing to pay top dollar for space.

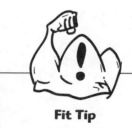

Fit Tip

Join a gym near your workplace and use it at least three times a week—before work, after work, or during your midday lunch break.

Fitness on the Road

Travel, especially for business, tends to throw people off their routine. Try not to let it happen. When your routine is off, so are you. Although exercising might be the last thing you feel like doing when you get back after a long day of travel, classes, or meetings, it probably is the best thing you can do for yourself. Always bring basic gear with you. Barbara Udell, director of Stress Management and Lifestyle at the Florida Pritikin Center, suggests packing your workout wear last, so that it's the first thing you see when you unzip your bag at your destination.

In addition to your workout clothes, shoes, and a bathing suit, which always should be on your to-bring list, you can take along such lightweight devices as a jump rope, rubber resistance bands, and perhaps even an aerobics video that you can use if your hotel room has a VCR. They don't take up much space in your suitcase. Keeping up with your fitness program can get your blood flowing, stretch out your muscles, help you sleep better in a strange bed, and even reduce stress. Your workout might not be up to your home standards, but consistency is still the key. Some workout is better than no workout.

Get a Plan

You can plan your workout schedule while you are on the plane or when you get to your hotel, and it can fit around your schedule of meetings, seminars, or classes. Write it in your scheduler as if it were a business appointment. Setting an exercise schedule increases the chances you will do it instead of finding an excuse not to.

Most hotels, especially those geared toward business travelers, have some type of fitness center on their premises. Some hotels have sizable, state-of-the-art workout facilities; others stash a treadmill and a weight machine in a guest room at the end of a long hallway. Hotel swimming pools are usually too small for swimming laps, but you can use yours to do some aquatic exercises. Inquire about your hotel's workout facility when you check in and check it out as part of the routine of getting settled. Be sure to note the facility's hours and make your plans accordingly. Depending on the size of the facility, keep in mind that other travelers probably have the same idea as you do.

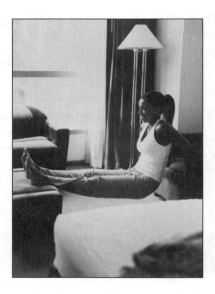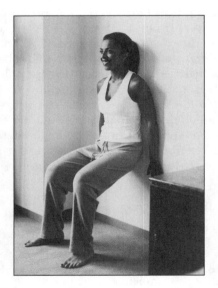

Unwind in your hotel room with some chair dips and wall-sits after a long day of meetings.

(Photos: Courtesy of Simonsen Says, Inc.)

A warm-up and 20 to 30 minutes of aerobics or strength-training is a good basic workout. Ask hotel employees to recommend good places nearby for a walk or a jog. If the weather is bad, try out your jump rope, hotel staircases, marching in place, or another activity you can think of to get your heart rate up a bit. You can alternate between any of these, repeating cycles until you have reached your time goals. Don't worry about what you look like strutting around the hotel's hallways and stairwells.

You are not the first and certainly will not be the last. Besides, all those other guests are strangers, so it really doesn't matter what they think. What they think might be admiration for your willpower and commitment.

Getting Down to Business

Working out in your room might be a choice, not a necessity. You might prefer to stay there for privacy, comfort, or to await an important phone call. Or your hotel may have no fitness center or a small, crowded one. Various sorts of exercises need no equipment at all, and a few use hotel furniture (see Chapter 8). You can ask a personal trainer to design an on-the-road workout routine that doesn't require any special equipment or that just requires a jump rope or an elastic exercise band or cord.

Because your room won't have an exercise mat, you can use a bath towel or a folded bedspread to cushion your hands and knees and to keep you off the carpet when you are doing floor work in a strange place. Any floor exercise you do on the floor at home or at the gym is fair game in your hotel room. You know how to do them, and if time is a problem, you can mix and match—but do something every day. Here are a few examples of in-room exercises:

Quote, Unquote

"I have never met an exercise obstacle I could not overcome .... Here's my travel formula: Pack an ordinary kitchen timer, place a hotel towel on the floor, park yourself in front of the radio or television, and set your clock for 3½ minutes per exercise. If you don't have much time, do a general warm-up followed by push-ups, abdominal crunches, gluteal squeezes, and a general cool-down."

—Margaret Richard, television host, *Body Electric*

➤ **Push-ups and crunches.** You know by now what these are. (If you have time for nothing else, crank out a couple sets of these basic exercises.)

➤ **Lunges.** This is another basic exercise that works your glutes, hamstrings, and quads and that requires no equipment at all. Stand with your hands on your hips, behind your neck, or hanging straight down and with your feet shoulder-width apart. Take a giant step forward and bend your knee to 90 degrees. (Your lower leg should be perpendicular to the floor.) Then push off again with the front leg and return to the starting position. Do four repetitions on each side, and then alternate.

➤ **Decline push-ups.** Use the desk chair in your room as a bench. Put your feet on the seat and your hands on the floor to do decline push-ups, which are an advanced and very effective workout for your chest, shoulders, and triceps.

➤ **Tricep dips.** Using the desk chair again, place both hands behind you on the seat and keep your feet under your knees. Lower your body until your butt is

231

just off the floor or straight out in front of you and your upper arms are parallel to the floor. Because this works your shoulders and triceps, it combines well with push-ups for a basic upper-body workout.

➤ **Back extension.** Stand with your feet shoulder-width apart and your hands behind your head. With your legs fairly straight (but without locking your knees) and your back straight, bend at the waist until your torso is parallel to the floor. Then slowly raise your torso from the hips. Alternatively, lie down prone (face down) on the floor, and simultaneously lift one arm and one leg a few inches off the floor, stretching rather than arching your back. Some people prefer raising the arm and leg on the same side, while others are more comfortable raising the opposite arm and leg. These no-equipment exercises stretch and strengthen your lower back, which is especially useful when you are traveling and have been carrying a heavy briefcase, a laptop, or carry-on luggage through airports and across sprawling parking lots.

➤ **Leg raises.** If you have an exercise band with you, put it around both ankles and lie on the floor on your side. Lean on one elbow or keep your torso on the floor. Raise your top leg slowly, as high as you can, and then lower it. Repeat on both sides. If you do not have a resistance band, try to improvise some type of ankle weight or put on the heaviest shoes you have with you and do the leg raises anyway. Just the weight of your own leg helps tone your outer and inner thighs.

➤ **Squats.** Stand with your legs shoulder-width apart and extend your arms straight out in front of you. Keep your arms in position and your heels on the ground as you bend your knees until your thighs are parallel with the ground.

➤ **Sit-ups.** Like crunches and push-ups, you can do sit-ups anywhere. Lie on the floor with your hands behind your neck. Sit up using your stomach muscles. Repeat and do any other version of sit-ups you have been practicing at home or in the gym.

➤ **Rope jumping.** A few minutes of jumping rope can rev up your heart and provide a quick cardio fix. You won't be able to do it in your room because of the low ceiling, but many suburban hotels have grassy lawns, and some high-rise city hotels have rooftop recreation facilities. If you jump rope around the pool, make sure that you find a nonslip surface to jump on—and remember that tiles don't give and are hard on the joints.

Another alternative for working out on the road is to see if your health club at home has any reciprocal memberships with clubs near your hotel. Check what the options are in your destination city before you depart. Some hotels make arrangements for you. Guests at The Phillips Club, a new boutique hotel in Manhattan, enjoy complimentary access to the nearby Reebok Sports Club/NY, a trendy 140,000-square-foot mega-club. The hotel's Fitness Package includes a one-hour private session with a personal trainer, eliminating any excuse not to work out while on business in the Big Apple, call 212-835-8800 or log on to www.phillipsclub.com. You'll probably be staying in a less-exclusive hotel, but wherever you are, the hotel concierge or front desk also will know if a nearby club offers day memberships to business travelers. YMCAs and recreation centers in many communities permit drop-ins, too.

According to a 1999 survey by Healthy Choice foods, American travelers found the following to be their greatest challenges for staying healthy while on the road: finding healthful foods at airports, 76 percent; maintaining normal eating habits, 61 percent; maintaining normal exercise routines, 59 percent; maintaining normal sleep routines, 59 percent; finding a time/place to exercise, 56 percent; finding healthful food at the destination, 54 percent. Fifty-nine percent of the respondents to *Travel & Leisure's* 1999 annual business travel survey said they use hotel gyms when traveling.

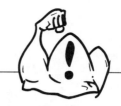

Fit Tip

Traveling on a plane tends to dehydrate your system. Resist the temptation to drink alcohol or caffeine on the plane and consume as much water as you can, even if it means wandering down the aisle to restrooms frequently.

The Least You Need to Know

➤ Set off on an exercise track with a fitness vacation, where you can have a program designed and get into the workout habit.

➤ Select equipment for your needs and establish a congenial environment to turn part of your home into a personal gym.

➤ Learn how to combine workouts with working to be more productive on the job and healthier in general.

➤ Build exercise into your business travel schedule to maintain your fitness level on the road.

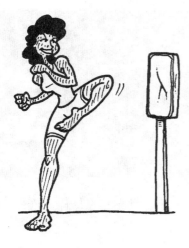

Chapter 17

Fight Your Way to Fitness

In This Chapter

➤ High interest in martial arts, thanks to Tae Bo's popularity

➤ The disciplined realm of traditional martial arts

➤ The demands of "real" boxing

➤ Fitness routines inspired by military training

Martial arts and fitness have a chicken-and-egg relationship. You need to be somewhat fit, strong, and flexible to get involved in most martial arts disciplines, yet practicing these programs will make you fitter, stronger, more focused, and more flexible. Martial arts have been around for centuries. They reflect warrior traditions as embodied in cultural rituals and military training in many Asian cultures. Karate, judo, and other disciplines have long had adherents in the West, but they were considered exotic by the general public.

The recent rise in popularity of Tae Bo, a dynamic kickboxing-inspired routine created by karate champ Billy Blanks, has put martial arts in the spotlight, and they now are in an unprecedented high position in the fitness world. Workouts based on boxing training, variations of aerobic kickboxing, and other routines are all the rage. They pack 'em in at health-club classes and sell videos like the proverbial hot cakes. These workouts tend to be so energetic that many aren't suitable for new exercisers just off the couch, but they provide interest and motivation to anyone in a fitness program—and in a rut.

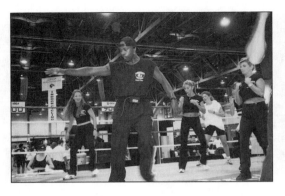
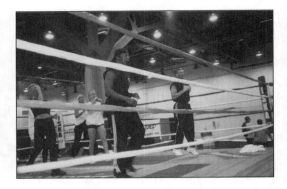

Former karate champ Billy Blanks created Tae Bo, the fitness craze he brought into the mainstream.

(Photos: Courtesy of Billy Blanks Tae Bo)

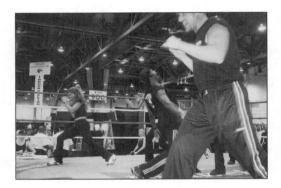

Aerobic kickboxing has become all the rage and is a good way for the fit to become fitter.

(Photo: Claire Walter)

How Martial Arts Can Improve Fitness

Fans claim that traditional and contemporary martial arts are good for just about everything from calorie-chomping, total-body workouts to spiritual enlightenment.

Martial arts have a long and honored tradition, especially in the Orient. Attention to physical and mental discipline is matched by the respect students have for masters and the ritual encounters with foes. Call them the original mind-body-spirit workouts. Some are ancient, with origins lost in the misty past. Others are more recent, even contemporary, and can be traced to specific masters who created them. Examination of the origins and intricacies of these disciplines is far beyond the scope of this book.

An Internet search of "martial arts" generated the following list of disciplines. Some of these are well-known; others are obscure. Just reading through them will give you an idea of how many varieties there are:

➤ Aikido

➤ Capoeira

➤ Choi Kwang-Do

➤ Chung Moo Doe

➤ Daito Ryu Aiki Bujutsu

➤ Gatka

➤ Hapkido

➤ Iaido

➤ Jeet Kune Do

➤ Judo

➤ Jujitsu

➤ Karate

➤ Kendo

➤ Krav Maga

➤ Kuk Sool Won

➤ Kumdo

➤ Kung Fu

➤ Kyudo

➤ Muay Thai

➤ Naginata

➤ Ninjutsu

➤ Pyong Hwa Do

➤ Savate

➤ Shintaido

➤ Shorinji Kempo

➤ Silat

➤ Tai Chi Chuan

➤ Tae Kwon Do

➤ Taido

➤ Tang Soo Do and Soo Bahk Do

➤ Vovinam Viet Vo Dao

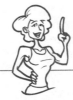

Fitness Fact

Three million Americans take classes in aikido, judo, karate, tae kwan do, and other disciplines in 18,000 martial arts schools, according to the Educational Funding Company.

Masters of these paths are strong of body, mind, and will, but getting there requires students to patiently travel a long and very specific road. If you want to learn self-defense, you might be a candidate to study traditional martial arts. You will get into shape step by step, but they all require more discipline to learn, more years of study to master, and more formality than many modern Americans are willing to invest. Millions of Americans have embarked on such arduous paths, but more of us look for excitement and quickly visible results. That's why the new breed of martial arts–based fitness programs is so popular.

An American Council on Exercise (ACE) handout says, "Kickboxing is a hybrid of boxing, martial arts, and aerobics that offers an intense cross-training and total-body workout. It blends a mixture of high-power exercise routines that strengthen the body and mind, decrease stress, and hone reflexes while increasing endurance and cardiovascular power. While kickboxing's roots are in full-contact fighting, it has found a safe and very effective niche in the fitness community."

Although some experts have embraced the invasion of these warrior ways overlaid with a hip-hop sassiness, others have reservations. The meteoric rise of aerobic kickboxing has been equaled by an increase in injuries, particularly various forms of back strain, hip problems, shoulder injuries, and other joint problems. Many people start doing aggressive moves before they are in shape for them, or they continue a routine when they should stop. Petra Robinson of the American Fitness Association characterizes aerobic kickboxing as "a program for the fitness elite. It's too intense for beginners."

Kickboxing

Most aerobic kickboxing classes begin with light stretches and a cardio warm-up before launching into the nitty-gritty. Typical routines include a series of repetitive punches, hand strikes, and kicks done rapidly to potent music, building to combinations of these three types of moves. Even though you are thrusting through the air rather than working against resistance, it qualifies as a total-body workout because it uses several muscle groups and is intensely aerobic. Classes end with a cool-down period.

The ACE cautions that "there are other important factors to consider before taking that first kick." Aerobic kickboxing can be effective and fun—if you're careful. Here are some tips for anyone embarking on this type of exercise program, but beginning exercisers need to be the most conservative of all:

➤ Consider your current level of fitness. Don't make an aggressive martial arts–based program your first foray into exercise.

➤ If you have arthritis, tight hamstrings, an inflexible back, or other physical limitations, you might not be a good candidate for aerobic kickboxing.

➤ Even if you are in good shape and participate in cross-training programs, take it easy until your body adapts to a new type of move.

➤ When you start, look for a beginner class, an introductory technique class, or a progressive class in which you learn the basic moves and do them until you are comfortable doing them at a moderate pace before putting them into fast combinations. If these classes are not available, at least find a class led by an instructor who includes beginner tips for all the moves and combinations.

➤ Among the basic moves are proper stance and how to punch and kick to avoid injury.

➤ If you use a tape to work out at home, start modestly and pay special attention to the instructions regarding proper form. Working out in a room with a mirror can help you see whether you are doing the moves correctly.

➤ Beginners especially should avoid high kicks until they get used to the routine and become more flexible.

➤ Do not lock your joints when throwing kicks or punches.

➤ Do not overextend kicks. Kick only as high as you can raise your leg while maintaining proper body alignment.

➤ Do not do too many repetitions of a single high-impact movement. Many experts consider eight one-foot hops to be the limit for most people.

➤ Do not wear weights or hold dumbbells when throwing punches; it jeopardizes your joints.

➤ Proper technique for each move is the key to injury prevention.

Quote, Unquote

"Any time that you strike the air with kicks or punches, you are working on speed and form. In order to develop the larger muscles, you have to have resistance. Hitting a heavy [punching] bag is similar to weight training because it provides resistance."

—Keith Vitall, former world karate champion

➤ Do not feel that you have to work out for the entire duration of a class. An hour is a long workout at such intensity.

➤ Do not give in to group peer pressure and exercise beyond fatigue.

Good Sense and Safety

Martial arts used for self-defense have a long history of time-tested training programs directed toward fighting an opponent. The newer and jazzier martial arts–inspired programs used for fitness are directed toward self-improvement, not besting an eventual opponent. When you participate in such a program to get in shape or lose weight, it might be choreographed, and in most, you have no opponent. This means you can practice the moves safely and in control with no surprises, which is a luxury that boxers in the ring and martial arts students don't have.

Because the energy of contemporary martial arts–based programs is so contagious and the promise of enhanced fitness so potent, people tend to get carried away. Even though these routines can help people get fit, doing too much, especially too soon, can cause injuries. Critics have warned of joint, ligament, and tendon damage. The key is to start these programs slowly and judiciously, focusing on proper body alignment. Before you make a move, set yourself up in a stable, balanced, and "rooted" position. Practice moves in slow motion, noting how each punch or kick originates by being drawn in to the core of your body. This readiness move is known as *chambering,* and it enables you to move strongly, accurately, cleanly, and with less chance of injury. The final step in each move is actually delivering the kick or punch to its real or visualized target. Ideally, a trained and knowledgeable instructor should correct you if you are doing a move in a way that might cause an injury.

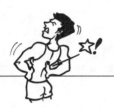

Achtung!

Ease into aerobic kickboxing programs. Stop when you are fatigued or if you feel twinges or pain where you shouldn't.

Basic Boxing and Martial Arts Moves

Like other forms of exercise, boxing and martial arts have their own moves. Here are some moves that might be wrapped into an exercise program based on various forms of fighting:

➤ Bobbing and weaving

➤ Punches with the right and left arms

➤ Hooks with the right and left arms, sometimes with a circular motion preliminary to the hook

➤ Uppercuts with the right and left arms

➤ Jabs with the right and left arms

➤ Combination punches

➤ Front kicks with the right and left legs

➤ Side kicks with the right and left legs

➤ Back kicks with the right and left legs

➤ Knee lifts or blocks with the right and left legs

➤ Combinations of punches and kicks

Tae One On

Tae Bo, undisputedly the hottest video workout of the late 1990s, was developed by charismatic martial artist Bill Blanks. Millions of videotapes have been sold, and a fleet of derivative workouts has been launched, but Blanks was no overnight sensation. He created the concept back in 1975, combining karate kicks and boxing jabs for his own training. Eventually, he added music to make the workout more fun, less martial, and more attractive to women.

The name Tae Bo comes from "tae," which means "leg" and relates to the kicks and lower-body aspect of the workout, and "bo," which is from "boxing" and relates to the punches and upper-body workout. It also is an acronym for Total Awareness Excellent Body Obedience.

Paula Abdul was the first celebrity to discover Tae Bo, but it soon was embraced by Hollywood stars and sports stars alike who flocked to Billy Blanks's World Training Center in Sherman Oaks, California. From there, it spread across the country via television infomercials, assimilation into health-club class rosters, and word of mouth. Drawing from such traditional martial arts as karate, kickboxing, and tae kwon do plus Western-style boxing, hip-hop, ballet, and weight training, this heavily promoted cardio and muscle workout changed the way people exercised at the very end of the twentieth century. Tae Bo is a sweat-raising exercise and is said to be as intense as step aerobics using an 8- to 12-inch bench. Its sharp, full-body moves also put it in the category of high-impact exercise. Blanks still teaches at his modest storefront studio, even though millions of Tae Bo tapes have been sold. For details, contact 1-800-22-TAE-BO or www.taebo.com.

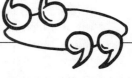

Quote, Unquote

"Tae Bo isn't a self-defense course and should never be considered a substitute for protection, but we use imaginary opponents as targets. Women get into shape and gain confidence and awareness that may not have existed before."

—Billy Blanks, Tae Bo creator

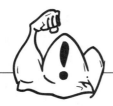

Fit Tip

Any class that uses the specific name "Tae Bo" must be taught by an instructor trained by Blanks. Others are out-and-out imitators or at least have drawn their inspiration from Blanks's program.

More Kicks from Kickboxing

Tae Bo is the brand name that first hit the public consciousness, but kickboxing and aerobic kickboxing are generic names for a whole family of derivative programs that combine boxing, martial arts, and aerobic training. The origins stem from full-contact fighting, but modern health-club renditions use some of the moves set to music to create a hip workout. Here is a small sampling of the programs you will find at gyms and on videotape:

➤ Cardio Athletic Kickbox, developed by fitness trainer Eversley Forte, combines boxing punches, martial arts kicks, and athletic drills in a workout with the motto "Play hard but play safe." For details, contact 1-800-599-9519 or www.behind-scenes.com.

➤ KickBox Fitness was developed by world heavyweight kickboxing *and* karate champion Joe Lewis and three partners. The routine is done to music and features a series of combination punches. When participants are ready, they can add bag work using 12-ounce gloves and a heavy bag. Rhythmic sparring, in which class members pretend to box with each other to music, rounds out the routine. Contact 1-877-333-KBOX or www.kickboxfitness.com.

➤ Kickbox Express is an aggressive aerobic kickboxing program that comes in three levels: basic, circuit training, and high-low. Creator Janis Snaffel spends time on biomechanics to stress proper technique and safety, both in classes and on tapes. Many women relate to tapes in which a woman demonstrates the moves. Contact 1-888-685-2608 or www.fitnessexpressintl.com.

➤ "Ichiban" means "number one" in Japanese, and it's the name of a group exercise program from Japan that melds various martial arts elements from several sources into one seamless routine. Combinations include four basic punches (jab, rear-cross, hook, and upper) and four basic kicks (knee kick, front kick, side kick, and hook kick) plus moves as performed in Western boxing, kickboxing, karate, tae kwan do, and kung fu. For details, e-mail yo-dragon@msc.biglobe.ne.jp.

These programs can be effective, because a 135-pound person is likely to burn 350 to 450 calories during a typical 50-minute kickboxing, aerobic boxing, cardio kickboxing, or similar class. A large man, working at a very high intensity, could burn up to 800 calories.

Plain Old Boxing—Without the Kick

On the surface, it doesn't seem as if boxing, with its three-minute rounds, could possibly require as much training and conditioning as a triathlon, a marathon, or other endurance activities. Boxing demands speed, strength, coordination, reflexes, and heart, however, and boxers are among the best-conditioned athletes. Remember Rocky Balboa running, shadow boxing, sparring—and ultimately triumphing? In fact, real boxers train even harder than Rocky, performing a variety of strength, power, aerobic, and coordination activities. Milton Lacroix of Supreme Team Boxing in New York starts newbies with such "basic moves" as throwing two-pound weights into the air and catching them as they move around in a circle. "After two or three minutes, they're dead—until they get used to it," says Lacroix.

In addition to training serious boxers, more gyms now offer their facilities and expertise to people who never intend to get into a ring but want to get in really good shape. A training program of boxing for fitness most likely will feature "bag work" (punching a heavy bag, speed bag, and double-ended bag), skipping rope, and shadow boxing. Bag work, in particular, provides both aerobic conditioning (because of the constant movement) and strength training (because the bag offers resistance for your muscles to work against with every punch you throw). Serious boxers do a lot of bag work, supplemented with jumping rope, running, agility training, and weightlifting. In other words, they are seriously into cross-training. They also practice fighting against an opponent, but if you're into this for fitness and not for the sport, such sparring is optional.

People who use boxer training moves for fitness often assert that punching is not only good exercise but also a dynamite stress-reliever. Slam Man is a new wrinkle on boxing's face. Marketed as a home product, this sand-filled, padded dummy consists of just a torso and a head with eight embedded lights as targets. It is preprogrammed with 15 workouts that are displayed as light combinations that you hit. Slam Man isn't a dancing doll but a stationary target. Therefore, it is useful for upper-body conditioning, coordination, and endurance, but it doesn't require the footwork of a punching bag.

Kathy Rivers, a six-foot beauty who is both a bathing-suit model and one of the country's few female professional boxers, works out three to four hours, six days a week. When she decided to give boxing a try, she began training seriously. Within three months, she went from size 14 to size 9. How? Her workout emphasizes strength training with and without weights as well as aerobic conditioning. Her daily regime includes abdominal, leg, and flexibility exercises without weights. She pumps iron three days a week, runs five to seven miles twice a week, and does bag work, wind sprints, and sparring with a partner the other days. Most people who exercise don't ever approach this level, but it is always instructive to learn what the pros do.

Military Training for Nonmilitary Types

Army drill sergeants are known for their ability to whip butterball privates into lean, mean machines in just eight weeks. Assorted fitness programs that draw their inspiration from military training—without the firearms—occasionally surface. They generally aren't for beginning exercisers, but they can be effective all-around workouts for veterans who are bored with their long-time programs. Outdoor survival skills and team-building courses frequently incorporate some of these elements. Here are some programs that incorporate military fitness training:

➤ Navy Seal Exercises, developed by Mark De Lisle, is a hard-body program that promises "no gyms, no equipment, no excuses." For details, call 1-800-281-SEAL (1-800-281-7325) or log on to www.sealfitness.com.

➤ Mitch Utterbeck, an Army Special Forces veteran, is the director of adventure training for Trident Adventures of San Diego. He has developed a workout featuring various exercises, each to be done for a specified amount of time rather than a certain number of reps. He created a regimen consisting of a stair run on a flight of 20 or more steps, a barbell lift, push-ups, double crunches, and several other exercises—in addition to a warm-up and cool-down. His recommendation is for novices to begin with 30 seconds of each exercise, working up to two minutes for each. Even if your fitness plan is totally different, you can incorporate the time method into virtually any program instead of counting reps and sets.

➤ Hurdles, ropes, cargo nets, and other obstacles are the staples at Lori Ann Lloyd's Overcoming Obstacles Fitness Camps. She also offers one-on-one training. Lloyd has been a world champion obstacle course warrior and gears her camps toward all levels from beginners to wannabe obstacle course competitors. For information, call 407-438-STAR (407-438-7827).

The Least You Need to Know

➤ Aerobic kickboxing can burn calories quickly.

➤ Start kickboxing slowly and gradually increase intensity to prevent injury.

➤ Martial arts can be used for defense as well as fitness.

➤ Rigorousness and discipline inspired by military training provide strong structure for several exercise programs.

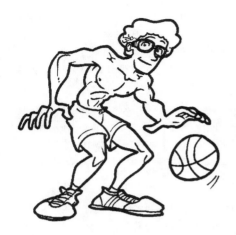

Playing Your Way to Fitness

The need for leading a healthy, active lifestyle is indeed serious, but exercise can be play as well as work. Keep in mind that most sports and games require movement. You can think of the benefits of participating in or training for a sport as the three Fs, because you'll often get *faster* and *fitter*—and you'll have *fun,* too. Actually, there are five Fs. Many of these activities are ideal for *families* and *friends* to do together.

Play with a Kid

Keeping up with children is a great way to mesh exercise with parenthood. When babies are small, parents move them and their paraphernalia all day. Carrying an infant, walking him or her when colic strikes, pushing a carriage and then a stroller, and even dealing with endless rounds of laundry keeps parents, especially moms, in motion. When children grow and become more self-reliant, parents take that as a cue to sit down and rest. Physical inactivity, however, takes its toll. If you think you are tired when babies and toddlers require constant attention and chores, it's just a prelude to the constant lethargy you will feel if you take it too easy when your children get older. Being an active participant in life sets an excellent example for your children, and participating in sports together can be a treasured family bond.

Here are some ways you can spend quality active time with your children while you rev up your metabolism and have fun, too:

➤ **Swimming.** Sign up infants and toddlers for baby swim classes. Not only are the classes designed to "drown-proof" your children, you also will get exercise because parents are in the pool with their little ones. Playing a game that includes lifting your child out of the water is nothing less than an upper-body workout for you.

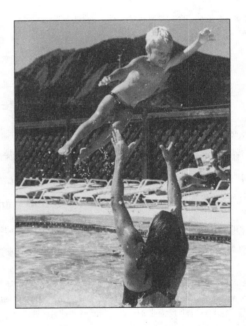

Outdoor pools offer refreshing summer recreation with your children.

(Photo: Anne W. Krause)

➤ **Beach time.** When you take children to the beach, don't just sit there. You can swim, of course, but many kids like to splash and parents like to watch them. Partner up with another parent and take turns watching the children. When you're off duty, take advantage of the time and go for a short walk. Just walking on resistant sand strengthens your shins, calves, and even the muscles in your feet. Walking barefoot on sand naturally sloughs and smoothes the skin on the bottom of your feet. Wading adds the resistance of water to your walking, as long as you keep moving and don't merely stand knee-deep in the water. Toss a beach ball around with your kids or help them build a sand castle. This isn't major exercise as much as just a fun time.

➤ **Bicycling.** Go for a family bike ride. When your children are little, you can hitch up a special bicycle trailer designed to hold a toddler or two. Pedaling yourself, your bike, the trailer, and the tyke can be a real workout. When your child gets old enough to pedal, you can hook a tandem behind you. Your youngster can pedal, but you're in control because you steer—and you're the only one with brakes.

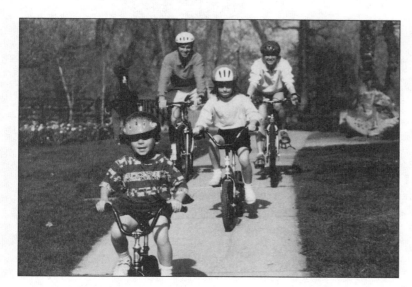

Bicycling with your children is good exercise for all, and it's fun, too.

(Photo: Anne W. Krause)

➤ **Hiking.** Plan family hiking or camping trips. A "hike" with a small child can be a short walk in the woods, and you might spend as much time carrying your little one as not. This imprints children with the idea of healthy outdoor activity in a natural setting from their earliest years. The same goes for camping. You probably will find it convenient to start by car camping when your children are small, but short backpacking trips are feasible when they are quite young. Because the scope and range of such outdoor activities grow as your children do, getting into the habit of such activities from the beginning is an investment in future family fitness.

➤ **Skating.** Ice skating, in-line, and roller skating are terrific sports for youngsters—and parents. Four or five is not too young for basic ice-skating lessons. Children are often a bit older when using skates with wheels rather than skates with blades. Some children are happy just skating around in circles at a rink, but others take to it so quickly that they soon ask for figure-skating lessons or to join a junior hockey program. In-line skaters can start at a playground, on the asphalt of a basketball court, or in some other confined area before graduating to sidewalk skating.

Tromping through the snow with your kid in tow makes relaxing by the fire well-deserved.

(Photo: Anne W. Krause)

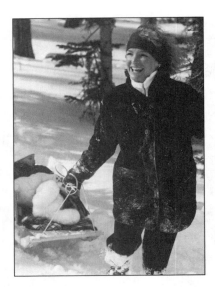

➤ **Coaching.** When your children become interested in team sports, such as soccer, basketball, and the like, keep them and yourself motivated by volunteering to coach or referee. To be a good coach or referee, you can't just stand around. Keeping the whole team focused, on track, and motivated requires you to move around, too. This, in turn, will keep you on track with your fitness program.

Many sports require *power,* which can be defined as a combination of strength and speed. Others require *agility,* which can be defined as nimbleness when starting, accelerating, decelerating, stopping, and changing direction quickly. Volleyball, tennis, racquetball, and basketball require both power and agility. If you get involved in these sports, you should train to improve both.

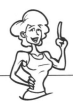

Fitness Fact

According to the National Sporting Goods Association, Americans' participation in the following activities showed the biggest percentage increases from 1993 to 1998: in-line roller skating, 118 percent; roller hockey, 106.2 percent; snowboarding, 102 percent; off-road mountain biking, 87.2 percent; backpacking and wilderness camping, 58.9 percent; on-road mountain biking, 45.6 percent; exercising with equipment, 32.2 percent; soccer, 27.8 percent; martial arts, 26.7 percent.

Play Like a Kid

Kids don't think about whether their heart rate is on the rise or how many calories they are burning. They just play. Give your fitness program a change in direction. Dredge back into memories from your own childhood for the games you loved most, or watch your kids play with their friends. Then grab a couple of friends and let the fun and laughs—and yes, the exercise—begin. You'll be surprised at how readily you'll get your heart rate going and how quickly the time flies. Here are a few ideas to get you started:

➤ **Team tag.** The person who is "it" holds a small ball with which he or she tries to tag any of the other members below the waist. When the "it" person tags someone, the person who was tagged is "it."

➤ **Hula hoop.** If your kids have a hula hoop (or if there's one in the attic), pull it out and give it a twirl.

➤ **Dodgeball.** Find an empty parking lot and a big rubber ball. Divide into teams and take turns trying to hit opposing players and being the targets. The object of the game, and the part that will really get you moving, is to dodge the ball (that is, not to get hit by the ball) when your team is the target.

➤ **Footbag.** Commonly known as Hacky Sack after a trademarked product, this little bag is a staple among college students looking for a diversion on a nice spring day.

➤ **Golf.** Although golf is not an aerobic sport, if you walk the course instead of using a golf cart, you gain the benefit of a long walk. Golf also improves hand-eye coordination, which can help with more energetic pursuits such as tennis or racquetball. Golf was not generally thought of as a family sport until Tiger Woods came on the scene. The pictures of the adorable preschooler with a golf club in his hand have inspired many parents to sign up their children for golf lessons.

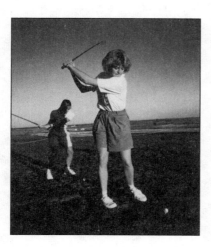

Walking a golf course and swinging at that tiny ball is a workout for both your legs and your hand-eye coordination.

(Photo: Anne W. Krause)

Encouraging Youngsters to Be Fit

Perhaps even more frightening than the picture of an increasingly overweight adult population are recent figures on childhood obesity in the United States. According to U.S. Department of Agriculture figures, the percentage of overweight children ages six to 17 has doubled since 1968. In addition to changing unhealthy eating habits, youngsters need to be more physically active. Here are some of the national initiatives that have been launched to target overweight and obese children:

➤ **Girl Sports.** A Girl Scout–sponsored program to encourage young girls to participate in sports at local and national levels. 1-800-GSUSA4U.

➤ **The President's Challenge.** Physical fitness testing program for children ages six through 17. 202-690-9000.

➤ **Skate-in-School.** A program to provide safe and affordable in-line skating opportunities for children. 808-213-7193, ext. 410.

➤ **Start Smart Sports Development Program.** This National Alliance for Youth Sports program focuses on building such fundamental sports skills as throwing, catching, and kicking. 1-800-729-2057.

The greatest gifts you can give your child are the gift of health and the habit of physical activity to sustain it, so that he or she is not a candidate for such programs for overweight youngsters.

How We Play

In 1998, the Sporting Goods Manufacturers Association (SGMA) commissioned American Sports Data, Inc. to survey Americans age six and older about sports participation during 1997. Eight of the top 10 most popular sports are still considered to be "recreational," while eight of the top 20 activities are considered to be "fitness." The 25 most popular activities of the 102 activities included in the survey, in terms of millions of participants who did each activity at least once, are

1. Recreational swimming: 94.4
2. Recreational walking: 80.9
3. Recreational bicycling: 54.6
4. Bowling: 50.6
5. Freshwater fishing: 45.8
6. Tent camping: 42.6
7. Basketball: 42.4
8. Free weights: 41.3
9. Billiards: 39.7

10. Day hiking: 38.6
11. Treadmill exercise: 37.1
12. Fitness walking: 36.4
13. Stretching exercise: 35.1
14. Running/jogging: 35.0
15. In-line skating: 32.0
16. Calisthenics: 31.0
17. Stationary cycling: 30.8
18. Golf: 30.0
19. Weight-resistance machine: 22.5
20. Darts: 21.8
21. Slow-pitch softball: 19.4
22. Ice skating: 18.7
23. Stairclimbing machine: 18.6
24. (tie) Soccer: 18.2
24. (tie) RV camping: 18.2

Take Me Out to the Ball Game

Group exercise predates aerobics classes and studio cycling. Team sports, which provide exercise done in a group, include volleyball, basketball, soccer, softball, hockey, and any other competitive sport you might have played in junior high and high school. With the passage of time, they might now seem like "lost" sports, but you might have a hankering to pick one of them up again. Go for it. They provide fitness benefits and camaraderie, and they do exist for adults.

Adult recreation leagues provide the framework many people need. You might be tempted to cut a fitness class, but you wouldn't dream of letting your teammates down. So you go and play and, therefore, get exercise. Because of scheduling problems or personal preference, however, you might be the type of person who prefers playing only when you feel like it, or you might travel on business frequently and not have a regular schedule. That's where pickup games come in. Gyms, rec centers, and skating arenas are among the venues that schedule first-come, first-play basketball, hockey, and other sports.

Volleyball

Didn't everybody play volleyball in high school gym class? Some people keep it up for years. The Midwest has a long history of indoor volleyball—the conventional kind in a gym—but more recently, beach volleyball has taken hold as well. Even in Chicago, with its storied cold and blustery winters, year-round beach volleyball has its adherents. Sand is trucked in from Indiana and is dumped in a former metalwork factory. Wisconsin, Michigan, and Minnesota all boast multicourt volleyball centers that host leagues, pickup play, and courtside coed socializing. These facilities offer more exercise and a more with-it scene than such regional recreational staples as bowling. What appeals to Midwesterners in the winter also appeals to Southerners in the summer, where air-conditioned beach volleyball facilities have also been developed.

You might not get a consistent aerobic workout when you play volleyball, but when you have to move, you *really* move. The game requires quick, explosive actions as you move to hit the ball over the net. It also is a good team-building sport, because you cannot win a volleyball game without teamwork. As with other team sports, the volleyball court is a good place to find companions who want to train to increase aerobic strength to help them on the court. This might net you a training partner, too. Volleyball leagues—whether in the gym or on an indoor "beach"—abound throughout the country. Call your local recreation center, Y, or health club to find a volleyball league near you. You also can contact USA Volleyball at 719-228-6800, or you can log on to www.usavolleyball.org/adult/main.htm to find nearby indoor and outdoor recreational league play.

Fitness Fact

Wallyball *is* similar to volleyball, but it is played in a racquetball court. Games are organized for men, women, and coed play.

Basketball

Basketball requires more constant running than volleyball or virtually any other sport. Like volleyball, basketball involves quick action and fast reactions, especially on defense. It also requires teamwork, so it is a good place to find companions for other fitness activities. Again, men's and women's pickup basketball and league play abound around the country. Call your local recreation center, YMCA, or health club to find a basketball league near you.

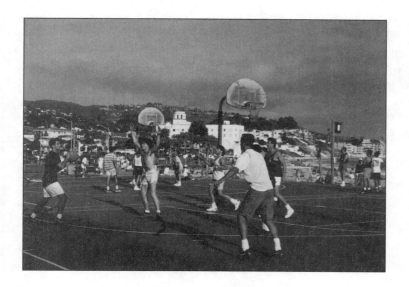

A pickup game of hoops with buddies is a fun way to get a workout.

(Photo: Anne W. Krause)

Beach basketball is a fast—and fast-growing—recreational sport that combines aspects of beach volleyball and playground basketball. It is played on a circular court with a single basket on a pole in the sand but without a backboard or an out-of-bounds area. For more information, contact World Beach Basketball at www.beachbasketball.com.

Soccer

Soccer is hot. Not since Pelé has it grown so much in popularity in the United States as in the late 1990s. The 1999 World Cup victory by the United States women's team raised soccer's profile, and the popularity of the favorite hometown star, Mia Hamm, and her teammates has fueled soccer's boom. A good soccer game requires a lot of running and agility. It will keep your heart pumping as you run up and down the playing field, and handling the soccer ball benefits motor coordination skills.

Men's and women's soccer leagues abound for all ages and ability levels. In some cities, you can even find indoor soccer leagues for year-round play. Your local recreation center, Y, or health club is a good place to inquire about adult soccer leagues in your area.

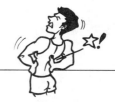

Achtung!

To help prevent ankle sprains and strains, wear high-top sports shoes to play basketball.

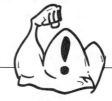

Fit Tip

Check www.cityhoops.com to find pickup basketball games all over the country.

Softball

When people play softball, they often identify it with baseball. This is why it has been a popular team sport for a long time. In the summer, adult softball games are played on diamonds around the country until well into the night. Many companies form teams, and the competition between teams can be fierce but always friendly. Injuries frequently occur because people go out for a softball team cold turkey without any training. Warm up before the softball season starts with some running, sprints, and throwing, as well as some flexibility exercises.

Take me to play at the ball game—and I get to run around the field.

(Photo: Anne W. Krause)

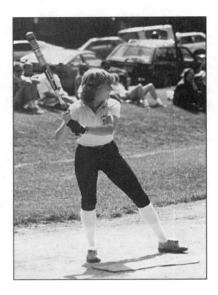

If you're interested in playing softball, check with your company's Human Resources department; take a look at the bulletin board in the coffee room; or inquire at your local recreation center, Y, or health club. For more information about leagues, rules, and tournaments, contact the Amateur Softball Association at 405-424-5266.

Hockey

With the increase in construction of new rinks around the country, recreational ice hockey is experiencing explosive growth. Look for league and pickup play for both men and women at a nearby rink. In-line skating has spawned in-line hockey, which still tends to be more pickup and less league in most locations. Ice hockey has migrated from being solely a Snowbelt sport to being a Sunbelt activity, too. It is a wonderful way to escape the heat, but in-line hockey remains mostly an outdoor activity.

Footbag

Remember Hacky Sack from your college days? One offshoot is a serious organized sport with several branches. Footbag Net is a fast singles or doubles court game that resembles elements of several sports: the court strategy of tennis, the set-and-spike tactics of volleyball, and the no-hands rule of soccer. Players use only their feet to kick the footbag over a 5-foot-high net. Freestyle Footbag is choreographed and set to music, much like high-level aerobic dance competitions. Footbag Golf features a course with nine or 18 "holes" that resemble funnels. For more information, check World-Wide Footbag Foundation's Web site at www.footbag.org.

Summing Up

YMCAs across the country provide a wide array of sports opportunities and fitness classes. A nationwide toll-free number—1-800-USA-YMCA (1-800-872-9622)—can help direct you to a convenient Y that offers suitable activities. In studying America's propensity for leisure-time physical activity (known in government lingo as LTPA), the National Center for Health Statistics found that 59 percent of American men and 49 percent of American women engage in "little or no physical activity" during their free time. Inactivity is particularly high among Mexican-American women (74 percent), non-Hispanic black women (67 percent), and Mexican-American men (65 percent). Among the activities that fall into the government's LTPA category are walking, jogging, golf, bowling, gardening, and dancing.

According to Chris Ballard, author of *Hoops Nation*, the country's top five spots for pickup basketball are West Fourth Street at Sixth Avenue in Manhattan, Houston's Fondé Recreation Center, the Venice Beach Courts in Los Angeles, Atlanta's Run N' Shoot Athletic Center, and Rocky River Courts in Rocky River, Ohio.

Where people live has a lot to do with which activities they're most likely to choose. Arizonans prefer hiking. New Yorkers would rather walk. People from Illinois like to bicycle, and South Dakotans are avid in-line skaters. In Washington, D.C., fitness classes are tops.

The Least You Need to Know

➤ Introduce your children to sports when they are young.

➤ Sports provide a good foundation for your children's lives, and keeping up with them can help you stay fit, too.

➤ Playing like you were a kid again provides fun, as well as fitness benefits.

➤ Rec centers, YMCAs, and health clubs are great family sports resources.

➤ Adult league sports are a great way to get in shape and meet new people.

➤ Teammates from recreational sports are good workout partners.

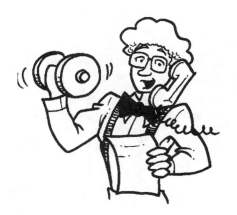

Weave Workouts into Your Life

You can organize your life so you have time to exercise, or you can rethink the things that you do so that physical movement is as automatic as breathing or swallowing— better yet, you can do both. Even as you embark on a fitness program, reasses your day-to-day tasks and try to make every day more physical. Even simple activity burns calories. Activity tones your body. Activity makes you feel good. Activity means *life* and *living*.

The Way Things Were

In the "old days," people didn't go to the gym. For all but the most pampered gentry, simply getting through the day was quite a workout. Housework, yardwork, and virtu- ally all factory jobs and trades involved constant physical labor. Back then, houses had cellars, main-floor parlors and kitchens, upstairs bedrooms, and way-upstairs attics, and all but the fanciest apartments were walkups. People didn't hop on stair- steppers. They used the stairs.

Housework was work. Homemakers used carpet sweepers, carpet beaters, brooms, rag mops, and elbow grease instead of chemicals or cleaning services to keep homes clean. Before the advent of the automobile, and even for years afterward, many people walked to the bus or the streetcar, climbed aboard, and then walked to their end destination. There were no drive-in banks, grocery shopping was a store-to-store expedition rather than a one-stop process (and there was no Internet or catalog shopping), and sending out a package meant a trip to the post office rather than a FedEx or UPS pickup.

Even after the advent of the automobile, drivers had to work the clutch, shift manually from one gear to another, and get out to jack up the car and change a flat. Even after automatic transmission came about, it was a long time before cars came with power steering, power brakes, power windows, and power-operated rearview mirrors. When people used to drive somewhere, they had to get out of the car to open and close the garage door, and they had to crank the wheel, push hard on the brakes, and do other manual tasks.

Labor-saving devices certainly have made life easier in many ways, but when it comes to our health, they haven't necessarily improved things for us physically. Quite the contrary, in fact. In many cases, we now have to create an artificial activity environment to mimic what once was natural. Some people can easily readjust their lives to be more physically active. Others have to pick and choose what is practical in "demodernizing" and "reactivating" their lives.

In many parts of the world, people still live in a simpler yet more physical way. "I am cycling down the Tibetan Highway in southern China," wrote Judith Mandelbaum-Schmid in *Walking* magazine. "Everywhere, there are people walking, lifting, and hauling. A woman crosses a field with a bundle of corn stalks strapped to her back. It's taller and wider than she is and must weigh a ton, but she seems unfazed. A man pedals a tricycle with a six-foot flatbed trailer attachment piled with a load of orange persimmons. He's older than I am, but definitely in better shape than me or most of my 26 traveling companions. Though we're on lightweight mountain bikes, he effortlessly passes us. In these surroundings, we might as well all be from Mars. For the country people who live here in the Yunnan Province, going on vacation to get some exercise is a ridiculous, if not alien concept. For them, exercise is as natural as breathing."

China is rapidly becoming a modern urban and industrialized society, but it isn't necessarily becoming physically soft. New apartment houses in cities are only required to have elevators if they are more than eight stories high. Not only do millions of Chinese practice tai chi every day, but just in going home—even empty-handed—residents of the upper floors of these buildings get more daily exercise than most Americans. No one suggests that the United States institute such draconian fitness policies, but the Chinese may be on to something when it comes to keeping active to stay strong and maintain good health.

According to a 1999 Opinion Research Corporation survey for a weight-loss program called Take Off Pounds Sensibly, not even half the adults in America exercise regularly during an average week. This is how levels of activity were distributed: intense activity (aerobics, running, swimming, biking), 19 percent; moderate activity (walking, yoga), 29 percent; light activity (housecleaning, gardening, golfing), 20 percent; no standard routine (but trying to do physical things during the course of the day), 13 percent; don't exercise regularly, 19 percent.

Start Your Day with a Stretch

When we wake up, our natural instinct is to take a good stretch. We tend to arch our back, open our arms, and stretch our spine—and most of us do this without even thinking about it. You can build on this natural tendency to help start your day right. Set your alarm five minutes earlier, and while you're lying in bed waking up, start your day with a conscious stretch. As you lie there, make yourself as long as you can by reaching your hands over your head, stretching your legs, and pointing your toes—even if it pulls your covers out of place or you have to lie at an angle on your bed. Next, curl up into the fetal position so your back is rounded to stretch your lower back, and then make yourself long again. It's amazing how good you will feel when you begin to loosen your muscles from whatever your sleeping position was and get the blood flowing.

Quote, Unquote

"Prior to 1950, the traditional design of communities in the United States allowed people to freely engage in walking and bicycling. Over the past half-century, development practices have discouraged the pedestrian."

—Richard Killingsworth, Centers for Disease Control

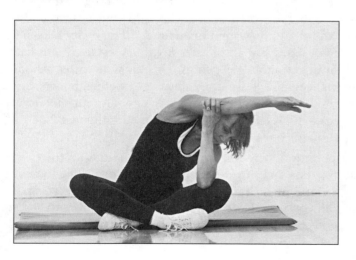

Start your day with some easy stretching to get your blood flowing.

(Photo: Anne W. Krause)

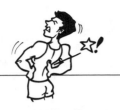

The shower is another great place to wake up your muscles. With warm water flowing over you, bend over gently toward your toes, let your arms drop in front of you, and stretch them, lengthening your body as much as you can. Then reach your arms overhead, stretch again, and breathe. The warm water helps loosen the muscles and makes them easier to stretch.

One of yoga's most basic moves is called the Salute to the Sun. This flowing series of energizing postures elongates the muscles, stretches the spine, and gets the blood pumping. Its name alone should tell you how it relates to stretching in the morning. (For the sequence of postures in this energizing morning ritual, see Chapter 9, "Other Paths to Stretching and Toning.")

Although it's not possible for people to fidget their way to fitness, some people manage to help control their weight this way. The National Institutes of Health discovered that people who fidget a lot, producing almost constant motion, burn anywhere from 138 to 685 more calories a day than physically quiet individuals.

All Day Long, All Day Strong

You can add many obvious and not-so-obvious activities to your day that will help make you more active. Whether you work odd hours, have a basic 9-to-5 schedule, or work out of your house, here are several ideas for integrating activity into your day:

➤ Walk or bike to work or on errands whenever feasible. According to the League of American Bicyclists, cycling to work not only can help your health, it also can save money. After an initial investment of about $750 for a city bike, a helmet, a lock, a rear reflector light, and a front headlight, a bicycle commuter can save up to $3,000 a year in automobile expenses. This includes lower insurance premiums, fewer parking fees, and less money spent on gasoline, repairs, and maintenance. Bike commuting helps the environment, too. A four-mile round-trip commute just three days a week for one year keeps an estimated 2,340 pounds of emission pollutants out of the air.

➤ If you use public transportation, perhaps you can walk to and from the train, bus, or subway on at least one end of your commute. You might like to rev up with a morning walk, or you might find an afternoon stroll to be relaxing. (If you dress up for work, all you need to do is wear socks and sneakers to and from work and carry your good shoes.)

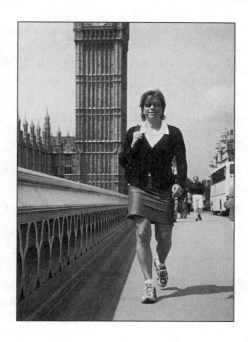

Don your sneakers and add an extra block or two on your way to work from the bus stop or train station.

(Photo: Anne W. Krause)

➤ If you must drive, park at the end of the lot farthest from the building and walk to the door. If the weather is nice and you have time, do a lap around the lot or the building before heading inside.

➤ If you are slave to your desk at work, try to devote your lunch hour to some sort of activity: a workout at the gym or at least a walk around the block—or several blocks. If you move briskly, you should be able to cover a mile in about 20 minutes, once you've gotten into the walking habit.

➤ Take the stairs instead of the elevator at your office, in department stores, in hotels, or in your building if you live in a high-rise.

➤ Stand up while talking on the phone to give yourself a break from your desk. Standing up helps stretch your muscles and enables you to breathe more deeply. This can help energize you throughout the workday.

➤ Even if your job keeps you tied to the telephone or chained to your computer terminal, the habit of getting up, walking around, and stretching for a few minutes (at least) once an hour does wonders for how you feel and your productivity.

➤ Be mindful of your posture throughout the day. It feels good to straighten your back and to push your shoulders back after you've been concentrating on a project for a period of time, perhaps hunched over your desk.

➤ Make it a practice to do simple stretches while sitting at your desk, and do so periodically throughout the day. Try reaching your hands over your head to stretch your arms and back, arching and rounding your back to loosen your spine, and rolling your head from side to side to stretch out your neck. If you work at a computer terminal, drop your arms to your sides, stretch your arms toward the floor, and extend your hands with palms down at right angles to your forearms.

➤ Be sure to drink water throughout the day. This is good for you (it keeps your body hydrated), and it also can mean extra trips to the water cooler and the restroom.

➤ If you need to contact a colleague, walk over to talk or drop off a memo whenever you can instead of relying on the phone, e-mail, or interoffice mail.

➤ Keep a big fit ball near your desk and use it as your chair as much as possible. The ball keeps your posture straight and prevents hunching over.

The amount of activity you slip into your routine might be minimal compared to a construction worker, a waiter or waitress, or a retail salesperson who is moving around all day. Even though these little trips seem like trivialities, they do add up—as long as you don't make the destination of those office walks the snack bar or the candy machine.

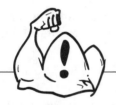

Fit Tip

Many companies sponsor employee teams in local races. T-shirts and company spirit are the rewards. Nearly 100 teams from competitive to casual enter the Bolder Boulder, for example, an annual 10-kilometer running and walking race in Colorado that attracts more than 40,000 participants. If there's a local race coming up and your company doesn't have a team, perhaps you can start one.

House and Garden Work

Since your grandma's era, the "work" has been removed from housework. In decades past, there were carpet beaters instead of vacuum cleaners—to say nothing of central vacuum systems that don't even require hauling the canister around the house. Wash day meant lifting baskets of wet laundry, bending and stretching to get it on and off the line, and ironing everything. If you can do without some of your labor-saving electric appliances, you'll help your body, your bankbook, and the environment.

In truth, most of us won't sacrifice major conveniences in the name of fitness. You can, however, at least think about a little kitchen exercise. Kneading bread makes for strong forearms, and even simple tasks such as opening a can, chopping an onion, and whisking egg whites use more calories than flipping a switch or pushing a button.

Likewise, garden chores also can help burn calories. An hour of gardening can burn 250 to 450 calories. Weeding, planting, trimming, and digging are comparable to brisk walking or jogging in terms of caloric expenditure. Mowing with a hand mower, or at least walking rather than riding while cutting grass, is beneficial to your health. It's a fine way to help keep your lawn and yourself trim at the same time.

Look at the following results from the American College of Sports Medicine's calculations of the caloric expenditure of a 150-pound person doing the following chores (a lighter person burns fewer calories, a heavier person burns more). It's no wonder that old-time lumberjacks were muscular moose!

Doing laundry	142
Washing dishes	165
Sweeping	178
Car repair	214
Clearing land (hauling branches)	357
Scrubbing the floor (on knees)	393
Chopping wood	429
Sawing trees (handsaw)	501
Carrying large logs	787
Chopping trees with an ax (fast)	1,217

Add Years to Your Life—and Life to Your Years

Study after study has indicated that staying physically active not only prolongs your life, it also improves the quality of your life. For example, the American Medical Association's Archives of Internal Medicine conducted a study indicating that adults who garden at least one hour a week are two thirds less likely to suffer heart attacks than sedentary people.

People who exercise their artistic expression at the same time as their body often enjoy robust good health into old age. Ever wonder why so many professional musicians and orchestra conductors live to such ripe old ages and are still active in music until the end? It's because playing an instrument or keeping the baton in motion is good exercise. It engages the mind as well as the

Quote, Unquote

"Clearing brush, chopping wood, stacking logs. That's the routine I used to become heavyweight champion of the world. In 1973, I did not lift one ounce of weight before becoming champ. I didn't even know what a rep was. There is no better workout than clearing brush."

—George Foreman, former world heavyweight champion, *USA Weekend* magazine body. There's also a lot to be said for the mental alertness that serious music requires. An Ohio State University study showed that playing the piano burns 140 calories an hour, playing the violin or cello burns 160 calories an hour, and playing the drums burns 230 calories an hour. So be grateful your parents insisted on music lessons, drag out that old instrument, and play away.

What if you're not musical but you're interested in artistic creation? Take a sketchpad or a camera and go for a walk in the park, a city neighborhood, or a pretty spot out of town. If you carry a camera, some lenses, and perhaps a tripod, you'll haul some extra weight as you walk. (Lowe Pro makes special backpacks with padded interiors for photographic gear, so you won't get lopsided from carrying your camera gear on one shoulder.)

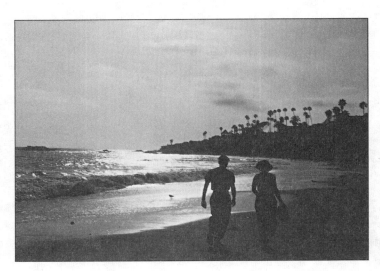

An evening stroll on the beach during a vacation can help work off those vacation meals.

(Photo: Anne W. Krause)

Working Activities into Your Program

Once you've committed to being at least moderately physically active, the next trick is to figure out what constitutes "moderate." The U.S. Surgeon General issued a report that included the following list of examples, each of which burns about 150 calories each time you do it but dramatically cuts the risk of heart disease, stroke, diabetes, hypertension, and colon cancer. Some of these activities are less vigorous but require more time (top of the list); others are more vigorous activities that take less time (bottom of the list).

266

Make it a habit to do at least one of the following activities, or something comparable, every day. The Surgeon General believes that "moderate" exercise includes the following:

➤ Washing and waxing a car, 45 to 60 minutes

➤ Washing windows or floors, 45 to 50 minutes

➤ Playing volleyball, 45 minutes

➤ Playing touch football, 30 to 45 minutes

➤ Gardening, 30 to 45 minutes

➤ Walking 1¾ miles, 35 minutes

➤ Basketball (shooting baskets), for 30 minutes

➤ Bicycling 5 miles, 30 minutes

➤ Social dancing (fast), 30 minutes

➤ Pushing a stroller 1½ miles, 30 minutes

➤ Raking leaves, 30 minutes

➤ Swimming laps, 20 minutes

➤ Basketball (playing a game), 15 to 20 minutes

➤ Bicycling 4 miles, 15 minutes

➤ Jumping rope, 15 minutes

➤ Shoveling snow, 15 minutes

➤ Stairwalking, 15 minutes

To get some exercise while doing a good deed, shovel an elderly neighbor's sidewalk when it snows. Some communities even have official "snow-shoveler" or "ice-buster" programs that make volunteers responsible for clearing particular walks.

Get Children Moving—on Their Feet

In an old comedy routine, Bill Cosby talked about his father walking five miles to school "uphill both ways." It's sad to say, but things have changed since Bill Cosby's dad's day. Many children no longer walk or ride their bikes to school—a sure-fire form of daily exercise. Instead, they rely on parental chauffeuring, school buses, and carpools. As soon as they're teenagers, they drive themselves to school. It is a logical progression that children who are driven become teenagers who drive who become adults who pop into their cars for even the shortest of errands.

If it is at all possible where you live, do your children, yourself, and your community's traffic and air quality a favor and get them started walking or riding their bikes to school when they are very young. If you accompany them when they're little, you'll get some exercise as well. Before America became car dependent, walking was part of our culture. Now we have to make a conscious effort to incorporate it into our lives. In September 1998, 100 schools across the country participated in the first annual National Walk Our Children to School Day. In some school districts, such as Laredo, Texas, where many children usually travel on buses, parent volunteers met youngsters at four drop-off areas and walked them to school. One day a year can only be considered a start. For information about inaugurating this type of program in your town, call 1-800-266-3312, ext. 929.

You don't have to wait until school days, however, to get outside with your little ones. Baby packs and carriages for infants, solid strollers for toddlers, and big-tired jogging strollers that are strong enough to haul a preschooler enable you to get out of the house for a walk or a run—and get your children into the fresh air and away from the television. For suggestions on how to coordinate your workouts with parenthood, see Chapter 24, "Special Situations."

The Least You Need to Know

➤ Reducing your reliance on modern conveniences will add physical activity to your life.

➤ Stretching makes your body more flexible.

➤ Taking a few minutes out of every hour of every workday to move around and stretch keeps you alert and is good for your body.

➤ Do house and garden work to get toned and burn calories.

➤ Teach your children to be active by setting a good example of daily physical activity.

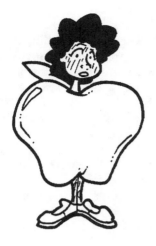

Chapter 20

You Are What You Eat

In This Chapter

➤ American Heart Association guidelines for good eating

➤ How to balance your intake for good nutrition

➤ Fad diets and fat–burning pills

➤ Creative ways to cut calories and eat healthy

Being fit is not simply about being thin. A slim, trim body is a worthy goal, but being fit is truly about being healthy, strong, and energetic. Thinking only of thinness, focusing on it, and obsessing about it can lead to nutritional imbalance, chronic health problems, and in extreme cases, eating disorders. Focusing on cardiovascular health and strength and seeking sensible ways for eating to help achieve this is what we all should strive for.

Many nutrition and sports-medicine experts, as well as the American Heart Association (AHA), agree that balance is the key to eating healthfully. In fact, "balance" has become something of a mantra. In all aspects of life, "balance" became the buzzword of the 1990s, and it will probably remain so as the twentieth century gives way to the twenty-first.

A Balancing Act for Good Health

Just what is "balance" in nutrition anyway? To understand current thinking, it is necessary to rewind to the 1980s, when it became clear that heart disease, diabetes, and certain types of cancer associated with high fat intake were on the rise. At that time, the American Heart Association's experts set some guidelines for intake of certain food groups, especially fat. They recommended that Americans cut their fat intake from the artery-clogging average of 42 percent to no more than 30 percent of their total daily calories. This, the experts believed, was realistic and was about as low as most Americans would go, although many experts would like to see people cut their fat consumption to not more than 20 percent of their daily caloric intake. More recent studies have broken this down to no more than 10 percent in the form of saturated fats (see the section "The Facts on Fat" later in this chapter, for information about the differences between saturated and unsaturated fats). What does this translate to? A person consuming 2,000 calories a day should take in no more than 65 grams of fat, which translates to half a tablespoon of butter or oil.

A balanced, healthy diet will keep you active as you grow older.

(Photo: Anne W. Krause)

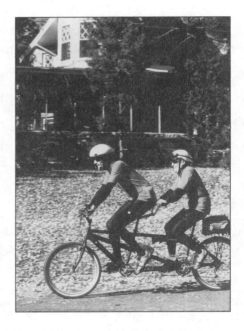

In addition, the AHA recommended that carbohydrates should make up about 55 to 60 percent and protein 10 to 15 percent of a healthy American's daily diet. Many people assumed these recommendations to be gospel, not guidelines. They took them to mean that every bite needed to fit into this formula, which is as much a setup for failure as is any diet. To fit into this bite-by-bite profile, your diet would cut out a lot of foods and would lack variety.

Balance means eating a variety of healthy foods, perhaps a little more of this or a little less of that on any given day, but generally aiming for the AHA's guidelines. "Balance" does not mean that every bite you put into your mouth has to be a perfect combination of carbohydrate, fat, and protein. A good balance takes these three food types into consideration over time. In the course of a week, your average intake of carbohydrates, fats, and proteins should be roughly in balance. Eating can be one of life's pleasures. When you put your life in balance, it should still be fun.

In the late 1990s, even as nutritionists were beating the drums for a high-carbohydrate, high-fiber, low-fat diet, The Zone, Dr. Atkins' New Diet Revolution, and Sugar Busters were flying off bookstore shelves and onto the bestseller list. Thus inspired, dieters returned to days that started with bacon and eggs and ended with T-bone steaks. Tales of shed pounds were told around office water coolers, park benches at playgrounds, and supermarket meat counters. The jury is still out on whether such plans will lead to long-term weight loss combined with good health—or result in thin but unfit people with clogged arteries, heart disease, and other ailments. American dieters have, once again, jumped on a quick-fix bandwagon, and nutritionists are very concerned.

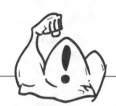

Fit Tip

Get out of the habit of eating processed foods, snack foods, and foods laden with artificial flavors and colors. The ingredient list on these foods reads like a chemistry lab report. Eating "health food" isn't nutty.

Pyramid Power

Sometimes words alone convey a potent message; sometimes it takes a picture to bring the message into sharp focus. The U.S. Departments of Agriculture and Health and Human Services have adopted the image of a pyramid to convey essentially the same message of a balanced diet that the American Heart Association promotes.

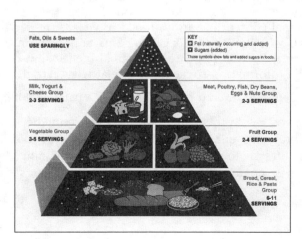

The food guide pyramid is a guide to daily food choices.

(Photo: U.S. Department of Agriculture, Human Nutrition Information Service, August 1992, Leaflet No. 1 572)

Using the food pyramid as a guideline for your daily intake, you can achieve a healthy, balanced eating lifestyle that includes the following:

➤ **Complex carbohydrates.** The foods that form the building blocks of your daily diet are at the bottom of the pyramid. These are six to 11 servings of grains, including bread, cereal, rice, and pasta. Be smart about this, too. Breads should be made with whole-grain flour, such as wheat, rye, or sourdough, and cereals should be natural and healthy—not sugar-coated, artificially colored, or flavored children's varieties.

➤ **Vegetables and fruits.** The tasty treasures from the produce department form the next levels, three to five servings from the vegetable group and two to four servings from the fruit group. Cruciferous vegetables such as broccoli, cauliflower, Brussels sprouts, and cabbage have been shown to carry additional cancer-preventing benefits.

➤ **Dairy.** Closer to the top of the food pyramid are two to three servings from the dairy group, which good sense dictates should be mostly low-fat or no-fat milk and yogurt and little from the all-fat or high-fat butter and cheese group.

➤ **Protein.** Two to three servings of protein, in the form of meat, poultry, fish, dry beans, soy products, eggs, and nuts, are recommended.

➤ **Fats and sugars.** Fats, oils, and sweets occupy the teensy point of the pyramid, indicating that they should be eaten sparingly. Fats that are eaten should be of the unsaturated kind, which are considered to be "good" fats and are actually essential to our diet. This hardly constitutes the typical American fast-food, snack-food diet!

Many people who look at this pyramid immediately think it is a license to pig out, especially on bread and pasta. A portion, as viewed by the AHA and the various U.S. government departments, is modest. It isn't a spaghetti mountain swimming in Alfredo sauce. It's half a cup of uncooked rice or pasta. When it comes to prepared foods, what constitutes a "serving" varies from food to food. You can get a good idea of the food values and nutritional content of various foods, as well as the serving size, by looking at the package, whether it's a milk carton, a pasta package, a cottage cheese container, a bread wrapper, or anything else. You can also check out the American Dietetic Association's information-packed Web site at www.eatright.org.

The following guidelines can help you in your quest to achieve a balanced diet:

➤ Keep a log of everything you eat, at least when you start out, and check it against the food group intake formula. (You can combine this with your exercise log and come up with a "lifestyle log" that tracks how you have changed your habits and what effects these changes have had on your weight, your strength, and your health.)

➤ When you're choosing a food to consume, consider what you ate at your last meal and what you expect to be eating at your next meal to try to attain balance.

➤ Look at your options. Do you really want that burger? Or would a grilled chicken sandwich taste just as good? Must you have ice cream? Or will nonfat sorbet or yogurt satisfy you? If you really want the burger or the ice cream, eat it and enjoy it. Just watch your fat and calorie intake for the next few meals.

➤ Make up your own guidelines that help you stick to the formula. For example, nutritionist Georgia Kostas, author of *The Balancing Act Nutrition and Weight Guide,* formulated the "three-quarters rule." Make your plate three quarters vegetables, beans, grains, and fruit, and make the other one quarter your entrée. When you indulge in one of your favorite food treats that's not really high in nutrition, try cutting your normal intake. Eat one scoop of ice cream instead of two.

➤ Take control of the size of the portions you eat. People generally eat way more than they need. Even if the food is healthy, there's too much of it. Eat only one half of the portion at the restaurant and save the rest for the next day. Buy indulgent snack foods in minibags so there's no temptation to eat more.

➤ Don't be sucked in by the "economy" of large packages of tempting snack foods when you are shopping or the suggestion to "super-size" your order in a fast-food restaurant (which you shouldn't be patronizing anyway).

➤ Dress up plain foods, such as pasta or baked potatoes, with toppings that are good for you, such as steamed and chopped broccoli, tomatoes, mushrooms, or your favorite spices or herbs mixed with a dollop of yogurt or reduced-fat sour cream.

➤ Stop eating when you are full or even a little before. Save your leftovers for the next day.

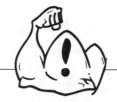

Fit Tip

When you eat pasta for dinner, chances are your dinner portion counts as two to three "servings." When you are dining in a restaurant that tries to impress you with its portion sizes, a dinner portion might be four or more "servings."

Once you get on the balance bandwagon, you'll find that it's easy to be realistic with yourself and your life. Every day and every week won't be nutritionally perfect. Maybe it's holiday time or you went to a few dinner parties. That's life, and you have to relax and enjoy it. When you begin to recognize the benefits—physical, emotional, and spiritual—of a balanced diet, it will be easier to keep on track most of the time and to enjoy the splurges without remorse.

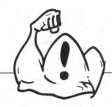

So-y Good for You

Many women, especially in their middle years, already know that eating soy products is immensely helpful in reducing the discomforts of menopause and in drastically reducing the risk of breast cancer and other cancers. New studies, however, are showing that soy products are beneficial to men as well. According to a 1999 report published in the *Archives of Internal Medicine,* researchers from the Wake Forest University School of Medicine found that eating soy foods—those rich in compounds called isoflavones (a plant estrogen)—might result in a significant decrease in blood cholesterol levels. After just nine weeks, participants in the study who consumed soy products with the greatest amounts of plant estrogens showed a marked drop in their levels of both lipoprotein (LDL, or "bad" cholesterol) and total cholesterol. The more isoflavones the soy product contained, the greater the benefit. Dr. John R. Crouse III led a team that studied 156 healthy men and women with blood cholesterol levels of 140 or higher. The people who started with the highest levels of cholesterol (164 or higher) derived the most benefit from a diet rich in soy-based isoflavones and showed the most dramatic decrease in cholesterol levels.

To Diet or Not to Diet?

In this day and age, the word "diet" has become synonymous with altered eating habits to result in weight loss, but "diet" actually is a word that refers to daily sustenance. Everyone is on a diet. Putting yourself on a weight-reducing diet is not a bad goal, but a healthy lifestyle, not just a weight-loss plan, is essential to reach and maintain your best weight. If your goal is to shed excess pounds, you must figure out the ideal combination of a well-balanced diet and physical activity for your body. Your lifestyle log can help you judge what works for you in all aspects of your being. Changes in diet and physical activity must become part of your life and not just a phase to lose weight.

You can go about reaching your goal to lose weight a number of ways. You can take the healthy route, which might seem long and arduous at times, or you can try the diet of the month, which probably will only give you a quick fix. In the long run, it will not maintain your ideal weight, nor will it necessarily be healthy for you. Despite popular diet-plan marketing ploys, there are no quick fixes to maintaining your ideal weight, and fad diets do more harm than good to your metabolism and health.

Now that any thoughts of trying quick-fix weight loss have been dispelled, here are some ideas to help you reach your weight-loss goals:

➤ Visit your doctor for a physical examination to determine whether there is anything you should take special care about, such as blood pressure, cholesterol, or additional physical activity.

➤ Determine your goals and decide whether you want to set up your own weight-loss program or work with a nutritionist and/or a personal trainer.

➤ Make sure your program follows a realistic timeline. Losing weight too fast is a sure-fire indication that you will gain it back and then some. This program is a lifestyle program and includes diet and exercise.

➤ Eating and exercising should be fun, so make sure you include some indulgences and rewards for a job well done.

➤ Keep a log or journal of your daily food intake and physical activity. Also note how you feel. Some days will be harder than others, and you might see a pattern that will help you revise and improve your program.

➤ Review your journal regularly to see your progress and to help keep yourself on track.

➤ Be good to yourself. If you don't do well one week because of a few parties, a vacation, or the holidays, don't despair. If you stick to a healthy, nutritious diet most of the time, a little indulgence is okay. Just remember to get back on track; you will feel better because of it.

Working with a nutritionist and/or a personal trainer can give you the discipline you need to get started on your weight-loss program. Because you will be paying for their expertise, you will be more likely to stick with the plan to get your money's worth. Get a recommendation from a trusted friend or interview several nutritionists/ personal trainers before committing to working with someone who will help reshape your body and your life.

Keep in mind that anyone who has become "morbidly obese"—a dangerous health situation in which someone is 45 percent or more above his or her ideal body weight for his or her height and age—needs to see a physician and perhaps go to an obesity clinic that specializes in radical behavior modification in activity and eating.

The following are several ideas for shaving about 100 calories off your daily intake without really trying:

➤ Instead of a handful of nuts, munch on a handful of pretzels.

➤ Use one less tablespoon of butter or oil per recipe.

➤ Add 6 ounces of seltzer or sparkling water to 4 ounces of juice instead of drinking 8 ounces of juice.

➤ Drink a wine spritzer (half wine and half seltzer) instead of a glass of wine.

➤ Drink 8 to 16 ounces of water about a half-hour before each meal and even before snacks. This not only will help keep you hydrated, it will make your hunger subside a bit. It makes you fill up more quickly so you have less room for food.

➤ Eat half a fistful less pasta (about a half cup) per portion.

➤ Dip chips in salsa instead of guacamole. Dip carrot, celery, or green pepper sticks instead of chips.

➤ Use mustard instead of mayonnaise on your sandwich.

➤ Eat a half scoop of ice cream with a half scoop of sorbet instead of one big scoop of ice cream.

➤ Treat yourself to filet mignon as opposed to a T-bone steak.

Women's magazines, food columns, and food and nutrition Web sites are full of calorie- and fat-paring eating tactics. You can come up with plenty of other little tricks like this to help you save calories during the course of the day or the week.

The Counting Game

Keeping track of how much fat, fiber, protein, and carbohydrates you take in is easy, thanks to nutrition labels on packaged foods. The trick is to pay attention to the serv-ing size. If you only eat the serving size listed on the package, your calorie and gram count will be quite accurate. Many times, however, the first half-cup, inch, or what-ever doesn't seem like enough of what you are eating. Americans tend to eat bigger portions than needed or recommended on the package. Then they wonder why the calories and grams they think they counted don't produce weight loss.

One of the food industry's modern triumphs is the development of reasonably palatable low-fat and no-fat foods. A dismal by-product of this development is that people have inferred that calorie consumption no longer matters when fat intake is lower. People seem to think they have the green light to ingest vast quantities of reduced-fat food and not gain weight. In fact, calories do count. In fact, by eating an excessive quantity of fat-free foods, people may be deluding themselves into thinking that they will lose weight.

Furthermore, some fat is necessary. It is the fat in foods that releases a hormone called cholecystokinin, which signals satiation, and by eating severely fat-reduced food, the hormone isn't released. Thus people keep eating and eating calorie-laden but fat-reduced meals and snacks, which add up to too many calories. In addition, some dietary fat is necessary for the body to process fat-soluble vitamins.

Don't use a workout program as an excuse to chow down on a huge steak every day. The recommended daily protein requirement is .8 gram per kilogram of body weight, which translates to a daily maximum of 60 grams for an average adult—just a shade over 2 ounces!

The Facts on Fat

It is important to watch your fat intake, but some fats are good, even essential to your well-being. The current fad of low-fat and no-fat foods does not delineate between good fats and bad fats. Another problem with the low-fat, no-fat craze is that foods marketed as low fat seem to invite some people to eat two or three instead of one of something or half a bag instead of a handful. This ends up adding calories to the bottom line and often calories that are high in sugar, sodium, and hydrogenated oils. If these ingested calories are not used for energy, they will be converted and stored as fat.

Experts agree that, when people try to completely eliminate fats, they often end up without enough "good fats," which have fatty acids that are essential for many of the body's properties and functions. "Bad fats" include saturated fats and transfats, and unsaturated fats include the essential fatty acids your body needs.

Quote, Unquote

"A popular sports-nutrition dietary fad revolves around the myth that high-carbohydrate diets impair athletic performance and make athletes fat. This dietary regime is based on case histories, testimonials, and unpublished, poorly controlled studies. Although athletes may be seeking a 'magic bullet,' a dietary cure-all does not exist. Following the diet (carbohydrate 40 percent, protein 30 percent, fat 30 percent) may actually impair performance because of inadequate dietary carbohydrate intake, and possibly calorie intake."

—Jane Houck, M.S., R.D.

What exactly does this mean in terms of what you can put into your mouth? Mono-unsaturated and polyunsaturated fats, those so-called "good fats," are found in such

Quote, Unquote

"It's really scary to apply the concept of not eating a low-fat diet to the public at large. Fat is so prevalent in the American diet that people should be aware of how much they are eating."

—Dr. Amy Roberts, coordinator of physiology at the Boulder Center for Sports Medicine and board member for the Boulder chapter of the American Heart Association, Colorado

Quote, Unquote

"If you don't get your nutritional needs met, those products [sports drinks and energy bars] aren't going to do much good. The athlete who is going to perform the best is the one who is best nourished."

—Linda Bonci, nutritionist for the Pittsburgh Steelers and the University of Pittsburgh Athletic Department

foods as nuts, seeds, and cold-pressed oils. Olive, canola, and peanut oils have the best reputation. Balance is the key to oil intake, even oils that are considered to be "good fats." These findings about types of fat do not constitute a green light for bathing everything in cold-pressed virgin olive oil, which adds a whopping 120 calories per tablespoon to your food intake.

Transfats, which are the worst fats, have no redeeming nutritional qualities and have the potential to do harm. These are fats made from hydrogenated oils and are most common in processed foods. Even among experts, the fat-intake controversy continues. All experts seem to agree, however, that some fats are just plain bad for you and that limiting your fat intake while eating a diet rich in the other important food groups will help you stay healthy. Some saturated fats, such as those from animal fat, do have nutritional value but are high in cholesterol. In contrast, fish oils are good for you in terms of both oil quality and the nutritional value of the fish they come with.

The fat-reduction message is getting through—sort of. The U.S. Department of Agriculture has disclosed that Americans reduced the percentage of fat in their diets from 45 percent to 34 percent between 1965 and 1995. That's the good news. The bad news is that Americans are ingesting far more calories and therefore more total grams of fat.

Consuming "Nonfood" Products

In addition to basic foods consumed at mealtime or in snacks, Americans have other opportunities to ingest products that they believe will make them thinner, healthier, stronger, smarter, and more alert. Some of these products work, and some of them don't.

Vitamins and Other Supplements

Some experts believe that vitamins and other supplements are not necessary if you consume a healthy, balanced diet. Others believe that a multivitamin rich in minerals and approaching 100 percent of the recommended daily allowance (RDA) is a smart strategy. In fact, a healthy diet is the best way to ingest your vitamins and minerals, and vitamins should be considered a supplement and not a substitute for a sound, balanced diet. Although some supplements may be good if you are not getting enough of something specific through your diet, virtually all experts agree that taking megadoses of vitamin and mineral supplements might actually be toxic to your body.

In addition to multivitamins, some situations call for specific nutritional supplements. Menstruating women, especially vegetarians, often are counseled to take supplementary iron. In addition, pre- or postmenopausal women are often advised to take a calcium supplement. B-complex vitamins might be recommended for someone under stress, and St. John's wort might be recommended for someone suffering from mild depression. These are all special supplements, however, for particular conditions. You should always consult your physician or a licensed nutritionist before dosing yourself with multivitamins or specific supplements.

Sports Drinks and Energy Bars

Sports drinks and energy bars can be a good way to supplement your diet once you become physically active, especially during rigorous athletic training or competition, but they are not a substitute for a healthy diet with the right combination of fruits, vegetables, grains, meat, and dairy products. Supplementing is the key, because these bars have a lot of calories. If you do not work off the calories, they will end up being stored as fat.

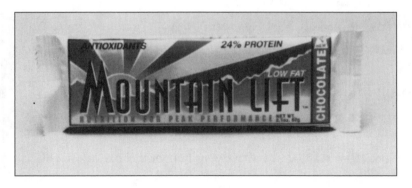

Supplement your diet with high-carbohydrate energy bars.

(Photo: Courtesy of the manufacturer)

If you like these products and they are part of your life, make sure they contain the percentages you need to supplement your diet. If you are using drinks and bars while you exercise, you are looking mainly for carbohydrates to fuel your muscles. A wide choice of bars is available today, and although most of them are high in carbohydrates and low in fat, a few have been developed with the high-protein, low-carbohydrate

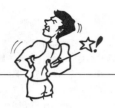

Achtung!

Fat-burning supplements (their technical name is thermogenic aids) comprise a $2 billion industry in this obese land of ours. Neither the supplements nor the claims made for them are governed by the Food and Drug Administration. Not only are many claims overblown, the side effects can be serious: diarrhea, jitters, insomnia, high blood pressure, heart disease, excess hair growth in women, and other problems.

philosophy in mind. Athletes often work with coaches, sports trainers, nutritionists, or sports physiologists to balance their intake of foods and supplements with their training and competition schedules, so as a new exerciser, it's wise to go slowly and cautiously when experimenting with these products.

The Importance of Water

Staying hydrated is essential, especially while you're exercising. Always drink before you are thirsty. Even if you like sports drinks, don't use them as a substitute for water. They should be a supplement to water. Sports drinks generally are lower in calories than juice and soda, but they do contain sodium, which might be all right, especially if you're exercising and perspiring a lot and need some sodium replenishment to prevent cramping. Sports drinks might not be good for you if you are on a sodium-restricted diet.

The most commonly overlooked aspect of good nutrition is proper hydration. If you are thirsty, you already are dehydrated. Your body needs at least 64 fluid ounces of water every day, more if you exercise regularly.

The Least You Need to Know

➤ A healthy, balanced diet is an essential component of your fitness program.

➤ Control your fat intake to reduce calories, but don't eliminate all fats from your diet.

➤ Too much low-fat food can still mean excess calories.

➤ There are no shortcuts to permanent weight loss, and fad diets can produce short-term weight loss but at a cost to your health.

➤ Think of creative ideas that really don't affect your hunger but cut calories and fat from your daily diet.

➤ Vitamins and other supplements are no substitute for a good diet.

➤ Drinking enough water is an important part of your daily intake.

Part 5

Other Essential Tips to Keep You Fit

This book is geared for new exercisers, for people just beginning to work out. Therefore, it emphasizes strength training, aerobic conditioning, and enhanced flexibility. Physical activities that help achieve these goals are important, but they are only a part of the big fitness picture. When you are embarking on a fitness program, there are many other things to know that can help you out—as well as some to watch out for. Some obstacles might make a fitness program seem unrealistic or difficult. Such obstacles include injury, illness, permanent disability, pregnancy, or advancing age.

Some of these—injury, illness, pregnancy—are temporary setbacks that you can work around. Others—disability, the passing of years—are permanent situations that you have to learn to live with. Fitness can help you do that, for none is a barrier to being as strong and healthy as you can be, given the temporary or permanent features of your life.

> *"Who gives today the best that in him lies*
> *will find the road that leads to clearer skies."*
>
> *—John Kendrick Bangs*

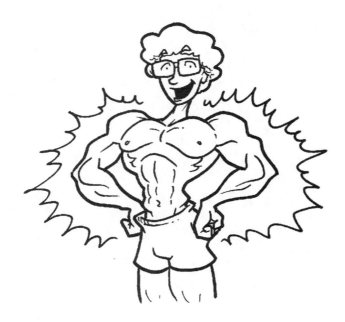

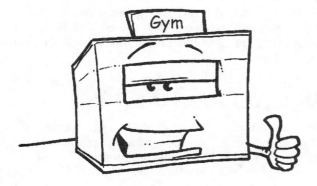

Chapter 21

A Primer on Gyms

In This Chapter

➤ Workout facilities for a variety of budgets and styles

➤ How to assess a workout facility that will work for you

➤ The costs involved in joining a gym

➤ Health club etiquette

In fitness circles, the words "gym" and "club" are synonymous with health club. When your exercising friends say they are going to "the gym" or "the club," they're not talking about the cavernous bleachers-and-hoops indoor sports venue of your old high school or a place to play golf. They are talking about the facility where they work out.

If you haven't been in a locker room since high school, and if you don't know what to expect or what's expected of you, anxiety and even intimidation might cut you out of the health-club experience. Don't let that happen. In truth, there's a gym format for everyone from the low-budget beginning exerciser who shows up in baggy sweats to the sleek gym rat who's as coordinated as he or she is attractive and who really looks good in Lycra. You know what else? The highly toned gym rats usually are so busy looking at themselves in the mirror that they won't bother paying attention to you or what you're wearing.

Still, it's nice to know that there are many options to suit a great range of exercisers. The range includes elaborate and expensive clubs offering a mind-boggling array of classes and programs in drop-dead-gorgeous settings to bare-bones and functional public gyms. All levels of gyms have some predictable characteristics in common—and some that vary widely. There are also private fitness studios where you work one-on-one with a trainer, or you can even hire a trainer to come to your home.

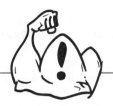

Fitness Fact

Regular gym attendees believe that joining and sticking to a program is good for their health. A study conducted for the International Health, Racquet & Sportsclub Association found that 28 percent of health-club members believe their health to be excellent. This is compared to 24 percent of people who exercise at home or participate in outdoor sports and only 11 percent of sedentary people. Gym rats who work out at least 150 days a year believe they are in the best health of all. Thirty-seven percent of people who go frequently to their clubs believe their health is excellent, compared to 28 percent of general exercisers.

All Gyms Are Not Alike

There are certain commonalities between gyms, whether they're public or private, independent or part of a franchised chain, or even "destination gyms" at spa resorts. No matter where you go to work out, you can expect to find rooms with an assortment of exercise apparatus, large and small studios for various scheduled classes, and locker rooms where you can shower and change. Studios are equipped with whatever equipment is needed for classes held there, such as aerobics benches, mats for floor exercises and stretching, hand weights, jump ropes, stretch bands, and other workout paraphernalia. And, of course, there are rooms for group cycling classes and its offshoots, such as studio rowing or stairclimbing.

Some clubs also offer tennis, racquetball, handball, basketball, or volleyball courts, and swimming pools for churning laps. There is often a sauna, a whirlpool, or a steambath—often all three, and perhaps more than one of each. Personnel include a cadre of weight-room attendants and exercise instructors, plus personal trainers and massage therapists whose time can be booked separately. These are common to virtually all gyms. Their size and variety, the degree of opulence, and the clientele are what differ. (The only version of a gym that often is significantly scaled-down might be a hotel's fitness center, which can be likened to a one-room gym with limited equipment and often no staff at all.)

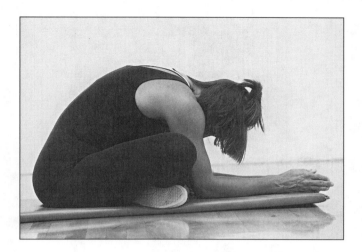

Gyms provide mats and space for floor exercises and stretching—an essential component of all workouts.

(Photo: Anne W. Krause)

Public

Public recreation facilities, as the name implies, generally are open to anyone who wants to use them. They include places such as your local YMCA and community recreation center. Usage tends to be available on a pay-as-you-go basis, by the day or by the activity, with a punch card or a monthly or annual membership that entitles you to use most amenities and classes without additional charge. Such public facilities usually don't require any kind of up-front initiation fee, and the rates are reasonable.

Community recreation centers are run by the specific city, town, or county where they are located. Colleges and universities also often have recreation centers for students and faculty, and some permit residents of the surrounding community to use them as well. Again, individual centers' facilities and programs will vary depending on the community's needs and budget. Residents of the city where the recreation center is located usually pay a slightly lower fee than nonresidents.

The YMCA, a nationwide, nonprofit, community-service organization, has independent facilities throughout the country. It offers community-based health, fitness, and aquatics programs and often a quality weight room as well. Each YMCA develops its own programs based on community needs. Because each YMCA is independent, facilities and programs vary from YMCA to YMCA. Call your local Y, or stop in for a visit to see if it fits your needs. It very well might, and it probably won't strain your budget.

Both of these types of public recreation centers are developed to appeal to the community as a whole, and they generally offer a wide variety of programs for adults and children. Their selection ranges from swim and gym classes for children and adults to aerobics and dance classes, after-school and summer camp programs for kids, and outdoor programs.

Gyms offer a variety of aerobics classes for different levels of fitness ability.

(Photo: Anne W. Krause)

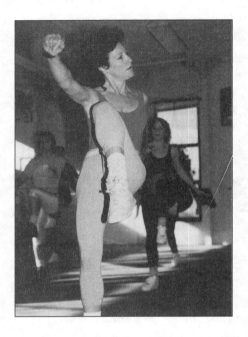

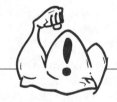

Fit Tip

Even if you belong to a private health club, you might find that the Y or rec center offers an interesting program that your private club doesn't. It's not an either–or situation. You can belong to a private club and also sign up for something specific at a public gym.

Public facilities do have downsides along the lines of "you get what you pay for." They might not have the latest models of apparatus or even as much equipment as a competitive private club. There probably will not be as many weight-room attendants. It probably doesn't matter a whole lot whether you're riding a new stationary bike or one that's few years old, as long as it's properly maintained, but you might be bothered if you always have to wait a long time for your turn at a cardio machine or strength-training station.

Private

Private health clubs and fitness centers are profit-making businesses. In well-populated cities and suburbs, they also are competitive with each other. In fitness-crazy communities where many people belong to clubs, they are *very* competitive with each other. Some gyms, such as Bally Total Fitness, 24-Hour Gym, or Gold's Gym, are franchises that belong to national chains. Others belong to local or regional chains. Still others are independent.

As you might expect, top clubs offer a full array of classes, from aerobics to yoga (or even Zen meditation) to Pilates, plus superlative weight rooms, swimming pools, indoor and outdoor ball courts, dance and martial arts studios, and more. They often have on-site retail shops (selling workout clothes, tennis balls, nifty sun visors, skin-care products, and so on), massage therapists, and even physical therapists and chiropractors—and perhaps even a hairstyling salon. Because many members' social lives revolve around the gym, the facilities might also include a lounge or a restaurant that generally serves healthy cuisine. Some gyms also offer childcare for tots while their parents' exercise plus kids' classes for older children.

Fitness Fact

Bally Total Fitness operates 335 fitness centers in 27 states and Canada, making it the largest national operator of commercial health clubs. Four million people belong to the chain's clubs, where they work out 110 million times a week. Bally's boasts 5,500 fitness instructors and 1,600 personal trainers.

Very Private

A new generation of "miniclubs" that might be considered very private are popping up in many cities and communities. These clubs generally are studios that offer totally individualized programs with one-on-one training. The advantages of a very private facility include privacy, the undivided attention of the trainer or instructor every time you work out, and no waiting for equipment. These clubs also come with hefty price tags, however, and they might not have as much equipment as big clubs. For the well-off, the shy, or someone recovering from an injury, however, they might be just the ticket.

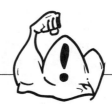

Fit Tip

New housing subdivisions often have some kind of common area that might have a swimming pool, tennis courts, and perhaps even a fitness room. Many apartment buildings have workout rooms as well. These facilities generally are open only to residents and perhaps their guests.

Specialized

A growing number of health clubs cater only to women, but there are far more specialized facilities than that. Your community might boast studios that specialize in just one discipline or activity, such as martial arts, boxing, music and dance programs, studio

Quote, Unquote

"Setting up a program for somebody and giving them a schedule is just the beginning. It's understanding what makes a person tick, what motivates them, and understanding what blocks that person from being the best athlete they can be."

—Lorraine Moeller, four-time Olympic marathoner and current running coach

cycling, yoga, Pilates, rock-climbing, and others. These facilities have several main advantages. First, their equipment is specialized and therefore is probably top of the line. Second, the staff and instructors are as specialized as the machines, so they can offer real expertise. Third, everyone using the facility has the same goal you do, which makes for a mutually supportive environment. Turning the tables, though, a staff and instructors that specialize in one activity might not be of great assistance if you are interested in a varied workout program. If you want to try out other activities or you want the option to cross-train, you can't meet your goals all in one place, which is the advantage of a multipurpose club.

In-Home Trainer

If you have set up your own home gym (see Chapter 16, "Where to Work Out"), you have a splendid opportunity to hire a trainer to work with you in your own home. This is the ultimate in personal attention, convenience, and privacy. It also is a great way to learn proper use of the expensive equipment you purchased. You can hire a trainer to work with you on an on-going basis, or you can just arrange a time or two to help you set up your program initially and then to tweak the program if you get bored or haven't progressed and need to push your workout to the next level. Word-of-mouth and recommendations at local health clubs are good ways to connect with a personal trainer, or you can log on to a nationwide directory at www.fit-net.com/trainers.

Personal fitness training services are available at a variety of gyms.

(Photo: Courtesy of Hyatt Regency Beaver Creek Resort and Spa)

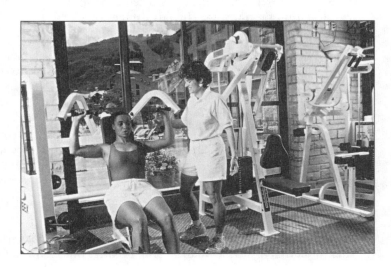

Destination Gyms

Some of the most elaborate facilities can be found at destination health spas, where guests pay top dollar for a week of exercising and relaxation. Not only are the gyms usually very attractive and equipped with top-of-the-line apparatus, they usually are in beautiful settings, such as the mountains, the desert, or near a seashore. (Again, see Chapter 16.) These gyms get a transient population, but their staffs and trainers are used to working with a changing stream of clients. Staff members are accustomed to evaluating people and working up a program for them, but they are not around for follow-up. In addition to excellent gym facilities, destination spas usually have an extensive menu of massage and aesthetic offerings.

The Bottom Line on Costs

There are as many cost figures as there are clubs, so use these figures only as a guideline. The best values tend to be public facilities, typically YMCAs or city recreation centers. Most sell an unlimited-use pass that is good for access to weight rooms, the swimming pool, tennis courts, and most classes. Studio cycling classes, running workshops, swimming or tennis instruction, and other specialized programs might cost extra—but the rates usually are modest. This makes them attractive not just to people on a budget, but also to new exercisers who are not ready to make a big monetary investment in a fitness program.

At public gyms, adult admission is under— sometimes well under—$5 per visit or $300 a year, and less-expensive children's or youth fees often are valid through age 18. In some communities, a low-priced youth or student pass also is available. In addition, many centers offer one-time entry fees and punch cards good for 10, 20, 50, or another specific number of visits. If you use the whole card, it generally is a good deal. Lockers are free.

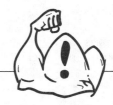

Fit Tip

Spa Finder, a glossy magazine, features an annual directory of categories such as "Fitness, Beauty, and Wellness," "Luxury Spa Destinations," "Weight Management Spas," "Adventure Spas," and more. If you can't find the magazine locally, call 212–924-6800 or check www. spafinders.com. Spa Finder is also a travel agency specializing in spa vacations and can be reached at 1–800–ALL-SPAS (1–800–255–7727).

The three most common cost components of private clubs are the initiation fee ($125 to $400), the monthly membership fee ($50 to $125 a month), and locker fees ($10 to $25 a month, which may be with or without towel and/or laundry service). Bally's Total Fitness, a huge national chain, comes in with near-public-gym costs. The company claims that most new members finance their initiation fees for up to 36 months. Initial monthly payments are $25 to $45 and drop to $6 to $15 after the initiation fee is paid off. The company also has a procedure for transferring membership from one location to another when a member moves.

There are ways to save money on health-club costs. Some clubs offer reduced-rate "matinee" or "early bird" memberships for people who can work out during slower times, such as weekdays between about 9 A.M. and 4 or 5 P.M. Other clubs periodically float two-for-one deals, which are excellent for couples, co-workers, or friends who want to shape up together. In competitive markets, at certain times of the year when many people prefer exercising outdoors or when a fancy new club opens nearby, some clubs offer good deals on memberships. Like public gyms, private ones might charge additional fees for some specialized classes. Clubs that don't include towel or laundry service might offer it as an add-on. Some clubs that are part of pricey destination resorts offer well-priced annual memberships for lucky locals.

In the past, health clubs earned a reputation for sales tactics such as lifetime memberships (now illegal in many states) and other high-pressure techniques. They are shaping up. According to the Council of Better Business Bureaus, consumer complaints against health clubs fell from 3,240 in 1991 to 263 in 1997. During that same time period, membership increased from 20,995,000 to 28,305,000.

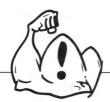

Fitness Fact

Studio- or gym-quality apparatus carry hefty price tags: up to $7,000 for a multifunction weight-stack machine, $6,000 for a treadmill, $4,000 for an elliptical trainer, and $3,000 for a stationary bike. This partially explains why health-club memberships are pricey—and why using a Y or rec center is such a good deal.

Joining a Private Gym or Health Club

You can always get a walk-through of any club that interests you. This provides you with a glimpse of the facilities and a sense of the atmosphere. A perky and enthusiastic membership representative probably will take you on your tour, and he or she is going to be very interested in getting you to sign on the dotted line right then. You might even be offered a good deal including a rate reduction or a lower initiation fee, for signing up that very day. Don't feel pressured to join a health club immediately. You often can accept the same offer or even negotiate a better one a few days later.

If you can, it is a good idea to do more than simply take a guided tour. Try to pay a test visit to the club to make sure it is a place you will be comfortable joining. Most clubs will let you try their facility for free, and some even will give you a complimentary week-long pass, but even a small charge is worth the investment. If this kind of offer is not mentioned during the tour and you think you might like the club, ask. It is important to see what the club is like during the time of day you will frequent it. You won't know whether you like the atmosphere until you've donned your workout gear and tested the place.

Like every business, private health and fitness centers occasionally offer sales or volume discounts. (Don't expect to find such deals offered by public facilities such as rec centers and Ys.) Here are some kinds of offers to watch for:

➤ **Seasonal specials.** In the North, you're most likely to find a good deal at a health club in the summer when many regulars prefer outdoor activities. In the South, value seasons might be spring and fall. "Summer Shape-Up" or other seasonal specials also might be promoted.

➤ **Volume discounts.** You also might want to check whether local clubs have corporate memberships available and see if your company is eligible. If a number of people from one company join a health club, savings often are available on membership fees and such.

➤ **Trial programs.** Some gyms lower their rates, lower the initiation fee, or come up with short-term, no-initiation-fee memberships.

If you've never joined a gym or health club, look for one that offers six- or 12-month introductory memberships and that has a cancellation clause in the agreement. Beware if a club insists on only a 24- or 36-month contract and extracts a heavy penalty for canceling. Two or three years is a long commitment. People who move, change jobs, or find a different workout site that suits them better should not be forced to keep an impossible or unsuitable long-term commitment to a club.

Good Gym Manners

Fitness-center etiquette can be divided into two categories: written rules and unwritten courtesies. When joining a gym, it is a good idea to find out the official rules and regulations of the facility, which might include hours of operation, check-in procedures, guest reservations, on-site smoking, policies for children, and so on. It won't be much fun if you show up to lift weights 15 minutes before

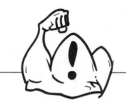

Fit Tip

You can tap into an online directory of more than 5,000 gyms nationwide at www.fit-net.com/gyms. This is useful if you are new to an area or are planning to move soon.

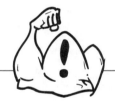

Fit Tip

Health clubs and gyms that are for-profit businesses often have aggressive sign-up campaigns, but they also want to keep you happy so you'll sign up for another time period. The good ones keep on top of things in terms of both equipment and staff to keep clients happy.

the club closes, and it won't be fun for other people working out if you let your young child into a part of the club where he or she is not allowed.

Following the Rules

When it comes to unwritten gym etiquette and good manners, keeping in mind the golden rule, "Do unto others as you would have them do unto you," is a good place to start. The spray bottle and towel are on the windowsill for a reason—so you can clean up your sweat after 45 minutes on the stairstepper. You don't want to use an apparatus that is still damp from another person's efforts, and no one else wants yours. If you hit the gym at a really busy time, you should be wiping down that sweat after only 30 minutes so someone else can have the opportunity to work out. In other words, don't hog one piece of equipment when there's a wait.

Other examples of unwritten rules might involve locker-room manners:

➤ At "rush hour," don't stay on a cardio machine for more than 30 minutes.

➤ Keep your grunting and groaning down in the weight room. Some body-builders try to impress others with how much they can lift, but the noise is more irritating than impressive.

➤ Don't stare in the locker room, no matter how great or bad someone else's body is. Give people their own space when they are changing clothes, and expect that you will be given the same consideration.

➤ Dispose of your used towels properly when you are done with them. Most clubs have towel bins in their locker rooms and/or at the front desk.

➤ If you use a paper cup for drinking water, toss it into the trash when you are finished.

➤ Don't leave gobs of shampoo on the shower walls, don't leave hair in the sink, and wipe down the vanity if you've made a mess.

➤ Dress appropriately so you don't make others feel uncomfortable. Provocative workout wear is not uncommon in some clubs, but it is frowned upon in others.

➤ Don't show up at the club polishing off your last crumbs of a hamburger and fries—or any food, for that matter.

➤ The major no-no in and around many clubs is smoking. After all, they are health clubs.

When you're in the gym, the locker room, or the weight room, be considerate of others. If you're not sure whether something you want to do is appropriate, trust your instincts. Wondering is a good sign that it might not be.

Foiling Foot Fungus

Athlete's foot can be an unfortunate by-product of going to the gym. This contagious fungal infection spreads like wildfire by direct contact with locker-room and bathroom floors. It appears that men are more susceptible than women and adults are more susceptible than children. Your toes know when you've caught it. Itching, burning, and cracked skin between your toes are the first symptoms.

To prevent athlete's foot, consider wearing shower sandals instead of walking barefoot in the locker room or in spa areas. Keep your feet clean and dry, perhaps even using a paper towel or a blow dryer (on cool) instead of a damp terrycloth towel. Wear cotton socks, change them often, and try not to wear wet sneakers. If you do get athlete's foot, over-the-counter antifungal creams can help cure the condition.

The Least You Need to Know

➤ All health clubs include a variety of exercise equipment and classes, a weight room, a locker room, and qualified fitness trainers.

➤ Workout facilities come in a variety of styles, from very basic to ultra elaborate and extensive.

➤ Workout facilities are available to accommodate all budgets.

➤ It is important to follow written policies, as well as unwritten common courtesy, at all clubs.

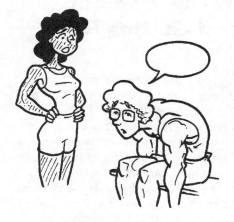

Chapter 22

When You've Hit the Workout Wall

In This Chapter

➤ Benefiting from an occasional day off without derailing your fitness program

➤ Telling "real tired" from "lazy tired"

➤ Rewarding yourself for what you've accomplished

➤ Consistency, the key to long-range fitness

"Whenever the urge to exercise comes upon me, I lie down for a while and it passes," said educator and author Robert Maynard Hutchins. He turned an antiexercising ethic into a catchy sentence often quoted by people who are looking for justification for being sedentary. Everybody, at some time or another, has a "Hutchins moment" when the will to work out is missing. Like every exerciser, at some point in your fitness program, you will be tired, discouraged, bored, or a combination of these. No matter how conscientious you are, you can expect it to happen. Your body and your brain will tell you that you just don't want to continue. It might be because you feel you've reached your goal, and you think your body will magically maintain that level of fitness and weight. Or you might experience the opposite emotion and feel that you'll *never* get there, so why bother?

When you hit the wall, you need to pull back, take a break for a day or two, treat yourself to something special, reassess your progress and your goals, and then plunge back in. The fitness you worked so hard to attain is not self-maintaining. You have to keep at it. If you haven't reached your goal yet, think about how much closer you are than when you started.

Falling Off the Workout Wagon (and Getting Right Back On)

For every day that you work out and eat right, you are one day closer to your goal. Every time you skip part of your program, especially early on when you are increasing rather than maintaining fitness, you are not nearing your goal. There are times, however, when that fudge sundae, that desire to sleep in rather than work out, or that magnetic pull of the television will win out over your workout. Missing a day when you are just beginning to exercise or even a week when you've been exercising for a while is not a tragedy. Using the missed day or week as an excuse to quit is.

When excuses become a frequent part of your vocabulary, words such as "tomorrow" and "later" are the first signs that you are about to fall off the workout wagon. Don't let it happen. Pull out every trick you know to get back on a program. A rider who falls off a horse gets back on. A skater or a gymnast who falls in the middle of a competition gets up and continues. A skier or a snowboarder who takes a tumble on the slopes gets up and keeps sliding. And that's how you should be when it comes to exercising and eating right.

No Excuse for Excuses

Here are some of the common excuses people—maybe even you—use to avoid a workout:

➤ "I'll start again tomorrow."

➤ "It's been a long day. I'll skip today and work out more tomorrow."

➤ "I'm too tired. I'll rest and then work out later."

➤ "I haven't had dinner yet. I'll go out later after I've eaten."

➤ "I'm too full. I'll let dinner settle and then go out later."

➤ "I just want to watch the news. Then I'll work out later."

➤ "It looks like rain. I'll go for a walk tomorrow."

➤ "It has just rained. Everything is wet. I'll go for a walk tomorrow."

➤ "I've got to get my oil (or tires) changed. I'll work out later."

➤ "I planned to go to the gym during my lunch hour, but my inbox is overflowing. I'll go later, after work, or tomorrow."

➤ "I have to get to the post office (or the bank or the dry cleaner) before it closes. I'll work out later."

Instead of looking for excuses *not* to work out, try to reprogram your thinking with reasons *to* exercise. The same incentives and motivations that got you started on the program are still there. Use them whenever you need them.

Be a Modifier, Not a Quitter

Sometimes all you need to do to start exercising again is tweak your program. If you stop because you are a beginner and you find it all too hard, don't quit. Instead, just work out at a less-ambitious level. If you stop because you are sore, give yourself time in a whirlpool or sauna or perhaps treat yourself to a massage. Then start again gently, perhaps with another form of exercise, and always remember to stretch after you've finished. As you become more accustomed to working out, soreness will not be a problem.

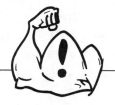

Fit Tip

The front of the Top 10 Exercise Excuses T-shirt features such clichés as "It's too hot," "It's too cold," "I'm too old," "It's too early," and "It's too late." The back triumphantly proclaims "DID IT ANYWAY." The shirt is available from the Babbling Brook Catalog at 1-800-765-3975.

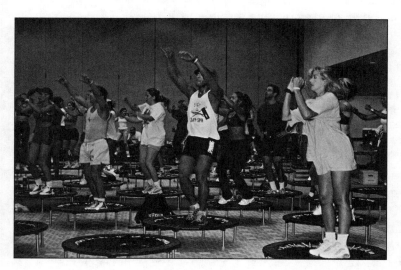

If you're feeling bored with your regular routine, try something new, like a Rebounding class.

(Photo: Claire Walter)

Even the most dedicated exercisers occasionally get bored with their routines. Here are some tricks—some of which fall into the category of cross-training—that you can try if you are tempted to stop working out because you are bored:

➤ Book a few sessions with a trainer to remotivate yourself and to develop a new routine.

➤ Try a new variation on your regular activity, such as cardio-funk, kickboxing, or any of the new hybrid cardio workouts instead of plain aerobics. You might want to try a different yoga program or go for a hike instead of a jog.

➤ Try a totally new exercise. If you're a runner, take a step class. If you're a swimmer, go for a bike ride. If you've been pumping iron, sign up for Pilates.

➤ Ask your spouse or partner to nudge you as a reminder to work out. You could even ask the person to come with you.

➤ Plan to work out with a friend. Even if one of you doesn't feel like exercising, the other one probably will.

➤ Don't let weather get you down. Invest in warm socks, rain gear, and deep-tread footwear for walking or running on snowy days. For exercising outdoors in the Sunbelt, purchase lightweight clothing and a brimmed hat with a ventilated crown.

➤ If the weather has turned really bad and you can't bear to exercise outdoors, head inside and try a class in aerobics, yoga, or martial arts. You can hop on a treadmill, a stationary bike, or another apparatus you haven't tried before.

➤ Even if you usually work out indoors, you can change your venue—and perhaps your outlook. Instead of exercising at home with free weights, go to a gym with a multistation machine or other strength-training devices. Or save yourself a trip to the gym and pop an exercise tape into the VCR.

Sharing the victories and defeats of your fitness regime with a friend will help keep you motivated.

(Photo: Courtesy of Keystone Resorts)

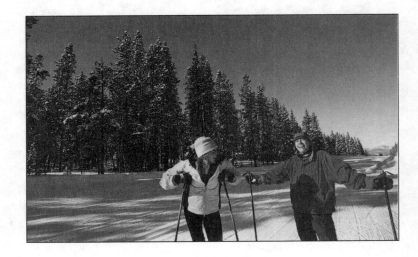

Sometimes it's simply frustration that causes people to quit exercising, and you might find yourself in that place, too. It often happens when you have reached a plateau and don't see yourself getting slimmer or stronger. Let's say you've put yourself on a one-year plan. About half of the strength gains come in the first three months. The smaller gains that follow might seem comparatively trivial. If this is the cause of your discouragement, drag out your "before" pictures or videotape or really pore over your workout log. You may have reached a plateau, but chances are it's far higher than your starting point. Revel in the progress you've made, congratulate yourself or give yourself a tangible reward, and rev up your routine for your next great leap.

Always remember that some exercise is better than no exercise, and once you have committed yourself to a fitness program, you will quickly become stronger and build endurance. A 15-minute walk seems like a marathon to someone who is really sedentary, and one-pound hand weights can feel like the world on Atlas's shoulders to a person with no muscle strength. Instead of giving up completely and returning to your old ways, set modest goals, post them where you can see them, and keep reminding yourself that you have no place to go but into a realm of greater strength and fitness.

Quote, Unquote

"Here's what I do [when I've lost interest in exercise]: I buy exercise equipment and put some money into it. Then I ask my wife and kids to get me up early in the morning and get me on the equipment. I've got a treadmill, a Nautilus chair crunch machine, a punching bag, and more. My garage is filled with that stuff, but I don't call it a waste because every one of those gadgets helped me when I needed it. If you can't afford equipment, buy running or hiking shoes and start walking."

—George Foreman, former world heavyweight boxing champion, in *USA Weekend* magazine

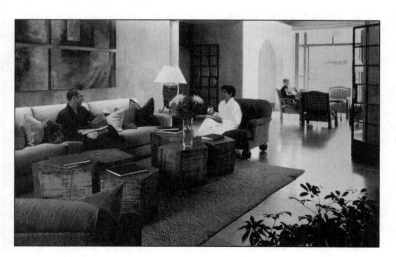

Promise yourself a trip to a spa when you reach a specific goal.

(Photo: Courtesy of Hyatt Regency Beaver Creek Resort and Spa)

Don't Be a Slave to Your Scale

What is it with people and scales? When we see one, our feet are drawn to it as if magnetically, and our eyes are riveted to the display. Up a pound? Down two? We shift our weight because we've learned that, on this scale, standing sideways or on one foot subtracts a pound. Silly, isn't it?

Certainly, weight is one indicator of fitness, and if you want to lose weight, that number might be all you care about. If you are on a true fitness program, however, you should understand that inches, muscle tone, strength, energy, and even factors such as blood pressure are far more important than a number on the scale. Therefore, if you know you have gotten stronger or more toned, if you get through the day more easily, or if your doctor gives you thumbs up instead of dire warnings, you know you're doing right by yourself, no matter what the scale reads.

Be Proud of How Far You've Come

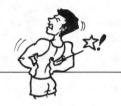

As previously mentioned, sometimes a workout routine can get frustrating if you don't see dramatic and tangible results on a regular basis. If you've been on a program to lose weight or to get fit for several months, look back to where you started. What were the goals you set when you first started? Pat yourself on the back for the goals you have reached. Congratulate yourself for keeping up with your program, even on days when you felt like giving up. Do you have more energy than you did when you started? Can you fit into a piece of clothing you never thought you'd wear again? Can you see the tone forming in your muscles? You deserve credit for every one of these accomplishments.

If just giving yourself a pat on the back doesn't do it for you, create a more tangible reward system for yourself. How often do you need a reward? If it's once a week, then at the end of each week without a skip in your workout routine, treat yourself to something small, like taking the time for a soak in the hot tub at the health club or an hour curled up reading a book. Promise yourself a bigger treat for each month you make it through your workout routine without a hitch. Think about being even more generous to yourself. Buy a new piece of workout clothing to wear to the gym or a new workout gadget, such as a heart-rate monitor; accessories for aquatic workouts; or safety equipment, such as a good light for your bike.

This system of self-rewards doesn't mean that you can't ever take a day off or that missing one or two workouts is a disaster. You are the final judge of your dedication, and you probably are your harshest critic. You also can develop a reward system with a workout buddy. It's easy to slack off or be hard on yourself, and your friend probably will have the same reactions. You can meet to work out together, or you can each follow your own routine but still help each other out. The two of you can share workout war stories to support each other, and this can be really motivational. Even if you and your friend are at different fitness levels, the support system between friends is important. If you don't exercise together, plan to talk with your friend once a week about how each of your routines is going. If both of you are on target, give yourselves a social event, such as getting together for breakfast or lunch once a month to congratulate yourselves your progress.

You might not see tangible progress every day, but once you begin working out regularly, you will be making progress whether you can see it or not. You will be getting stronger and more fit. You will lose weight if that is your goal, and your body will become firmer and more toned even if weight loss is not your goal. Always try to remember that your exercise program is leading you to a healthier, more active lifestyle.

Listen to Your Body

If you've been following your new fitness program with diligence and consistency, your workout wall might be just plain fatigue. The human body is smart. If a workout that has become easy is dragging, your body might be telling you it's tired. The longer you follow a workout routine, the better you will get to know your body and what it *really* is feeling. You can't maintain fitness without regular workouts, but your muscles won't dissolve into flab if you skip a day now and again.

Your body knows the difference between being "really tired" and being "excuse tired" or "lazy tired." Listen to your body when you feel weary. Perhaps you've been working late every day, you've got a dynamite social life and stay up too late too many nights in a row, or your child has been up every night because of nightmares or a tummy ache—yet you've still been working out on a regular basis. Maybe you've just pushed your workout routine to a higher level. If you think you feel tired, you probably are. Still, try not to use this tired feeling as a reason to stop working out or to go on a junk-food binge. Take a day off if you need to, or take a 15-minute walk instead of pushing through that 30-minute jog. You'll probably feel a lot better the next day.

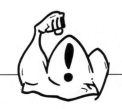

Fit Tip

Your body needs rest and recovery to get stronger, especially before and after a race and after intense weight work. Hard weight workouts break down muscle fibers. Rest builds them back up again and increases their strength. Pushing through a hard workout when your muscles are truly fatigued is not beneficial and can even cause injury.

Consistency Is the Key to Success

You probably brush your teeth every day and go to the dentist once or twice a year. The importance of regular dental hygiene is comparable to the importance of consistency in a workout regime. If you don't brush your teeth every day, you might not notice it right away, but over time, your teeth and gums will become unhealthy. At some point, you will have let them go too far, and you might eventually have root-canal surgery or even get false teeth. Likewise, if you don't work out regularly, you might not notice right away, but over time, you will have less energy, you might gain weight, and your doctor might report that you have high blood pressure or high cholesterol. To reach your fitness goals and lead a healthier lifestyle, a regular fitness routine is essential. Make physical activity a fun, important, and addictive part of your daily life.

Other Problems

Slacking off on a fitness program, or even being tempted to quit, isn't always a mere matter of the blahs—something that the power of positive thinking, self-congratulations, or a reward often can cure. Some people slow down or stop working out for various other reasons. Michael Gerrish, a personal trainer in Newburyport, Massachusetts, has identified various physical, emotional, and even nutritional conditions that prevent people from carrying on with their planned programs. He calls them UFOs—unidentified fitness obstacles. Such UFOs to working out, which you can deal with once you have identified them, include:

➤ Mild depression and depression-induced physical lethargy

➤ Genetic limitations or previous injuries

➤ Societal pressure or embarrassment about appearance

➤ Misaligned joints or joint pain from embarking on too ambitious a workout too quickly without adequate strength training

➤ Mood-altering medications or clashing prescription drugs

➤ Time pressure

➤ Attention deficit disorder (ADD)

➤ Poor nutrition, poor food combinations, or poor timing in eating and exercising

➤ Premenstrual syndrome (PMS)

➤ Allergies or allergy medications

➤ Overestimating workout or underestimating food intake

➤ Obsession with weight or calorie burning

➤ Chronic Fatigue Syndrome

If you suspect any of these problems, consult a medical practitioner. It might indeed be "all in your head," but then again, perhaps your problems are real and are based on physical or biochemical conditions. If so, traditional and alternative remedies have been known to help people overcome such hurdles to achieve their fitness goals.

Looking Ahead

Everyone has different interests and goals, and these interests and goals generally shift over time. This also is true of your fitness program. As with any goal or interest, lifelong fitness requires constant reevaluation and looking ahead. If you started your program for a certain reason and then attained that goal or no longer are interested in that goal, it's time to reassess.

If you started your fitness program to lose weight, for example, and you have reached that desired weight, you probably need a tangible reason to keep going. Perhaps in your quest to lose weight you came to really enjoy walking. Look at your newfound hobby and see where you can take it. Perhaps you can try jogging, or maybe you want to travel to a new destination, explore an exciting city on foot, or take a walking tour through beautiful scenery. It's thrilling to know that you now have the stamina for such adventures, and you might want your next one to be a trek someplace really exotic.

Maybe your fitness goal started because of your children. Perhaps you wanted to do more activities with them without getting too tired. During

Quote, Unquote

"It's not because you're lazy or lack willpower. There's something wrong with you, per se, but each individual has obstacles, and each person must identify them and cope with them."

—Michael Gerrish, personal trainer and author of *When Working Out Isn't Working Out*

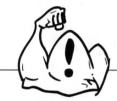

Fit Tip

Extra, extra ... read all about it! There are a multitude of magazines and books about almost every sport. When you need inspiration or how-to ideas, go to a bookstore or library to find a new book or magazine. For on-going stimulation, subscribe to a magazine about your favorite activity. If you can't find the one you want, log on to the Web and search for information about your new sport. Chances are there is a publication, or several, that covers it.

the process, maybe you learned to love bicycling. Maybe you want to try a one-day cycling tour or find a multiday tour that you and your children can do together. Perhaps you started swimming when you took your youngsters to the pool or the beach. Your next goal might be to become a better swimmer yourself, so you might enjoy an adult or masters' swimming class.

As you have learned in this book, you can participate in many activities that provide fitness benefits. Keep this book as a resource for ideas when you start to get bored or fall off the workout wagon. In addition, there are many other resources for finding new fitness outlets and people to work out with. The most important part of the road to fitness is keeping yourself interested so you develop consistency in working out. Working out doesn't have to be all work, so to speak. You are developing a lifestyle, so make sure you have along the way.

The Least You Need to Know

➤ Don't make excuses to yourself or others for not working out.

➤ Be encouraged by your accomplishments, not discouraged because you haven't attained your goals.

➤ If you take an occasional day off or pull back a little, you won't lose all you've gained.

➤ Reward yourself for your accomplishments.

➤ Your body will tell you when you need to rest.

➤ Relative consistency is an essential ingredient to a fitness program.

➤ As with any goals, your fitness goals will need ongoing reassessment.

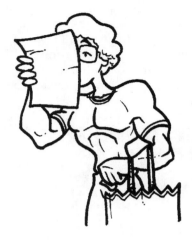

Chapter 23

Shape-Up Shopping List

In This Chapter

➤ Proper footwear, your most important fitness program purchase

➤ Exercise in what you have, or buy specialized workout wear

➤ Wear layers to stay comfortable while exercising outdoors

➤ Some exercise products that are a waste of money

Whether you exercise at home or in a gym, you need comfortable, functional exercise garments and appropriate, well-fitting footwear. In the beginning of an exercise program, you might feel that sweats or shorts, a T-shirt, and all-purpose athletic footwear is all you need in the way of equipment. In the beginning, this might be true. As you spend more time in the gym, start to walk or ride a bicycle, or engage in other fitness activities, however, you might feel the need to buy some specialized equipment or clothing. Water aerobics, for example, requires a swimsuit. If you add other sports to your program, you'll need suitable gear, garments, and footwear. Tennis, golf, running, cycling, and team sports are just a few of the activities for which gearing up is the first step.

Fitness Footwear

We all know the great stories about the renowned East African runners who won Olympic medals barefoot, and the Tarahumara Indians from Mexico's Copper Canyon who competed in—and often won—Colorado's grueling Leadville Trail 100 wearing sandals made from discarded automotive tires. Remember too that the fitness gurus of the late 1970s and early 1980s worked out with sweatbands on their foreheads rather than supportive workout shoes on their feet. So why is footwear all that important? It's important for keeping our joints from absorbing the impact of running, walking, sports, or fitness classes. Remember, the Africans and Tarahumara didn't grow up wearing Western shoes, and those early fitness leaders didn't know any better at that time. Now they all wear specialized footwear.

Find the shoe that's right for you and your activity, and think about a safety accessory that holds identification information for walks, runs, and hikes.

(Photo: Courtesy of SOSAlert)

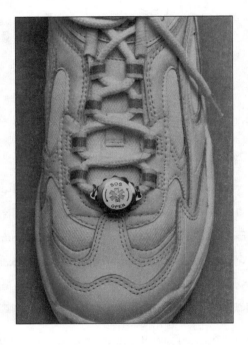

There's no such simplicity for today's exerciser! Even the simple days of the all-purpose sneaker—high-tops for basketball players and low-cut styles for the rest of us—are gone. Footwear designers now churn out shoes for a variety of activities. There are shoes designed especially for aerobics, walking on pavement, "rugged walking" on smooth but unpaved trails, running, trail running, cross-training, day hiking, biking, mountain-biking, tennis, and water aerobics. There are even short flippers for swimmers and approach shoes for rock-climbers to get to the site where they will change to their climbing shoes.

This is not just a marketing ploy: Different activities do require different lateral support, flex patterns, and cushioning. Perhaps this wasn't such an issue in the past. Specialized shoes for particular activities are arguably more important now because footwear has to accommodate exercisers who are older, heavier, and more injury-prone than the young kids who were once virtually the only people who wore sneakers.

Before you go into the store, know what kind of fitness activity you'll be doing and buy well-fitting, properly functioning footwear for it. Not only does your activity direct your purchase, so do your feet. A high or low arch, pronation, supination, or flat-footedness can impact every move you make and can cause discomfort or even injury if you have ill-fitting athletic shoes. Proper and stable footwear can make a huge difference in your performance, comfort, safety from injury, and even in the way you enjoy an activity.

Good athletic-shoe store employees will ask you questions about the activity in which you participate or are planning to participate. They will want to look at old shoes to see how they have worn, and they might put you on a treadmill to watch you walk or run. In addition, they should encourage you to walk around the store, the parking lot, or the mall in the shoes before you purchase them, and they should encourage you to try the shoes out at home or in the gym once or twice with the option to bring them back. You need to make sure they feel right after you get them out of the store. Be prepared to replace walking shoes every 1,000 miles, running shoes every 350 to 500 miles, and aerobics shoes after six to nine months of use.

Workout Wear

First and foremost, the clothes you work out in should be comfortable, not only in terms of how they feel but how they *make you* feel. Some people might be comfortable in skimpy short-shorts and a sports bra; others might rather die than be seen in anything but a baggy T-shirt and shorts or sweatpants. In that regard, choose whatever you are comfortable in, considering the environment in which you exercise and what others wear there. Depending on the activity you choose, there probably are preferred garments designed especially for that sport. People seem to dress differently in a weight room than in a yoga studio. Although these garments are not mandatory, they might make your workout more enjoyable because you will be more comfortable.

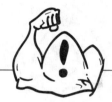

Fit Tip

In some circumstances, custom orthotics, which are specially molded to fit your feet and are inserted beneath the soles of your shoes, can improve your comfort and performance.

Just as men should wear an athletic supporter for many activities, women should plan to wear a sports bra any time they might be bouncing around. Sports bras usually are made from a Lycra blend that stretches comfortably through various arm and body movements and that prevents the discomfort, and perhaps embarrassment, of bouncing breasts. Sports bras come in pullover or hook-closure styles. They all have wide shoulder straps, and many come in T-back designs for additional comfort and support. Large-breasted women can look for harness or underwire styles. In addition to being comfortable and supportive, many sports bras are breathable and wick moisture away from your skin.

Workout wear comes in many shapes, sizes, and colors. Working out in clothes you feel comfortable in will make your workout better.

(Photo: Claire Walter)

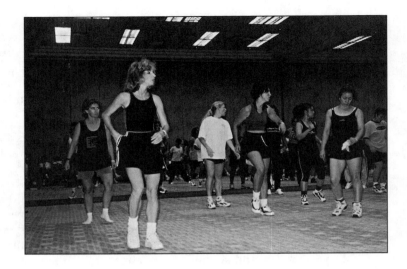

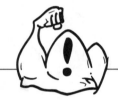

Fit Tip

When you are trying on a sports bra, check its comfort by replicating the movements of the exercises or sports for which you will wear it. If you wear a C-cup or larger, investigate a "harness" bra that supports each breast individually.

If you are a gym person, you probably can get away with shorts and short-sleeved shirts all the time. Many people find a T-shirt and sports shorts made of a breathable synthetic material to be just fine. If you want to get a little more elaborate, a breathable synthetic shirt also is comfortable and makes you look like a serious exerciser. If you don't feel comfortable in shorts, you might prefer to wear calf-length or full-length tights or sweatpants in the gym.

Clothing designed for special aerobics classes generally is similar to dancewear. Leotards and tights are popular but not essential, especially if you don't want to appear in public in tight-fitting attire. However, when you trim down, you'll be ready for outfits that suit the activity and the spirit of aerobics. Big loose T-shirts over Lycra or Lycra-cotton blend tights and a sports bra is a popular look that is functional and also disguises some extra poundage. Yoga classes call for bare feet; long, loose pants; and a long- or short-sleeved shirt. Many martial arts programs have their own type of togs. When you sign up, you'll be told what to wear and where to get it.

Outdoor activities are another story. Nature's "climate control" is more fickle than the gym's heating and cooling systems. For running and walking, the same basic shorts/shirt apparel that you wear indoors works well, as long as the days are moderate. In cool or inclement weather, avoid cotton, because once it gets wet, it stays wet, and it will get cold quickly as well. Synthetic fibers such as polypropylene, Capilene, and Supplex wick moisture away from your skin, dry quickly, and therefore do not make you chilly when you stop. Gore-Tex is used as outerwear in rainy, snowy weather. It sheds water and allows perspiration wicked from the skin to pass through the outer shell.

Layers are your ticket to the outside in cold weather, whether you are running, cycling, winter hiking, snowshoeing, or cross-country skiing. Everyone has different sensitivities to the cold, so you'll have to judge what will work best for you based on the following guidelines:

➤ **Base layer.** Against your skin, wear a soft layer of synthetic fabric, such as polypropylene or Capilene. This layer can be a full set of long underwear, tights, or a shirt.

➤ **Middle layer.** Depending on the temperature, you might want to add a middle layer, such as a wool sweater or a synthetic fleece jacket or vest.

➤ **Outer layer.** On wet, windy, or very cold days, some type of shell layer will be needed as an outer layer to repel wind, water, or both.

➤ **Accessories.** Protect your extremities with gloves or mittens and something for your head, such as a headband or a hat. Remember that up to 50 percent of the body's heat loss is through the head, so if your head is cold, the rest of you will be, too. These accessories also should be made from synthetic fiber to wick away moisture and to keep you from getting cold. On your feet, you need a good pair of synthetic, wool, or wool-blend socks to keep your feet warm.

For cycling, a bike helmet is essential to protect your head. You also might want to invest in Lycra bike shorts or long pants with padding in the crotch for cold-weather rides. Although you can wear regular shorts, you will find the styles designed specifically for cycling to be a lot more comfortable and worth the investment. Cycling gloves with padding on the palms are another item that makes cycling more comfortable, and they offer good protection for your hands. When the weather is inclement, plan to layer over your cycling shorts using garments similar to those previously described. Cycling feels colder than running or walking, because you are going faster on a bike, which creates wind chill.

If you exercise in a pool, either doing water aerobics or swimming laps, invest in a comfortable one-piece tank suit that doesn't ride up in the back or fall off your shoulders—unless you are a male, in which case the style of your choice works fine. A swim cap can somewhat protect your hair from chlorine, though many women who are aquatic exercisers prefer to just pull their hair back and off their necks and faces. If you swim outdoors in a cold climate, it is important to wear a swim cap for warmth.

Swim goggles protect your eyes from becoming irritated by the chlorine, and they help you see better while you are underwater. Fit is important when buying goggles, because they won't do you much good if they leak. Try them on in the store before you buy. Pay special attention to the seal around your eyes without having the strap around the back of your head. Although you will not want to swim without the strap, you can check the seal of the goggles this way to determine if there's proper suction around your eyes and if the goggles are likely to leak while you are swimming.

A myriad of other sports might have clothing designed specifically for them, but these basics should get you started for just about any sport you want to try. If you plan to play pickup volleyball, basketball, or soccer, for example, gym clothes should work just fine. If you eventually join a team, however, you might have to get a uniform. If you are going to go rock-climbing, gym clothes can get you started, but if you plan to go regularly, you'll soon want tights. You'll also probably want your own rock shoes and harness instead of rentals. If you start in-line skating, pads in the proper places—elbows and knees plus wristguards and a helmet—are mandatory.

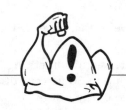

Fit Tip

If you get hooked on a particular sport, check out other clothing you might want to invest in. Sometimes you can get good deals at garage sales, through classified ads, or at a sporting-goods resale shop.

A mail-order catalog containing workout and sports clothes for women, including sports bras for the hard-to-fit and large-busted, is available from Title Nine Sports at 1-800-609-0092 or www.title9sports.com. Venerable L.L. Bean issues a catalog of women's outdoor gear and clothing culled from its vast inventory. As of this writing, some orders qualify for a free trial subscription to *Walking* magazine. You can order a catalog from 1-800-221-4221 or www.llbean.com.

Water Bottles and Hydration Systems

Staying hydrated all the time is important, but it becomes especially critical when you are exercising. Dehydration not only will affect how you feel and how you perform, it is not good for your general health. If you feel thirsty, you already are dehydrated, and the risk of dehydration increases as the temperature rises. Fortunately, many different versions of the water bottle make hydration easy.

Unbreakable plastic sports bottles easily fit into bottle holders on stationary bikes and other aerobics machines in gyms. You don't even have to bring water to the gym. Most gyms make it easy for you to stay hydrated while working out by placing water fountains throughout the facilities, including weight rooms and some aerobics studios. Make it a habit, though, to carry a water bottle with you wherever you work out. Stash it next to the cardiovascular apparatus or weight machine, next to your bench in a step class, or at the edge of the pool during an aquatic exercise class.

When you are outdoors walking, jogging, or cycling, there are several options for staying hydrated. You can buy a waistbelt or a fanny pack with a holder specifically for your water bottle. If you're cycling, make sure you have at least one metal or plastic water-bottle cage installed on your bike. Sports bottles fit right in. Insulated water bottles help keep water cool longer on hot days and keep it from freezing in the winter. Hydration systems also have become popular. Camelbak started the trend with a backpack style lined with an inner bladder to hold water, and many slight variations now exist. What they have in common is a flexible tube with a nipple on the end that goes over your shoulder and is always handy for a quick sip. What should you drink? It can't be emphasized enough that water is the best liquid to keep you hydrated, but it can be supplemented with sports drinks, juices, and herbal teas. Skip caffeinated and carbonated drinks before and just after your workout. If you're counting calories, it's good to know that water is calorie-free. To stay hydrated for a hard exercise session, you should try to follow these guidelines:

➤ Drink at least 16 ounces two hours before you exercise.

➤ Drink at least 8 ounces one hour before you exercise.

➤ Drink at least 4 to 8 ounces every 15 to 20 minutes while exercising.

➤ Drink at least 16 ounces an hour after exercising.

➤ Drink at least 64 ounces throughout the day, whether or not it is an exercise day.

Obviously, if you are going for a leisurely walk or bike ride on a mild day, taking a gentle yoga class, or doing any other short, light workout, you won't need much more water than your normal amount. Obviously, too, a large man will need more water than a petite woman, even if both are exercising at comparable intensities.

At-Home Exercise Equipment

If you want to work out at home, you might embark on something as complicated and costly as setting up an entire gym, or you can simply buy a few inexpensive items to making exercising want easier.

Mats

If you wantexercise at home, you probably won't want to lie on the bare floor, you certainly won't want to stretch out on hard tile, and you might not even want to be that close to a padded carpet. If you are going to be doing any floor work, such as crunches or leg raises, you probably will want a real exercise mat—sooner rather than later. Mats come in a number of different styles, sizes, and colors. You can buy mats specifically designed for yoga or exercise, and you can select from styles that roll up, fold up, or stay flat for storage. They usually are made from some type of foam encased in a flexible plastic covering that wipes off easily.

Mats generally are about two feet wide, but they come in a variety of lengths, thicknesses, and heights. If you want to be able to stretch out and fit all or most of your

311

body on the mat, you will need a longer one. If you don't mind having your legs and feet off the end of the mat, look for one as short as three feet. Even that length should cushion your head. Thickness varies from as thin as ³⁄₈ inch to as thick as two inches. If you are buying a mat for home use, these are all criteria you will have to consider. Decisions should be based on where you will be using the mat, how hard the floor is in that area, and how much space you have to store a mat when it's not in use.

Home Weights

If you want to buy weights to use at home, you have a number of options. Hand weights or dumbbells, similar to those you might use at the gym, are available in pairs in a variety of weights ranging from one pound to 110 pounds. You can buy them vinyl-coated, which gives them a better appearance, makes them easier to clean, and is more forgiving on a wood floor if you drop them. In addition to hand weights, you can purchase leg weights. These generally are made from some type of heavy Cordura with straps and Velcro to attach them to your wrists or ankles.

Other Workout Gadgets and Gear

Swiss balls, want also known as fit balls, improve balance and coordination, tone and strengthen muscles, and are fun and interesting to use. They are also good for rehab when recovering from an injury. These large, inflatable rubber balls come in different diameters in 10-centimeter (about 2½ inches) increments. For effective and comfortable exercising, you need to order the right fit.

User's Height	Diameter of Swiss Ball
Under 5'0"	45 centimeters
5'1" to 5'6"	55 centimeters
5'7" to 5'11"	65 centimeters
6'0" to 6'3"	75 centimeters
Over 6'3"	85 centimeters

If you have trouble balancing on a sphere, you might be happier with a Physio-Ball, which resembles a rubber peanut and therefore rolls only backward and forward, and not in any random direction. Whichever product you choose, you also might want to invest in a pump to keep it inflated to your comfort level.

There are many other products you can buy to enhance your workouts, such as heart-rate monitors, jump ropes, balance boards, resistance tubes and bands, aerobics steps, muscle and exercise charts, exercise videos, and more. These were discussed in the chapters on strength training and aerobic conditioning in Parts 2 and 3 of the book.

Buying Home Gear

Fitness gear is available in fitness and sports stores, through direct-mail catalogs, and over the Web. Here are a few places you can check out:

➤ Fitness Wholesale direct mail catalog, 1-888-FW-ORDER

➤ SPRI Products Inc. fitness products catalog, 1-800-222-7774 or www. fitnessonline.com/shop/spri

➤ Fitness First direct mail catalog, 1-800-421-1791 or www.fitness1st.com

➤ Fitness Factory Outlet direct mail catalog, 1-800-383-9300

Spend Wisely

Joan Price, co-author of *The Complete Idiot's Guide to Online Health and Fitness* and author of *The Complete Idiot's Guide to Online Medical Resources* and *Joan Price says Yes, You CAN Get in Shape!*, compiled a list of what she called "money-wasters." She wrote in her online column at www.fitnesslink.com, that the criteria are simple: "the machine or gadget doesn't do much; it especially doesn't do what it's supposed to do; and/or it allows you to do what you could do perfectly well without it. In general, any item that claims it 'spot reduces' is pulling your leg, because spot reducing is a myth. Any machine that claims fat-burning or aerobic training but doesn't let you get in your higher-intensity heart rate range is also a loser."

Here's her list of items that people waste their money on in an effort to shape up or lose weight—and her comments on why they are such a waste:

➤ **Ab rollers.** These hot sellers promise you perfect crunches. Well, duhhh—you can do perfect crunches just as well on your own. In fact, you can do them better without the assistance, because rollers don't train the upper, lower and transverse abdominal muscles in the specific ways you can without the device, says Marc Evans, former U.S. triathlon team coach and author of *Endurance Athlete's Edge* (Human Kinetics, $20). That's because the roller assists the curl, taking away the activation of those

Quote, Unquote

"I am often asked if I do exercises in addition to the ones I offer on *Body Electric*. My answer is an emphatic 'no!' My routine is this. I teach a one-hour muscle-toning class in the gym twice each week plus an additional hour at home, a total of three hours of muscle toning a week. I take a brisk 30- to 45-minute walk most days. My home gym includes an exercise mat or a towel and several sets of hand-held weights in different weight increments, which can be combined for more of a challenge. And don't forget the television."

—Margaret Richard, television host, *Body Electric*

specific muscles that would engage if you weren't hanging onto the bar. Plus it limits the variety of abdominal exercises you can do. Bottom line: learn good form and do it on your own.

➤ **ThighMaster.** Much worse than the lowly adductor/abductor machines is this best-selling piece of plastic that promises inner thighs of a star. Raspberries also go to Bun Blaster, BunMaster and any and all press-this-flab-and-the-fat-will-go-away gimmicks and gizmos. You can't exercise one part of the body and expect to lose fat in that area. Repeat after me: There's no such thing as spot reducing!

➤ **Aerobic rider.** Despite the inflated calorie-burning and full-body-workout claims, these riders only deliver if you're a beginner. In a study sponsored by the American Council on Exercise (ACE) and conducted by California State University at Northridge, aerobic-rider exercisers following manufacturers' guidelines burned only 50 percent or fewer calories than on a treadmill. Even when they pushed to the most strenuous workouts possible, the rider exercisers still burned about 25 percent fewer calories than on a treadmill. The only muscles consistently exercised on all brands were the hamstrings.

➤ **Aerobic glider.** This gives you the delusion you're getting a workout. "You stand on it, your hips move back and forth," says Edmund R. Burke, Ph.D., sport scientist at the University of Colorado at Colorado Springs and former Olympic coach. The glider, one of the fitness industry's top-selling infomercial products, rates lower than walking for a fit exerciser. Researchers at California State University at Northridge found that moderately-fit males, ages 23 to 29, couldn't get their heart rates up over 155 bpm on these devices, no matter how much they exerted themselves. They should have been able to reach a heart rate of 194 bpm during a peak-performance test.

If you have exercise gadgets sitting in your closet that never fulfilled their claims, you may have some fitness money-wasters to add to Joan Price's list. And next time you see some celebrity touting another magic machine on late-night television, remember that you might just add it to the collection in the closet.

The Least You Need to Know

➤ Purchase footwear that fits and functions correctly to enhance performance and prevent injury.

➤ Workout wear can be as simple and comfortable as shorts and a T-shirt or as specialized as an outfit made for cycling, martial arts, or other routines.

➤ Drink plenty of water before, during, and after a workout to stay hydrated for peak performance.

➤ Simple and basic equipment, such as hand weights and stretch bands, suffices for exercising at home.

➤ There is no such thing as a fitness fast fix; therefore, gadgets that make inflated promises are consumer rip-offs.

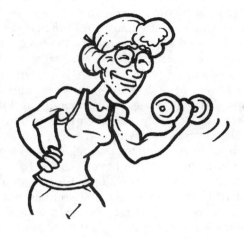

Chapter 24

Special Situations

In This Chapter

➤ Modifying an exercise program during pregnancy

➤ Getting back on track after childbirth or surgery

➤ Staying healthy during menopause

➤ Exercising into old age

Most fitness advice is of the one-size-fits-all variety—no matter what size you happen to be at the outset. Other than the blanket advice to consult your physician before beginning an exercise program, much of the advice addresses young, or youngish, adults in good health. Overweight? Perhaps. Out of shape? Probably. Willpower-impaired or simply confused? Most certainly. Other than that, however, the assumption is that there are no other roadblocks to exercising. That's quite an assumption. At various times in your life, your exercise program must be tailored to fit particular circumstances. And in many cases, physical challenges to exercise are permanent or chronic and must be overcome with modified, often customized, workout programs.

Pregnancy Exercising

Women often wonder whether it's safe to exercise while pregnant. A very general answer is "yes" with some caveats. It usually is all right to work out if you already are fit when you become pregnant. You also must be careful, conservative, and have your

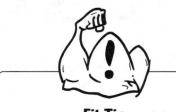

Fit Tip

The longer you were on a fitness program before becoming pregnant, the more attuned you are to your body when you are expecting.

doctor's approval. Exercise can help ease some of pregnancy's discomforts, such as shortness of breath, dizziness, fatigue, and even the nausea that many women experience during their first trimester. Research shows that women who exercise while they're pregnant feel strong, fit, and energetic. In addition, they tend to experience fewer of the discomforts that abound late in pregnancy, they gain slightly less weight, and they bounce back more quickly after their baby is born. Therefore, if you aren't working out when you are thinking about having a baby, prepregnancy is a good time to get into shape. If you haven't done that, take nice long walks or join a fitness class for pregnant women, alerting your instructor that you had not been exercising before, and get into a real workout routine afterward. Pregnancy is no time to start an on-and-off program of sporadic exercises.

How Much Is Too Much?

How much can a pregnant woman exercise? You should be able to keep up with your prepregnancy fitness routine as long as your body feels okay. Here are a few guidelines for planning your pregnancy fitness plan:

➤ **Stick to a schedule.** Regular exercise is better for you than sporadic workouts.

Sticking to a workout during pregnancy will make you feel better and can aid in recovery after pregnancy.

(Photo: Anne W. Krause)

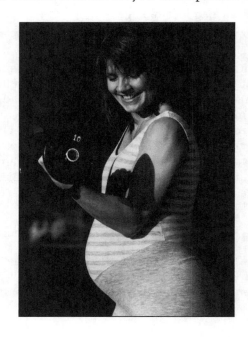

➤ **Stay in your comfort zone.** Try to keep up your prepregnancy fitness plan as long as you feel comfortable doing so. If necessary, break a daily workout into two shorter workouts and reduce the speed or intensity.

➤ **Lessen your intensity.** Try to limit your overall exercise intensity to at least 50 percent of your prepregnancy intensity. Watch your breathing, and stop exercising if you're winded. Keep your heart rate below 140 bpm to avoid depriving the baby of oxygen. As you get further along in your pregnancy, you will get tired and winded more quickly.

➤ **Stay off your back (and off your feet).** Avoid exercises that require you to lie on your back after the first trimester, because the pressure of the growing fetus restricts blood flow back to your heart. In addition, don't stand still for long periods of time; the excess weight of pregnancy can cause varicose veins. Jog, walk, or go snowshoeing as long as such activities feel good. Swimming and aquatic classes also are excellent workouts. Swimming is the only time you can lay prone (on your tummy) for an extended period of time, and it gives your back a well-deserved break.

➤ **Be alert to your center of gravity.** As your body shape changes, so does your center of gravity. Activities that are fine and comfortable early on might not be later in your pregnancy. In your third trimester, you should avoid sports that require balance or that put you in danger of abdominal trauma.

➤ **Wear comfortable workout clothes.** Loose, nonconstricting clothes are important for the pregnant exerciser. When activity becomes uncomfortable, try wearing extra breast or abdominal support, or switch to non-weight-bearing exercises, such as swimming, water walking, water aerobics, stairstepping, an elliptical trainer, or recumbent or stationary cycling.

➤ **Continue strength training with some nodifications.** You probably shouldn't be on a body-building routine when you're pregnant, but keeping your muscles toned and firm will ease you through pregnancy, childbirth, and recovery. Continue strength training with weights and exercise bands, but avoid exercises that require you to lie on your back (as previously mentioned).

➤ **Eat right.** Be sure to eat healthy foods and to eat enough—but not too much. Remember, you're eating for two, not four (unless you are expecting triplets). Pregnant women need an additional 300 calories a day. Alcohol and caffeine should be consumed sparingly, if at all, during pregnancy.

➤ **Be aware of overheating.** Pregnant women generate extra heat, especially in the first trimester when important fetal organ formation is happening. For this reason, you need to drink plenty of water and avoid situations in which you might overheat. Raise the red flag on exercising hard in hot weather, soaking in the hot tub, and sitting in a sauna or steamroom, especially during your first trimester. Overheating can cause the temperature of the amniotic fluid in the uterus to rise too high, which can seriously harm your baby.

319

Main Goal: Deliver a Healthy Baby

If you were not following a regular fitness routine before you got pregnant, now is not the time to train for a race or to take on new activities that are more strenuous than what you were doing before. Use the guidelines previously listed and keep in mind that your workout goals should be modest. Your main goal is to deliver a healthy baby. Don't even think about pushing yourself the way you might if you were not pregnant. Stay on your routine and modify it as your pregnancy progresses. If you haven't been active, taking easy walks on a regular basis or enrolling in a beginner exercise class geared toward pregnant women will probably make you feel better throughout your pregnancy and ease the birthing process.

As with anything else during your pregnancy, if you ever have any questions about your fitness routine, contact your prenatal care provider to discuss it with him or her. Don't sit around and worry. Trust your instincts and don't do anything physical that makes you feel uncomfortable.

Proper shoes are important for all fitness activities, especially while you are expecting. You will be tougher on your shoes, and your feet might change size during pregnancy—lengthening, widening, or both. Be sure to check the size of your feet every trimester to ensure proper fit.

As you get closer to your due date, ligaments get looser to help get the body ready to open up for birth. Stability of certain joint areas, specifically the groin, sacrum, pubis symphisis, and lower back, might be at risk. Cut back on the weight you lift when you are doing exercises that involve these susceptible areas and do not overstretch. Many health clubs and hospitals offer fitness classes for pregnant women. These are excellent for staying fit without overdoing it and harming yourself or your baby.

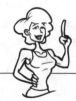

Fitness Fact

Studies have found that babies born to active mothers are more alert, more interested in their surroundings, and less demanding of their mother's attention than babies born to sedentary women.

After the Baby Arrives

After delivery, the first question naturally is, "How is my baby?" The second question asked by workout-aholics often is, "When can I begin exercising now that I've given birth?" There are no clear-cut answers to this question. You can ask your doctor about when he or she feels you are ready to begin exercising, and restarting your regime also will depend somewhat on how you feel. (This is another time when it is a good idea to listen to your body.) Unless you had a particularly complicated delivery, walking probably can begin fairly soon after giving birth. Taking as little as 15 to 30 minutes while Dad watches the newborn so you can get some fresh air, plus a little time to yourself, will probably be one of the best things you can do shortly after having a baby. When your infant is a little older, taking him or her with you on your walks will be good for both of you. As long as the weather cooperates, put the baby in a Snuggli or a stroller and get out of the house.

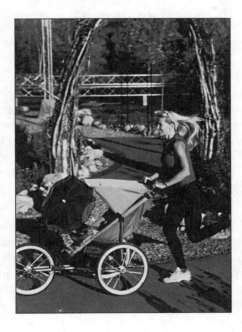

Baby-joggers—strollers designed specifically for jogging—can help parents with toddlers stay in shape.

(Photo: Anne W. Krause)

Save a more regimented fitness program until your physician gives you the green light and you have the time and energy to work out. When you start out, remember that your body has just gone through major physical changes—don't push yourself too hard. Begin by working out for about 30 minutes a session, three days a week. Try for an intensity level of about 50 percent of your prepregnancy workouts. Gradually build in duration, intensity, and frequency.

A baby backpack offers exercise and quality time with your toddler.

(Photo: Anne W. Krause)

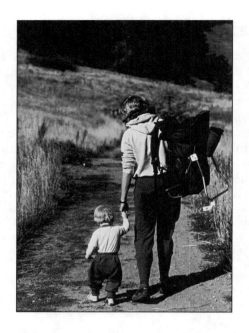

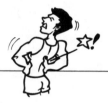

Achtung!

If you are breast-feeding, keep your exercise intensity low to prevent the accumulation of excess lactic acid in your milk.

As with your prepregnancy regime—in fact, as with any good program—postpartum workouts should always include a warm-up period and a stretching and cool-down phase. Remember to drink lots of water to stay hydrated. Most important, have fun and don't fatigue yourself so much that you cannot enjoy your new baby.

Perhaps you were not into fitness before your pregnancy, but you have become interested in starting a program now that you've looked at yourself in the mirror. It's good to start your new life as a mother with healthy new habits. As with any startup program, a trip to the physician is essential before you begin. Find out what your fitness baseline is, and set realistic goals that you will have the time and energy to meet. Refer to Chapters 1 through 3 for guidelines about setting up your fitness plan. If you want to work with a personal trainer to set up a postpartum workout program, signing up with a woman who has had a child and has gone through the same thing you have is a good idea. She will be an empathetic expert.

Toddler Time

As children grow, just keeping up with them can be a workout in itself. Including your baby in your fitness routine can be a rewarding experience, and it can add some challenge to the workout. Most babies love to be pushed along in a stroller. They love the motion. The fresh air is good for them, and the sights and sounds are stimulating. That being true, use your baby as an excuse for taking long walks or even jogs rather than as an excuse *not* to exercise outdoors. Nowadays, sturdy jogging-strollers are built with three wheels and a heavy-duty design. They can be pushed on uneven sidewalks or unpaved paths while walking or jogging. Regular strollers are sturdy and work well for walks along paved paths.

Even many health clubs accommodate mothers with small children. Some offer "mom-and-me" classes and feature exercises that include the baby. Not only do you not lose the precious time you like to spend with your child, these classes also will give you some ideas for at-home exercises that are good for you and fun for your child, too. Some health clubs and recreation centers offer childcare for infants while moms work out. Although you might not want to leave a small infant in childcare for too long, this break will give you the opportunity to take an aerobics class, to do some strength training, and to work on your abdominal muscles to firm them back up after being stretched from pregnancy.

If you need the motivation of an exercise buddy, the companionship and incentive of another mom to work out with is that much more helpful. If you're feeling the need for adult company, chances are there are other new mothers out there looking for the same thing. In addition to walks with other moms, you can plan picnics in the park and pool or beach get-togethers as your children grow. You also can take turns watching the kids. One of you can do some workouts at home while the other baby-sits and then trade places.

Family Fitness

As your children grow, weave physical activities into the family's social structure. Make regular walks, hikes, bicycle rides, and active games part of what you and your kids do together. This will not only set an example for the importance of a fitness routine as the kids get older, it will be a healthy and fun way for your family to spend time together.

If your children begin to participate in organized sports, be supportive. Make sure they have the proper gear, that they are able to get to practice easily, and that you are there to be their cheerleader. You could even go so far as to volunteer to help coach or organize team functions.

A healthy diet should also be part of your family's fitness regime. Cook healthy meals, and keep

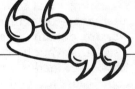

Quote, Unquote

"I have three personal trainers: Sam, John, and Joe [with baby Daniel not yet born when this interview with *Walking* magazine was conducted]. I'm always carrying them up and down the stairs. When I take my walks, I'm pushing a double stroller, which makes things a lot more strenuous."

—Jennifer Heaton, actress

healthy snacks around the house. Teach your kids to make their lunch before school and help prepare the evening meals. Make sure that at least a few evenings a week, dinner together is a fun and relaxing event.

Fitness Fact

A 130-pound woman can burn about 350 calories per hour by toting a baby in a backpack, according to *Shape* magazine. This equates to about an hour of doubles tennis, hiking, or weightlifting.

Sick Leave

Once you're on an exercise roll and you see and feel the benefits, you might feel reluctant to take time off even if you are not feeling 100 percent. You can exercise if you have the sniffles or a cold without a fever, and some research indicates that you can work out at your normal pace. The cold still needs to run its course, however, so exercising won't shorten its duration. When you are ready to start exercising again after you've been ill, start slowly and monitor your pulse rate. Experts caution against working out any time you have a body temperature of 99.5 degrees or higher. Fever is a sign that your body is fighting a virus, which is enough of a "workout." At the very least, fever increases the chance of dehydration; more seriously, exercising vigorously could cause the virus to invade your heart or the surrounding muscle.

It's okay to work out with the sniffles, but take it at a slower pace.

(Photo: Courtesy of Telluride Visitor Services)

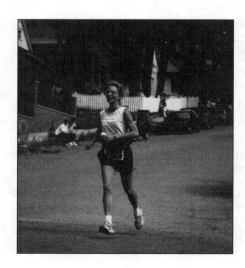

In addition to the numbers that pop up on the thermometer, be mindful of other signs that you might be too sick to exercise. Muscle aches can signal viral illness. A sore throat and a persistent, hacking cough could mean an infection. If you have any lingering problems or aches and pains beyond the norm, consult your physician or at least use common sense and take it easy if you have any doubts. If you feel the need to do something, try some gentle indoor stretches, and remember to drink plenty of liquids, such as water, hot herbal tea, or broth to avoid dehydration. If you have any bronchial problems, do not work out. This can bring the virus into your lungs and create worse problems.

To assess whether you're ready to begin working out again after an illness, take your resting pulse first thing in the morning. If it is 10 beats or more above normal, you still might be fighting an infection and should not exercise that day.

Postoperative Exercising

It used to be that, after surgery, patients were instructed to stay in bed and rest until they were too weak to move because of prolonged inactivity. Today, many operations that formerly required a hospital stay are outpatient surgery, and most doctors want their patients up and about as soon as feasible after surgery. Even when hospitalization is required, postoperative patients are encouraged to shuffle along the corridor, perhaps accompanied by saline solution on a rolling IV stand. In the past, they would have been bed-bound for days.

> **Quote, Unquote**
>
> "You can't 'sweat out' a cold. Whether you exercise or not, the duration of a cold is the same."
>
> —Thomas G. Wiedner, Ph.D., Ball State University, Muncie, Indiana

In fact, the types of surgeries that correct problems athletes often suffer from have seen some of the most dramatic changes. In the past, after knee surgery, the patient's entire leg was immobilized for weeks. Today, doctors have patients stretching and strengthening within days. Even after joint or back surgery, patients usually get the green light for some activity to get their muscles moving so that they do not atrophy during the healing period. Every individual case is different, so consult your doctor or surgeon to see what he or she suggests for postoperative activity and fitness recovery. If you were on a fitness routine before surgery, the doctor probably will have you up and moving as soon as possible.

Exercise Equals Osteoporosis Prevention

A broken hip. Ankle or wrist fractures. Dowager's hump. Simple frailty. These are the nightmares of a menopausal or postmenopausal woman who sees the fate of her grandmother or an elderly neighbor lady in her own future. Such injuries come with osteoporosis, most commonly caused when the female body ceases to produce estrogen and calcium is leached from the bones.

Walk frequently to help prevent osteoporosis.

(Photo: Anne W. Krause)

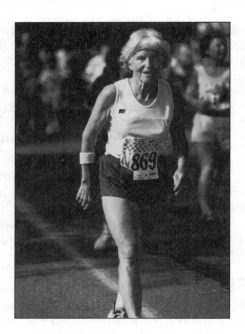

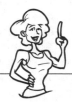

Fitness Fact

Studies have shown that women can lose 40 percent of their bone mass within seven years of menopause. Unless they do something about it, half of all women over 50 will suffer some kind of osteoporosis-related bone fracture at some time in their lives. (This isn't just a female disease, however. It is estimated that osteoporosis now affects eight million women and two million men.)

Osteoporosis can be prevented, mitigated, and even reversed. Conscientiously taking calcium (1,200 to 1,500 milligrams a day) and exercising properly can slow down or even reverse this debilitating loss of bone density. (Whether a woman additionally takes estrogen is a decision she and her physician must make.) A program with alternating days of resistance training, such as weightlifting, and walking is recommended. If you've never worked with weights, start slowly and preferably under supervision. Use light weights until you get accustomed to lifting. Walk at least 30 to 40 minutes every other day.

Disability Is No Bar to Fitness

As wheelchair athletes have shown, disability is no bar to fitness. In fact, the muscles some people use to compensate for those they cannot use are stronger than other people's. Think of the arm, shoulder, and chest strength of people who use crutches to walk. People in wheelchairs also use their upper bodies to move in and out of the chair. To obtain free exercise guides for people with special needs, call the National Center on Physical Ability and Disability at 1-800-900-8086.

Because fitness is more than just strength, other kinds of workouts can build aerobic strength, too. Physical therapists and physiologists with special training related to the disabled can help draw up a fitness program. For some people, swimming or other aquatic programs are suitable. Others might work out using special racing chairs. Still others enjoy playing wheelchair basketball or tennis. In fact, the U.S. Surgeon General's report recommending "moderate" daily exercise for good health even includes wheeling oneself in a wheelchair for 30 to 40 minutes or playing wheelchair basketball for 20 minutes on a list of examples of moderate-level activity.

Menopause Matters

The hormonal shifts that cause women to cease menstruating also cause other changes in their bodies, one of which is an unhealthy weight gain. Fat redistribution to the abdominal area can impact factors such as internal organ functioning, insulin sensitivity, increased cholesterol levels, and other problems. In her book *The Menopause Diet,* Dr. Larrian Gillespie pays particular attention to the accumulation of intra-abdominal fat (that is, fat stored within the abdominal cavity rather than subcutaneous fat stored just beneath the skin) as a risk factor in the following areas:

➤ Arthritis

➤ Hypertension

➤ Cancer of the breast, endometrium, and kidneys

➤ Incontinence

➤ Coronary heart disease

➤ Kidney failure

➤ Chronic lung disease

➤ Kidney stones

➤ Diabetes

➤ Polycystic ovarian disease

➤ Gallstones

➤ Sleep apnea

➤ Stroke

Much research has been done in these areas—beyond the scope of this book—but it all points to eating well, controlling your weight, and becoming or remaining physically active through and beyond your menopausal years.

Fitness and the Older Body

No matter what the definition of "older" is, no one is too old to exercise. The American Association of Retired Persons begins recruiting new members when they turn 50, which is a statistical turning point in physical fitness. Unless they do something proactive to counteract natural aging, from about age 20 to 49, people lose half-a-pound of muscle mass every year. After age 50, that loss changes to one pound a year. The result is decreased strength, coordination, balance, flexibility, and more. Nearly 40 percent of Americans over the age of 55 report that they participate in no leisure-time physical activity.

Even for people who have not previously exercised, these losses can be counteracted—astonishingly, at any age. In the mid 1980s, Dr. Walter Frontera, a scientist at the Tufts Center on Aging, performed a study with 60- and 70-year-olds. Some were put on an exercise program; others were not. Within 12 weeks, the exercisers were 100 to 175 percent stronger than their sedentary contemporaries. In a follow-up study, Dr. Maria Fiatarone, also of the Tufts Center on Aging, recruited volunteers aged 86 to 96 in a nursing home. Subjects in the study participated in a high-intensity strength-training workout, starting out at a safe level and progressing gradually. In just eight weeks, these frail, elderly men and women had increased their strength an average of 175 percent. In a test of walking, their speed and balance showed an average improvement of 48 percent.

Exercise for older people is not just an end unto itself. It helps many of them remain independent far longer, enhancing their feelings of dignity and self-worth. Other benefits include improved mood and sleep patterns and reduced risk of heart disease, diabetes, cancer, arthritis, and other potentially debilitating conditions. In addition, most older folks who start to exercise become more limber and often notice decreases in chronic aches and pains.

Exercise is good for both the body and spirit, and seniors' classes increasingly are incorporating the social interaction that so many live-alone seniors need. For example, Terry Ferebee Eckmann designed the steps and sequences of a program called Lines, Circles, and Squares with an easy-to-follow combination of pattern walking and simple moves from ethnic, social, and country line dancing specifically to add a social component to physical activity.

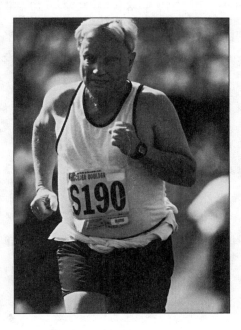

People who exercise into their later years stay independent longer.

(Photo: Anne W. Krause)

If you feel you fit into the category of "older" and you are not sure how to get started on an exercise program, first check with your doctor and get his or her approval before beginning an exercise program. Even folks with heart disease, osteoporosis, or other chronic conditions can exercise and will find it beneficial. Make sure you are aware of any restrictions the doctor would like you to put on your program. If you have any health issues, set up a time a few months down the road to go back so your doctor can monitor your progress.

When you get the go-ahead, set some fitness goals for yourself. No matter what exercise you pick,

Quote, Unquote

"People don't stop exercising because they grow old. They grow old because they stop exercising."

—Covert Bailey, author, motivational speaker, and founder of Covert Bailey Fitness start slowly and gradually progress. Pick an activity you know you will enjoy. Here are a few ideas for activities to get you started:

➤ Call your local recreation center, Y, health club, or senior center. Many facilities offer classes geared specifically toward the older, more mature population—often with sessions such as strength training, aqua aerobics, and low-impact aerobics.

➤ Walking is for everyone and is an excellent way to enjoy the outdoors. Start out with a warm-up of walking slowly or stretching for five to 10 minutes. For your walk, begin with a short distance, work up to walking for about 20 minutes, and then go for longer distances. Find a companion to walk with if you can.

➤ Bicycling also is a great exercise, either outdoors or on a stationary bicycle, especially if you have knee problems.

Fitness Fact

From age 65 to 84, the average decline in strength equals 1.5 percent a year. Physical inactivity accelerates the age–related decline in strength.

The Least You Need to Know

➤ Exercising during pregnancy can mean an easier birth, a more alert baby, and faster recovery.

➤ When you start a postpartum exercise program, include your baby in your quest to get back in shape.

➤ Set an example for your children by creating a fun and healthy fitness program for your entire family.

➤ Doctors often encourage patients to start easy exercise programs very soon after surgery, and exercise programs can be tailored for disabled people, too.

➤ Exercise programs for the disabled are on the rise.

➤ Women in midlife and beyond can exercise to prevent postmenopausal bone loss.

➤ Weight training increases strength in the elderly, allowing them to be independent for longer and therefore adding to their quality of life.

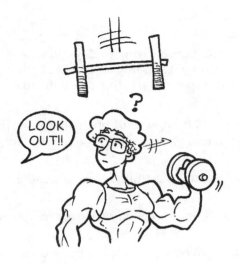

Chapter 25

Injury Alert

In This Chapter

➤ Risk factors for injury

➤ Definitions of common sports injuries

➤ When to self-treat an injury and when to seek medical help

➤ Surviving rehabilitation after a serious sports injury

You are determined to become active and fit to make your life better, not worse. Like anyone who embarks on a fitness program or participates in an active sport, you are to be congratulated for your new attitude. No one wants to get hurt. No one plans to get hurt. Many of us are not gracious about being hurt. However, with the active lifestyle that makes us stronger comes the risk of injury. Before you use this as an excuse to close this book and flip on the television from the "safety" of your sofa, remember that, in the long run, sedentary people are more likely to become ill—in fact, *seriously ill*—and to suffer certain kinds of injury than their active friends. So weigh the risks of injury, but more important, reap the rewards that come from fitness and good health.

Who Gets Hurt

Fitness activities are supposed to be good for you, but sometimes things go wrong and you actually get injured while you are exercising. High-impact exercise and excess weights are the main causes of injury, and specific factors increase the likelihood of getting hurt:

➤ **Too much, too hard, too intense, too soon.** Injuries most often are caused by these factors. In sports or fitness participation, gradual progression of *anything* you do is essential.

➤ **Age.** The older you are, the more likely you are to get hurt while exercising, especially if you are just starting out.

➤ **Previous level of activity.** If you previously were sedentary or inactive, you are more likely to get injured.

➤ **Weight and body composition.** The more overweight you are, the greater your chances of injury.

➤ **Gender.** Men and women get injured for different reasons. Men often are out to "impress" because ego plays a role in their exercise and makes them not always smart about their protocol. Women's greatest concern is osteoporosis.

➤ **Amount of exercise.** The more exercise you do, the more likely you are to get hurt from overtraining or simply based on the law of averages (similar to the likelihood of being involved in an automobile accident by increasing the amount you drive).

This is not meant to frighten or discourage you; it is simply meant to alert you. After all, many of the same factors that increase the likelihood of injury also indicate the need to exercise. You can't make yourself younger, and you probably won't change your gender, but as you rev up your activity level and shed extra pounds, your odds of getting hurt will decrease. A solid and sound fitness program—if you begin slowly, rev up gradually, and avoid the temptation to overdo it—will decrease your chances of injury. If you do get injured, the severity is likely to be less and your recovery is likely to be faster if you have a stronger body to begin with.

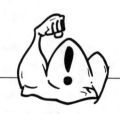

Fit Tip

Your notebook or logbook can be invaluable if you get injured, because you, your trainer, and your physician can see what you did during your workout that might have caused the injury.

Common Injuries

Most sports and overuse injuries are more annoying than life-threatening, although some can actually be severe or chronic enough that you might have to give up one activity and substitute another. Perhaps you'll switch to PowerWalking instead of running, low-impact aerobics instead of kickboxing, and so on.

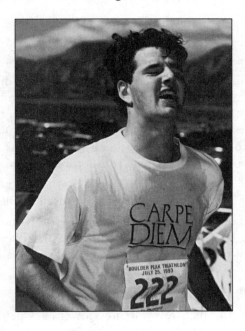

If you feel a sharp pain, which can indicate injury, stop and evaluate before continuing your activity.

(Photo: Anne W. Krause)

The Smart Guide to Sports Medicine offers a list of some common athletic injuries. Here's what they mean in lay terms:

➤ **Bone spur.** A calcium deposit on the bone, particularly on the heels, although it can happen on any bone.

➤ **Bruise.** Discoloration of the skin caused by broken blood vessels. A bone bruise is a deep bruise accompanied by deep-tissue tenderness.

➤ **Bursitis.** An inflammation of the fluid-filled sacs that enable muscles, tendons, and ligaments to slide over bone.

➤ **Chondromalacia.** A roughening under the kneecap where the cartilage is thinning out and tearing. It sounds like walking on gravel when the knee is bending.

➤ **Contusion.** A skin scrape.

➤ **Dislocation.** A joint injury in which the bones that are supposed to be connected by cartilage are offset from their normal positions.

➤ **Fracture.** A milder way of saying "break." A compound fracture is one in which broken bone pierces the skin. Stress fractures are "cracks" rather than "breaks" in the bone and are caused by excessive impact.

➤ **Laceration.** A cut in the skin.

➤ **Plantar fascitis.** Pain in the arch caused by an inflammation of the connective tissue between the heel and the ball of the foot.

➤ **Sesamoiditis.** Inflammation or even fractures of the metatarsal bones under the forefoot.

➤ **Shin splints.** Inflammation of the muscles and tendons of the shins.

➤ **Sprain and strain.** Related injuries that involve stretching, tearing, or even rupturing soft tissue such as ligaments, tendons, and muscle fibers. Sprains happen to ligaments that connect bones to bones. Tendons connect muscles to bones. Doctors categorize these injuries as follows: Grade I is a relatively mild injury involving one quarter or less of the affected muscle fibers. Grade II is a tear of one quarter to three quarters of the fibers. Grade III is a total rupture of the fibers.

➤ **Subungual hematoma.** Discoloration under the toenail caused by bleeding.

➤ **Tendonitis.** An inflammation or tenderness of the ropy tendon tissue connecting muscle to bone. This goes by various specialty names. Tennis players, for example, refer to tendonitis of the elbow as "tennis elbow;" basketball players refer to tendonitis of the knee as "jumper's knee."

The most common injuries and complaints for various activities follow:

➤ **Aerobics.** Plantar fascitis, shin splints, stress fractures, lower-back pain, Achilles tendonitis, calf strains, sesamoiditis

➤ **Basketball.** Dislocated or fractured fingers, stress fractures, shin splints, tendonitis of the Achilles, plantar fascitis, jumper's knee, ankle sprains

➤ **Bicycling.** Pulled hamstrings, knee and ankle pains and strains, handlebar palsy, genital discomfort, cervical and lower-lumbar vertebral pain

➤ **In-line skating.** Sprains, fractures, miscellaneous scrapes, head injuries, dislocation of the wrists, knees, or elbows

➤ **Swimming.** Rotator cuff tendonitis and tears, swimmer's ear (water trapped in the ear canal)

➤ **Tennis.** Plantar fascitis, ankle sprains, tennis elbow, tennis toe, shin splints, stress fractures, blisters

Fitness Fact

According to the American Academy of Orthopedic Surgeons, the following are the 10 recreational activities that were the leading causes of emergency room visits in a recent year: basketball, 693,933; bicycling, 599,874; football, 390,180; skiing, 330,389; skating, 322,311 (of which 192,377 were in-line skating); baseball, 219,023; soccer, 157,251; softball, 155,873; volleyball, 86,603; hockey, 77,140.

Feeling the Burn—or Really Hurt?

You've been running five days a week for several weeks, and you're feeling great except for that nagging pain in your shin. Or maybe after a hard hike up a steeper mountain trail than you'd ever ascended or a new workout the day before, you woke up one morning elated at your accomplishment but with a sharp ache in your gluteal muscles. Maybe lifting weights has left your biceps and triceps muscles aching, and one of your elbow joints is sore when you bend it. Are these normal aches and pains? Or are they an indication that you have a real injury that needs treatment? Sometimes it's hard to know. An injury can occur suddenly, but it also can be brought on over time by overuse.

The best "cure" for injury is prevention. Begin your exercise program conservatively, build gradually, and don't go overboard with your workouts. "Things" can happen, however, even if you are cautious. A strain, a sprain, a funny movement, or a misstep can throw something out of whack. When you have a nagging ache or pain, it generally is a good idea to give that muscle or joint a break for a few days to see if it goes away. Icing the injured area until it is numb can be helpful for a new injury, because it reduces swelling and pain. An over-the-counter pain medication—with or without an anti-inflammatory ingredient—might be all you

Quote, Unquote

"To prevent injuries, start out with what seems at first to be a ridiculously easy amount of exertion. Then make sure your body can handle the same amount of exertion on several different occasions."

—Dr. Lee Rice, D.O., medical director of San Diego Sports Medicine and Family Health need to get past the roughest period. If the pain does not go away, interferes with your daily routine, or is accompanied by swelling that does not go down, you probably need to see a doctor.

When to Seek Help

You can be your own medical practitioner when it comes to dealing with certain small injuries, such as minor strains, sprains, and overuse aches, that have not developed into anything serious—and the more you exercise, the more capable you will be of telling real injuries from trivial ones. The first thing to do when you injure yourself is to stop the activity that caused the problem in the first place. Dip into the medicine cabinet for an over-the-counter pain killer. If you choose to switch to another activity in an effort to remain on some kind of program, do not select one that uses the same injured muscle or joint.

The Rose Medical Center in Denver, Colorado, and the Columbia/HCA Healthcare Corporation's Sports Medicine Page suggest that you ask yourself the following questions when attempting to evaluate soreness versus pain and whether you need to see a doctor:

➤ Is the pain mild, moderate, or severe? Is it becoming worse?

➤ Does motion, however slight, increase the pain?

➤ Is a bone protruding from the skin?

➤ Is the area swelling?

➤ Is the area black and blue?

➤ Can you walk or move the injured part?

➤ Does the injury feel numb?

➤ Does the area below the injury feel cold or numb? Is it white in color?

If you answer "yes" to some or most of these questions, it is wise to seek medical attention as soon as possible. If your pain is relatively minimal, is not getting worse, and you can move the affected area without serious pain, you probably can start with an over-the-counter pain killer and basic self-treatment.

Quote, Unquote

"The first warning signal an athlete gets indicating something is wrong is pain. He must then decide whether the pain is just soreness from exercise or whether it's sharp sensation coming from a joint. If the joint hurts while playing or becomes worse, he should have an evaluation by a physician. The second symptom to pay attention to is swelling. Is he experiencing just puffiness that disappears quickly, or is the swelling occurring in the joint? If it's the latter, the injury could be serious and must be examined by a health professional."

—Dr. Thomas Wickiewicz, M.D., orthopedic surgeon and chief of the Sports Medicine department at the Hospital for Special Surgery, New York

The Rule of RICE

Self-treatment involves RICE, which stands for **Rest, Ice, Compression, Elevation**. Rest the injured limb—this means don't exercise it. Apply ice to the injured or sore area for 20 minutes every two to three hours for the first 24 to 48 hours. Compression will help slow down bleeding and swelling. Apply an elastic bandage to a sore joint, being careful not to cut off circulation, or a firm bandage to a scrape or cut. Elevate the affected area higher than the level of your heart.

When the swelling has gone down following the "ice" part of the treatment, heat can provide pain relief and relax your muscles. You can use a hot towel or a heating pad three times a day for about 30 minutes. Stay off or don't use the injured area for a few days after the swelling goes down and the pain goes away. These steps should help a minor strain or overuse injury heal. If the ice and heat treatments are not working or if the pain worsens, contact your doctor.

Always start back on an exercise program carefully. After all, you don't want to reinjure what has just healed. When you begin exercising again, start with heat to warm up the tissue before each workout. After each workout, icing should take down any swelling or inflammation. You might want to start back with an alternative exercise that puts little stress on the injured area. Reestablish range of motion of the injured area and then work on strengthening the muscles around the injured area.

Serious Stuff

Some injuries require medical attention right away. Don't fool around if you or your exercise partner is in any of the following situations.

Head injuries. If you get hit in the head with a ball, fall off your bike, or run into someone or something and hit your head, you might have a head injury. Even if you feel fine immediately after the event occurs, stop your activity for the day and watch for the following symptoms for the first 24 hours:

➤ Loss of consciousness

➤ Change in vision, including blurred or double vision

➤ Confusion, change in normal speech, memory loss

➤ Severe headache

➤ Vomiting

➤ Convulsions

Hand injuries. If you injure the bones or tendons in your hand during a sport such as boxing, basketball, rock-climbing, or in-line skating and you cannot move your hand or joints properly, you might want to have your hand checked right away. Surgical treatments for tendon repairs are much more successful soon after the injury occurs.

If you're recovering from a hand injury, EZ Grip can help you continue your weight-training regime.

(Photo: Claire Walter)

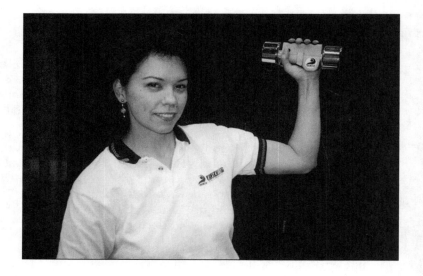

Knee injuries. If your knee swells up or is difficult to move or get around on, first ice it. Also make an appointment to see a doctor right away. A strain can stretch or tear ligaments around the joint and can damage cartilage between bones. X-rays or arthroscopy might be needed to diagnose the damage and perform minor repairs.

Other injuries. If you hurt yourself when you are working out and you feel dizzy or nauseous for an extended period of time, if you lose all range of motion, or if you have obviously broken a bone, see a doctor or go to an emergency room right away. Even if the injury doesn't turn out to be serious, the insurance of knowing is better than letting a serious injury get worse.

Working with a Physical Therapist

Physical therapy can be helpful if you are coming back from an injury or if you have any chronic, nagging pains that seem to recur continually. A physical therapist will assess your condition and provide specific, targeted exercises to assist in your recovery. Often there are opposing muscles (to the injured muscle) that can be strengthened to help the injured muscle recover.

Although they are not physicians, physical therapists go through rigorous schooling to learn about the musculoskeletal system, and they are licensed to recommend a variety of techniques to assist in the healing of many injuries. Physical therapy is available through private physical therapy practices, health clubs, hospitals, and sports medicine clinics, to name a few places.

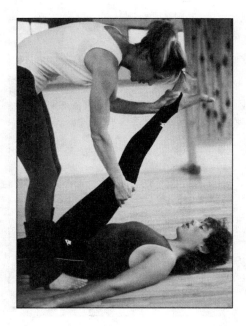

A physical therapist offers specific stretches and exercises to heal your injury.

(Photo: Anne W. Krause)

Coming Back from an Injury

In-water workouts are effective during the beginning of your recuperation process. In fact, physical therapists consider a warm pool to be one of the best rehabilitation environments. Water provides the resistance you need to maintain your muscle strength, but because you are buoyant in water, you will not stress the affected area— nor will you injury another body part while favoring the part you hurt. Some people become so enchanted by the comfort of working out in water that they stick with it even after the injury has healed.

For a serious athlete, emotionally surviving the rehabilitation process often is more difficult than physically overcoming the injury. The mental challenge of coming back from an injury often is the most difficult part of an athlete's recovery. Athletes in recovery mode often feel depressed, deprived of their familiar ways to relieve stress, and crushed by a sense of loss of participation in their sport. This phenomenon has been frequently documented. When a high-profile professional athlete comes back from long and difficult recuperation and rehabilitation to compete and triumph again, it makes headlines and often makes the athlete legendary. Think about 1999 Tour de France winner and cancer survivor Lance Armstrong or U.S. Ski Team star Picabo Street, who recovered from a devastating leg fracture to race to Olympic gold.

Water provides a no-resistance exercise environment, and it often is the first place for the recovering exerciser to work out in.

(Photo: Courtesy of Aquatic Exercise Association)

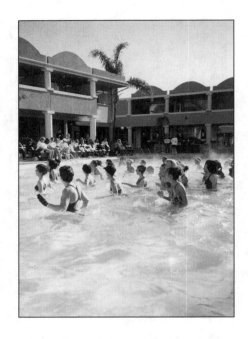

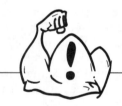

Fit Tip

Keep in contact with your regular workout partner while you are recovering. Even going out to a movie or for a smoothie once in a while is good for you.

Recreational athletes and people who have finally mastered a regular fitness program often have this same angst, even if they don't make the headlines. No matter what level you attain in your fitness quest, if you become injured, you will suffer a physical setback—and probably an emotional one, too. Therefore, as part of your rehabilitation, you need to boost yourself mentally while your body is healing physically. You might have to adjust your goals from your preinjury expectations. Although it might seem like you are downgrading, it is important not to be too ambitious and end up reinjured and back at ground zero again. Depending on the seriousness of your injury, you might need to make your goal a recovery goal, such as increasing your muscle strength by a certain amount by the end of the month instead of doing that race you planned on.

Think of your recovery time as part of your training. You can even keep a rehabilitation log just as you learned to maintain a workout log. Your rehab log could include entries such as the number and frequency of leg lifts you did on your recovering knee. Perhaps you also can find a partner—maybe the trainer or physical therapist you worked with in rehab or even another injured exerciser or athlete—with which to do your rehabilitation workouts.

If you got hurt participating in a sport you love, volunteer to help with a youth team or even to act as a scorekeeper, course marshal, or other official at a sporting event. In addition to helping you stay connected, volunteering is good for your bruised soul. As you are recovering, you might not be able to work out at your previous intensity, and you might even have to cut back your workout, but you still can help others. Special Olympics, local programs for the developmentally or physically disabled, senior centers, and preschool or elementary school programs have places for volunteers in fitness or sports programs. If that doesn't work, you might be able to help at an arts or cultural event. Plenty of places need volunteers, so find one that interests you.

Keep positive thoughts flowing. When you're feeling down, regardless of whether it's due to an injury, it can be hard to keep your attitude bright. Take five or 10 minutes every day—a few minutes when you wake up, at midday if you need it, and before you go to bed at night. Remind yourself of the things you're doing to heal yourself and to help others, and remind yourself that it all takes time.

The Least You Need to Know

➤ Be aware of risk factors for common injuries that affect participants in the activities you like.

➤ Maintain your workout log during recovery and rehab to track your comeback.

➤ Learn the difference between minor and serious injuries and how to identify their symptoms.

➤ Maintain a positive attitude during rehabilitation.

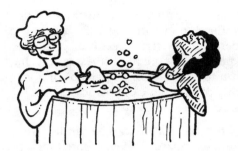

Stress-Busters

We all know people who use food, alcohol, or tobacco to forget their worries and problems, and we all know some who pound stress and tension out of their lives by going to a gym for a tough workout, running long distances, or swinging at a punching bag. This might work for some people, but you don't need to overindulge or engage in heroic physical battles to combat stress, and you don't need to bend an elbow at the pub in place of exercise. It turns out that even mild physical exercise—less than bag-punching but more than elbow-bending—can tame the tension within you. Getting away for a brief period of moderate activity can provide the break you need to disengage enough to relax.

Stress relief also can come from quieter, more introspective choices. You can relieve physical and psychological tension with a dip in the hot tub, a sit in the sauna, some meditative time, deep-breathing exercises, or a massage. You also can just consciously think positive thoughts about all the good aspects of your life.

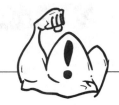

Fit Tip

A common American stress point is the neck and shoulders, because we tend to slouch our shoulders forward unconsciously while sitting and while working at a computer. This shortens our chest muscles. To help alleviate these stress points, clasp your hands behind your back, squeeze your shoulder blades together, and hold for 20 seconds.

The Biochemistry of Exercise and Stress

What we call "stress" is really a biochemical reaction involving the production of cortisol by the adrenal gland. Some experts believe that stress is a contributing factor in 80 percent of all major illnesses and that stress is the reason for more than 75 percent of doctor's visitors. Stress costs American businesses up to $300 million annually.

However, some stress in your life can be productive, in that it keeps you energized, prevents boredom, and even helps you stay focused. After all, for many people, an imminent deadline is great motivation. Some people, such as psychologist James E. Loehr, author of *Stress for Success*, make a case for stress as an antiaging factor. Most experts agree, however, that too much stress can be detrimental to your health. People who are constantly stressed out are more prone to suffer physical or psychological illnesses than people who also build relaxation time into their lives. Stress is linked to chronic pain, headaches, allergies, and insomnia, as well as more serious ailments such as hypertension, heart attacks, diabetes, and asthma.

Quote, Unquote

"One of the best ways to reduce stress is to exercise."

—Covert Bailey, author, motivational speaker, and founder of Covert Bailey Fitness

Effective ways to combat stress include getting enough sleep, eating right, talking and interacting with others, having a good laugh, taking charge rather than ignoring a stressful situation, and—to no one's surprise—exercising. Exercise raises the body's endorphin level and stimulates the production of opioids. Endorphins are chemicals in the brain that lift your mood; opioids seem to block the release of stress hormones.

Some Like It Hot

Heat therapy increases blood flow throughout the body, enabling the body to relax. There are a number of options for heat therapy including a good old-fashioned bubble bath in your own home. Light a few candles, put on some soft music, fill up the tub, hop in, and relax. If the phone rings, let someone else answer it, let the answering machine pick it up, or better yet, turn off the ringer before you get into the tub.

If you can't create a relaxing mood—even for a short time—because the kids are screaming or the dog is barking, find a health club or spa nearby that offers hot tubs, saunas, or steam baths. A hot tub resembles an oversized bathtub and usually is filled with hot water ranging from about 95 to 102 degrees Fahrenheit. It has benches on which to sit and relax and jets that can be turned on to provide water movement. You also can direct any sore muscles onto the force of the water coming from the jets for specific relief.

Fitness Fact

The American College of Sports Medicine's *Medicine & Science in Sports & Exercise* published a report indicating that women who cycled for just 20 minutes at a mere 40 percent of their maximum heart rate were less stressed and less anxious than a control group.

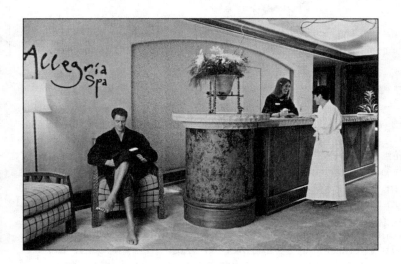

You deserve the ultimate stress-buster! A trip to a spa offers a combination of stress-relieving treatments, such as hot tubs, saunas, massage, aromatherapy, and more.

(Photo: Courtesy of Hyatt Regency Beaver Creek Resort and Spa)

Hot water soothes aching muscles and aching minds.

(Photo: Courtesy of the manufacturer)

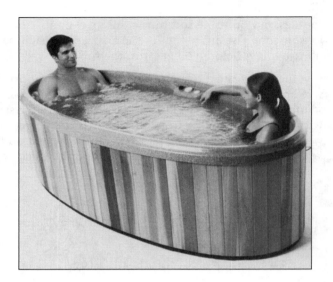

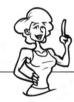

Fitness Fact

Jacuzzi is the trade name for the first commercially successful hot-tub brand. This name often is used interchangeably with the generic term "hot tub." Another common name is whirlpool.

Saunas, which were developed in Scandinavia, have become popular in America for relaxing. A sauna is a small room made completely of aromatic natural wood—the floor, the walls, the ceiling, even the door. A small private sauna resembles a cedar closet and can hold two to four people; a large one at a resort or gym accommodates more people. You sit or lie on a wooden bench as you bask in the dry heat that soothes the muscles and enables you to sweat out anything that ails you. If you like it very hot, choose an upper bench. If you prefer moderate heat, you'll find the lower benches to be more comfortable. Steady heat is transmitted into the sauna enclosure through a pile of hot rocks encased in a small wooden frame. If a wooden water bucket has been placed next to the frame, it is customary to periodically throw a ladleful of water on the rocks to add a brief burst of moisture to the dry air.

Saunas are meant to be used in the nude. In Europe, this is the practice even for coed saunas. (A towel to sit or lie on prevents your privates from frying on the hot wood.)

In the United States, people might use a sauna in the nude if it is specifically part of the men's or women's locker room, but they virtually always wear bathing suits in a coed sauna.

A traditional Scandinavian sauna often will have a bucket of water with birch or oak branches placed in it. These branches are used by sauna goers to "spank" one another lightly to increase blood circulation. Another traditional Scandinavian ritual is to roll in the snow, or even jump into a cold lake or an ocean, which many Scandinavian saunas are located next to. This is done right after emerging from the sauna, and it does get the blood flowing. In the United States, this cold plunge often is achieved with a cold shower.

A steam room is a fully tiled room that resembles an oversized shower stall, but it has tiled benches to sit or lie on. Nozzles around the room intermittently emit very moist heat into the air. The steam is so dense that it looks like a cloud or a thick fog, but it's hot enough to feel even in your lungs. Sometimes eucalyptus oil is sprayed onto the nozzles, and this helps open up your sinuses. Many people find the wet heat and hissing bursts of steam to be particularly soothing.

These heat treatments provide stress relief as well as physical relaxation. Perspiring, which your body does naturally in the intense heat, helps sweat toxins out of your body. In the early part of a sauna session, the dry air evaporates perspiration from your skin. Only after sitting in the dry heat for a while will moisture begin to form on your skin. In a steam room, the moist air masks your own perspiration.

Remember to stay hydrated while you are enjoying these forms of stress relief. Drink water before entering, and bring a water bottle along with you to remind you to keep sipping. If you lie down in the sauna or steam room, remember to sit up slowly and to sit for a minute before standing up and walking out. In addition, do not stay in the heat for too long. Twenty minutes a shot is usually the recommended maximum.

Hands Heal—the Soothing Touch of Massage

Are you sore and tired from a hectic week that probably involved work, family, commuting, working out, or a wickedly stressful combination of these elements? Do you get nagging knots in your neck as a result of a hectic lifestyle or too many hours in front of the computer screen? If your answer to either of these questions is "yes," there's nothing like a massage to relieve your miscellaneous aches and tension-caused kinks.

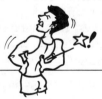

Achtung!

Pregnant women, especially women in their first trimester, should not even think about using a hot tub, sauna, or steam room. The heat can raise the body's core temperature and possibly harm the developing fetus.

Relax and have your stress rubbed away with a soothing massage.

(Photo: Courtesy of the Resort at Summerlin)

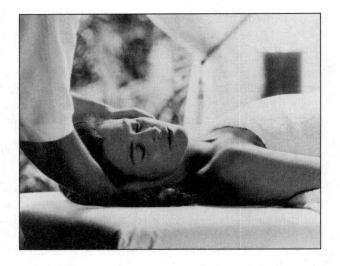

Touch is considered to be a healing art, and it is one of the oldest. The magic touch of massage is a centuries-old form of body work that includes kneading, stroking, and pressing along your entire body to relax all your muscles. Swedish massage, developed by Per Henrik Ling in the early 1800s, is the most common form practiced in the West today.

A massage therapist will use his or her palms, hands, thumbs, and forearms in kneading and stroking movements to work the muscles of your neck, back, arms, shoulders, legs, hands, and feet. Massage provides overall relaxation of the muscles and increases circulation. For Swedish and most other massages, you undress to the level of your comfort. (Most people prefer to be nude so the massage therapist can work unrestricted.) The massage therapist will drape a sheet or blanket over you and will expose only the body part he or she is working on. Your private parts will stay covered at all times. The therapist also will want to make sure that your body temperature is comfortable at all times and will adjust the room temperature and/or blankets at your request.

Other massage specialties include

➤ **NST.** Normalization of soft tissue (NST) is used to restore neutral body alignment by manipulating the muscles and joints to release and lengthen them. NST is used to treat overused injuries and chronic pain.

➤ **Deep-tissue massage.** This is a form of Swedish massage in which the massage therapist works deeper into the muscles and soft tissue.

➤ **Lymphatic or visceral drainage.** This is a detoxifying massage to tone and revitalize the organs through drainage of the lymph fluid.

➤ **Shiatsu and acupressure.** Often used for pain relief, these Asian healing treatments use manual pressure on the body's acupuncture meridians. These types of treatments work on physical and physiological levels as well as mental and emotional levels. They are done with your clothes on, so they are a good place to start if you are uncomfortable with undressing.

➤ **Watsu.** This is a variation of shiatsu that is done in water. The water is at least 98 degrees, and the movements in the water are very relaxing and soothing.

➤ **Myofascial release.** This type of massage restores movement to the myofascial tissue between the skin and the muscle.

➤ **Cranial-sacral massage.** This massage type provides tension relief by realigning the cranial sutures and spinal column.

➤ **Reflexology.** This treatment consists of manipulation and massage of the feet and the hands.

➤ **Sports massage.** This form of Swedish massage for athletes works on specific muscles. Sports massage uses lots of shaking to loosen up the muscles and stretching techniques to restore proper range of motion, speed up recovery from workouts and competition, and prevent injuries.

➤ **Pregnancy and postpartum massage.** Pre- and postnatal massage can help women prepare for and recover from childbirth.

➤ **Body scrub.** This type of massage exfoliates the skin and increases circulation. The therapist might use a loofah, a brush, salt, or another mildly abrasive object or substance.

➤ **Hydrotherapeutic massage.** This underwater massage is done in a deep tub instead of on a table. While a massage therapist can only work one part of the body at a time, water from nozzles on the bottom and sides of the tub plays over the entire body at the same time.

➤ **Integrative massage.** This form of massage integrates deep breathing with long strokes overlapping the joints. Deep breathing is an important part of relaxing the body and soul.

➤ **Thai massage.** This deep massage limbers the joints and stretches muscles. It is done fully clothed, and the therapist sometimes uses his or her feet to massage.

➤ **Chinese massage.** The therapist works each muscle perpendicular to, rather than along, its length, which helps release the myofascia. Also, a thin cotton towel is placed between the client and the therapist's hands.

Massages usually range in length from about 30 to 90 minutes, and they usually cost between $40 and $100, depending on where you go and how long the massage lasts. Remember that you are the client. When you go in for your massage, let your therapist know if you have any specific areas of soreness. He or she can pay particular attention to certain areas and can spend a little extra time working out the knots. Massages generally are available through therapists in private practice or at massage centers, health clubs, sports medicine clinics, and day or destination spas.

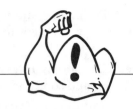

Fit Tip

For a massage on a budget, check to see whether a local massage therapy school offers inexpensive massages by students.

To get the maximum benefit from your massage, try to plan for extra time at the massage center before and after your treatment. If you leave yourself time for a leisurely shower and some quiet meditation before and an opportunity to relax afterward, you will enhance the benefits of the massage itself.

Meditation Can Move Emotional Mountains

Meditation is a form of mental relaxation in which you sit and consciously concentrate on nothing. "Nothing" can be breathing, a specific image, or a single repeated word or phrase (often called a *mantra,* which is a Sanskrit word). Although there is significant formal training for different types of meditation, particularly those that are part of religious practices, it doesn't take much training to derive some relaxation from withdrawing and focusing your attention inward.

To benefit from meditation, all you need to do is sit and focus on your breathing or on a specific word or phrase for 5 or 10 minutes at a time. Sit comfortably or lie on your back. Close your eyes or focus on a still and tranquil object, such as a candle, a flower, or a soothing pattern or image. Make each breath count. Inhale through your nose and fill your lungs deeply, then slowly exhale through your mouth. Let your rib cage and stomach expand and contract in synchrony with your steady, rhythmic breathing. Breathing into the stomach with the help of your diaphragm is what relaxes you.

Quote, Unquote

"When I meditate, the image I have in my mind is of a frog on a lily pad, resting but ready to move."

—Phil Jackson, former Chicago Bulls basketball coach

Upper-chest breathing (paradoxal breathing) is shallow and forces the neck muscles to work excessively. This, in turn, causes tense neck and shoulder muscles. If you like, you can think of a word or a phrase to play over and over in your mind. While you are meditating, do not let your mind wander back to your everyday stresses. The stresses will still be there when you're done, but you'll be better equipped to deal with them. As with anything else, meditation takes practice. When you get into the habit, though, you'll be amazed at how quickly you can zone out and how refreshed you'll feel after a very short time.

Breathing is an important element of all branches of yoga. Meditation also is a key element, because one of its goals is to keep the mind focused and quiet, even as the body adopts different postures. Chapter 9, "Other Paths to Stretching and Toning," contains more information about yoga.

"Music hath charms to soothe the savage beast."

So goes an old saying, and it holds true today. Sitting and listening to your favorite music often is a good way to get away from it all and relax. New Age music, some Eastern music, and European ecclesiastical music such as the Gregorian chants were composed for this very purpose, but some people prefer to relax with chamber music, light jazz, mellow "elevator music," and other soothing, nonintrusive styles.

As with meditation, the trick to using music for stress relief is to sit or lie down, relax, and focus on the sound. Don't try to sing along, and above all, don't let the problems you're stressing about creep into your mind. Instead, use the sound to help block them out.

Fitness Fact

When people are in stressful situations, those accompanied by their dogs showed the least amount of tension, according to a study conducted by the State University of New York at Buffalo Medical School. Stress levels were highest among people who were in stressful situations with their spouses.

Ah-h-h-romatherapy

Essential oils—seductive, aromatic fragrances drawn from natural plant sources—have charms to soothe even the most jittery souls. Some oils reputedly help you stay alert; others help you get to sleep. In its simplest form, aromatherapy can mean placing a bowl of potpourri in your bathroom or a bouquet of fresh flowers on your desk. There's more to aromatherapy, however, than just being in a room with something that smells good. You can find essential oils or have them custom-blended to stimulate a desired body response. Lavender, chamomile, clary sage, and neroli oils are reputed to promote relaxation or sleep. Other refreshing aromas you might try include sandalwood and orange. Aromatherapy—alone or in conjunction with massage using complementary botanical oils—promotes and enhances relaxation. You can benefit from these aromas as candles or oils that you can drop onto your pillow, add to a warm bath, or drip onto an aromatherapy ring for a light bulb.

The Least You Need to Know

➤ Even mild exercise can be an effective stress-buster.

➤ Meditation, music, and massage are the three Ms of tension relief.

➤ Massage relieves muscle tension and soreness while also relaxing you emotionally.

➤ Breath control, which is derived from yoga practices, also is very relaxing.

➤ Aromatherapy, which involves soothing through your sense of smell, is another relaxation practice.

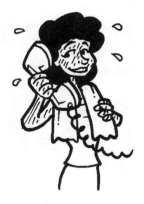

Resources

Books

American Heart Association. *Fitting in Fitness*. New York: Random House, 1997.

Andes, Karen. *A Woman's Book of Strength: An Empowering Guide to Total Mind/Body Fitness*. New York: Berkley Publishing Group, 1995.

Baechler, Thomas R., and Barney R. Groves. *Weight Training Steps to Success*. Champaign, IL: Human Kinetics, 1998.

Bean, Anita. *The Complete Guide to Strength Training*. London: A&C Black, 1997.

Birch, Beryl Bender. *Power Yoga: The Total Strength and Flexibility Workout*. New York: Macmillan Books, 1995.

Bodger, Carole. *Smart Guide to Getting Strong and Fit*. New York: John Wiley & Sons, Inc., 1999.

Bookspan, Jolie. *Health and Fitness in Plain English*. New York: Kensington Books, 1998.

Brungardt, Kurt. *The Complete Book of Abs*. New York: Villard Books, 1988.

Burke, Edmund, ed. *Complete Home Fitness Handbook*. Champaign, IL: Human Kinetics, 1996.

Colton, Katherine. *Smart Guide to Getting Thin and Healthy.* New York: John Wiley and Sons, Inc., 1999.

Curry, Lisa. *Get Up and Go.* New York: HarperCollins, 1998.

Darden, Ellington. *A Flat Stomach ASAP.* New York: Pocket Books, 1998.

Edwards, Sally. *Heart Zone Training.* Holbrook, MA: Adams Media, 1998.

Eshref, Hussein. *Easy Exercises to Relieve Stress.* Holbrook, MA: Adams Media, 1997.

Evans, Mark. *Instant Stretches.* New York: Lorenz Books, 1998.

Fahey, Thomas B. *Basic Weight Training for Men and Women.* Mountainview, CA: Mayfield Publishing, 1997.

Fitness Magazine Editors with Karen Andes. *The Complete Book of Fitness.* New York: Three Rivers Press, 1999.

Fletcher, Anne M. *Eating Thin for Life.* Boston: Houghton Mifflin, 1997.

———— *Thin for Life.* Shelburne, VT: Chapters Publishing, 1994.

Fletcher, Colin. *The Complete Walker III.* New York: Alfred A. Knopf, Inc., 1984.

Gillespie, Larrian. *The Menopause Diet.* Beverly Hills, CA: Healthy Life Publications, 1999.

Gosselin, Chantal. *The Ultimate Guide to Fitness.* New York: Crescent Books, 1995.

Iedwab, Claudio, and Roxanne L. Standefer. *The Secret Art of Health & Fitness.* New York: Weatherill, 1999.

Ikonian, Therese. *Fitness Walking.* Champaign, IL: Human Kinetics, 1995.

Karon, Stephanie, and Anthony L. Rankin. *Workouts With Weights.* New York: Sterling Publishing, 1993.

Katz, Jane. *The New W.E.T. Workout.* New York: Checkmark Books, 1996.

LeMond, Greg, and Kent Gordis. *Greg LeMond's Complete Book of Bicycling.* New York: Putnam Publishing, 1988.

Levin-Gervasi, Stephanie. *Smart Guide to Yoga*. New York: John Wiley & Sons, Inc., 1999.

Lieberman, Lori, and Andrea Bilger. *The Foldout Book of Tai Chi Chuan*. Trumbull, CT: Weatherill, 1998.

Mac Donnell, Michèle. *Alexander Technique*. New York: Lorenz Books, 1999.

Maisel, Edward. *Tai Chi for Health*. Trumbull, CT: Weatherill, 1998.

Malkin, Mort. *Aerobic Walking, the Weight-Loss Exercise: A Complete Program to Reduce Weight, Stress and Hypertension*. New York: John Wiley & Sons, Inc., 1995.

Pearl, Bill. *Getting Stronger*. Bolinas, CA: Shelter Publications, 1986.

Powers, Scott, and Stephen L. Dodd. *Total Fitness*. Boston: Allyn & Bacon, 1999.

Robinson, Lynne, Gordon Thomson and Joseph Pilates. *Body Control: Using Techniques Developed by Joseph H. Pilates*. New York: BainBridge Books, 1998.

Rodiger, Margit, and Sabine Saberlein. *Problem Zones*. New York: Sterling Publications, 1998.

Schatz, Mary Pullig, M.D. *Back Care Basics: A Doctor's Gentle Yoga Program*. Berkeley, CA: Rodmell Press, 1992.

Shimer, Porter. *Keeping Fitness Simple*. Pownal, VT: Storey Communications, 1998.

Sloan, Jim. *Staying Fit Over 50*. Seattle: Mountaineers Books, 1999.

Smith, Kathy, and Susanna Levin. *Kathy Smith's Walkfit for a Better Body*. New York: Warner Books, 1994.

Sobel, Sheila. *Smart Guide to Sports Medicine*. New York: John Wiley & Sons, Inc., 1999.

Tucker, Paul. *Tai Chi: Flowing Movements for Harmony and Balance*. New York: Lorenz Books, 1997.

Wharton, Jim and Phil. *The Stretch Book*. New York: Times Books/Random House, 1996.

Wharton, Jim and Phil. *The Whartons' Strength Book*. New York: Times Books/Random House, 1999.

Winsor, Mari, with Mark Laska. *The Pilates Powerhouse*. Reading, MA: Perseus Books, 1999.

Yates, Michael, Ph.D. *Body Shaping*. Emmaus, PA: Rodale Books, 1994.

Fitness Equipment by Mail or from the Web

Big Fitness Exercise Equipment Warehouse
560 Mineral Spring Avenue
Pawtucket, RI 02860
888-292-1807
www.bigfitness.com

Body Trends Health & Fitness
P.O. Box 3588
Santa Barbara, CA 93130
805-564-5063
www.bodytrends.com

Dynabody
4084 Michigan Avenue
Cleveland, TN 37321
1-800-950-3488
www.dynabody.com

Fit@Home
P.O. Box 5121
Buffalo Grove, IL 60089
888-999-FITT
www.fitathome.com

Fitness Factory Outlet
2875 South 25th Avenue
Broadview, IL 60153-9908
1-800-383-9300
www.fitnessfactory.com

Fitness Wholesale
895-A Hampshire Road
Suite A
Stow, OH 44224-1121
888-FW-ORDER
www.fwonline.com

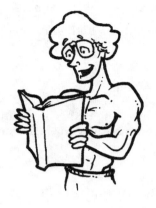

Glossary

abs   Nickname for the abdominal muscles and also for exercises that strengthen them.

aerobic   An adjective describing any steady and repetitive activity that challenges the cardiorespiratory system—that is, the heart and lungs—to make it stronger.

aerobic kickboxing   Type of fitness program based on martial arts moves, choreographed to music.

aerobic zone   Working at 70 to 80 percent of your maximum heart rate.

aerobics   A form of fitness routine based on dance and performed to music with enough intensity to elevate the heart rate.

agility   Nimbleness to start, accelerate, decelerate, stop, and change direction quickly.

anaerobic   An adjective describing the highest intensity level of exercise when the cardiorespiratory system can no longer deliver enough oxygen to the muscles to sustain further activity without tapping into the body's reserve.

anaerobic endurance   The ability of a muscle or muscle group to sustain intense activity for a relatively short period of time. Also known as muscle endurance.

anaerobic threshold   The point at which your body no longer processes sufficient oxygen for sustained activity, causing you to begin drawing on reserves.

anaerobic zone   Working at 80 to 100 percent of your maximum heart rate.

apple   A body shape characterized by the tendency to carry any extra weight around the waist.

asana   Sanskrit for "pose" or "position." This term is used in yoga classes.

ballistic stretch   A movement-induced stretch, such as an arm or leg swing.

barbells   A five-foot supporting bar with removable weights on both ends that is designed to be used with two hands.

BIA   *See* bioelectrical impedance analysis.

biceps   The muscle group on the front of the upper arm.

bioelectrical impedance analysis (BIA)   A method of assessing body composition by passing electricity though the body. Electricity passes more easily through muscle than fat, so a lower number is more desirable.

BMI   *See* body-mass index.

body composition test   The process of measuring body-mass index (BMI).

Body-mass index (BMI)   The percentage of fat as a part of total body weight.

calisthenics   Basic body-toning exercises generally done without the use of apparatus.

cardio   Relating to the heart.

cardiorespiratory endurance   The body's ability to deliver oxygen and nutrients to the tissues and to remove waste during a period of sustained physical activity.

circuit   Sequential use of all the machines in a weight room.

core   The center of the torso.

curl   A strength exercise in which the elbow or knee joint bends, as in an arm curl or leg curl.

delts   Nickname for the deltoid or shoulder muscles.

dumbbells   Relatively small weights designed to be held in one hand and usually used in pairs. Also called hand weights.

ectomorph   The longest and leanest of the three basic body types. *See also* endomorph and mesomorph.

endomorph   The roundest of the three basic body types. *See also* ectomorph and mesomorph.

exercise bar   Balanced, weighted bar used by itself, without plates, for strength training.

exertube   An exercise tube with a handle at each end.

fat-burning zone   Working at 60 to 70 percent of your maximum heart rate.

fat mass   Actual weight, in pounds, of fat in the body.

fat percentage   Fat mass as a percentage of body weight.

fit ball   A large, inflated rubber ball used for strength, flexibility, and balance conditioning. Also called a Swiss ball or physiology ball.

flexibility   The ability to move joints and use muscles through their full range of motion.

free weights   Barbells and dumbbells.

glutes   Nickname for the gluteal muscles of the posterior.

hand weights   *See* dumbbells.

heart rate   The number of times per minute that your heart beats. Also known as your pulse.

impedance   An electrical impulse measurement used in a body-composition test called bioelectrical impedance analysis (BIA).

jogging   A slow, recreational form of running.

lats   Nickname for the latissimi dorsi, the muscles on the back.

lean body mass (LBM)   Actual weight, in pounds, of the body's muscle, bones, and organs.

maximum heart rate (MHR)   The most beats per minute that the heart can possibly produce.

mesomorph   The most squarely built of the three basic body types. *See also* ectomorph and endomorph.

MHR   *See* maximum heart rate.

muscular endurance   A muscle's ability to contract repeatedly, to sustain strength, or to hold a fixed muscular contraction over time.

muscular strength   A muscle's ability to exert force for a brief period of time, or the maximum force that a muscle or muscle group can exert.

overload   In the context of strength training, making muscles work harder than usual to make them stronger.

pear   A body shape characterized by the tendency to carry any extra weight on the abdomen, hips, thighs, and buttocks.

pelvic tilt   Tucking the buttocks and contracting the abdomen to tilt the pelvis forward, a position suggested in several exercises to protect the lower back.

physical fitness   The condition that enables you to look well, feel good, endure stress, and perform daily tasks vigorously with energy left over. It involves cardio-respiratory endurance, muscular strength, muscular endurance, and flexibility.

physiology ball   *See* fit ball.

Pilates   Fitness program, developed for rehabilitation and embraced by dancers, which strengthens and elongates the muscles via mat exercises or specialized apparatus.

plates   Flat iron weights, usually 10 pounds each, on weight machines.

power   The combination of strength and speed.

quads   Nickname for quadriceps, the muscle group on the front of the thigh.

racking   Setting a weight machine to capture the entire weight stack.

range of motion   The fullest extent to which a joint can move mechanically. Range of motion is impaired by tight muscles and ligaments.

rating of perceived exertion (RPE)   A subjective assessment, rated from 1 to 10 (or 1 to 20 on some scales), of how hard you think you have worked aerobically.

recovery heart rate   The heart rate one or two minutes after stopping aerobic exercise.

recumbent bike   A stationary or street bike that you pedal while sitting back with your feet extended in front of you rather than in an upright or hunched-forward position.

rehab   Physical therapy or rehabilitation from a sports injury.

rep   Short for "repetition." One complete weight exercise done from the beginning of the movement to the end. Reps are grouped into sets.

resistance exercise   Activities that overload the muscles to make them stronger. These activities include weight training and other devices and actions.

resistance training   Weight training and other forms of strengthening exercises that build muscles because they work against some kind of resistance.

resting heart rate   The number of times per minute that your heart beats while you are at rest. Ideally, this is your morning heart rate before you have even gotten out of bed. Practically, in fitness situations, it is taken while you are sitting and have been relaxed for at least five minutes.

retro walking   Walking backward on a treadmill.

RPE   *See* rating of perceived exertion.

runner's knee   Degeneration of the underside of the kneecap caused by the constant impact of the foot and leg on pavement.

set   The number of completed exercises, or reps, between rests.

Spinning   Trademark name for a studio cycling class using Schwinn bikes.

stack   On a weight machine, plates of identical weight that are piled one on top of the other. They move on a track or on a cable and can be lifted in any quantity, from just one to the entire stack, depending on the desired weight.

stairclimber   *See* stairstepper.

stairstepper   An aerobic machine with variable-resistance pedals that enable you to mimic the motion of climbing stairs. Also called a stairclimber or stepper.

static stretch   Stretch without movement in which the muscle is held stationary at its greatest possible length.

stationary bike   An aerobic machine that resembles a bicycle without wheels.

stepper   *See* stairstepper.

strength training   Weight training and other resistance exercises.

stretch reflex   A muscle's initial reaction to a stretch—contracting to resist that stretch.

studio cycling   Class in which participants on stationary bikes follow an instructor's directions for intensity.

Swiss ball   *See* fit ball.

Tae Bo   The trade name of a cardio and muscle workout program that combines aerobic kickboxing, martial arts, dance, and weight work.

tai chi   A series of slow-motion movements, begun in China, to reduce stress, keep the mind sharp, and maintain the body's suppleness and muscular strength by moving the chi, or energy, through the body.

target heart rate (THR)   The heart rate that should be maintained for at least 20 minutes during aerobic exercise to improve cardio fitness.

target heart rate zone   The range within which you should be exercising aerobically.

TBW   *See* total body water.

THR   *See* target heart rate.

total body water (TBW)   Total amount of body water.

total body workout   Exercising to work the upper and lower body simultaneously.

treadmill   A motorized aerobic apparatus on which you walk, jog, or run on a moving belt.

triceps   The muscle group on the back of the upper arm.

VO2max Oxygen consumption.

weight training Weightlifting using either free weights or weight machines. Also called strength training.

yoga A mind-body philosophy from India that strengthens and tones the body, calms the mind, increases flexibility, and enhances introspection. It has numerous branches that meet these goals through different combinations of postures and movements.

Index

C

373

U

V

387